SickKids Handbook of Pediatric Thrombosis and Hemostasis

SickKids Handbook of Pediatric Thrombosis and Hemostasis

Editors
Victor S. Blanchette, Toronto, Ont., Canada
Vicky R. Breakey, Hamilton, Ont., Canada
Shoshana Revel-Vilk, Jerusalem, Israel

23 figures, 9 in color, 9 algorithms, and 59 tables, 2013

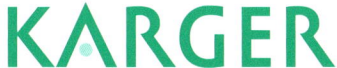

Basel · Freiburg · Paris · London · New York · New Delhi · Bangkok ·
Beijing · Tokyo · Kuala Lumpur · Singapore · Sydney

WS 300 .S566 2013

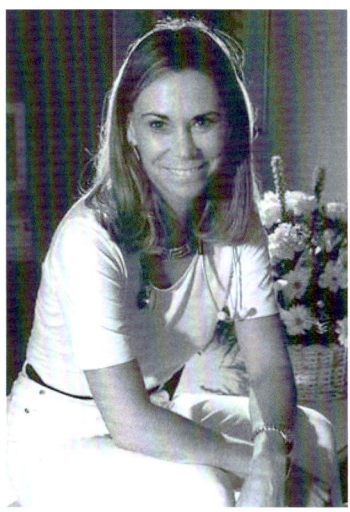

We dedicate this book in memory of Maureen Andrew, a skilled clinician, valued mentor, respected researcher and a pioneer in pediatric thrombosis. For many of the authors she was a colleague and friend. For those who didn't know her personally, she remains an inspiration.

'The great physician is one who not only uses what is known but also recognizes what is not known and what is needed in her patients. Maureen was a great physician.'   A. Zipursky, 2001.

Victor S. Blanchette, MA, MB BChir(Cantab), FRCP(C), FRCP
Professor of Pediatrics, University of Toronto
Medical Director, Pediatric Thrombosis and Hemostasis Program
Division of Hematology/Oncology, The Hospital for Sick Children
Toronto, Ont., Canada

Vicky R. Breakey, MD, MEd, FRCPC
Pediatric Hematologist/Oncologist, Assistant Professor
Division of Pediatric Hematology/Oncology, McMaster Children's Hospital
McMaster University
Hamilton, Ont., Canada

Shoshana Revel-Vilk, MD, MSc
Director, Pediatric Hematology Center
Senior Lecturer of Pediatrics, Hadassah Hebrew-University Medical School
Department of Pediatric Hematology/Oncology, Hadassah Hebrew-University Hospital
Jerusalem, Israel

Library of Congress Cataloging-in-Publication Data

SickKids handbook of pediatric thrombosis and hemostasis /
editors, Victor S. Blanchette, Vicky R. Breakey, Shoshana Revel-Vilk.
   p. ; cm.
  Pediatric thrombosis and hemostasis
  Includes bibliographical references and index.
  ISBN 978-3-318-02197-4 (hard cover : alk. paper) -- ISBN 978-3-318-02198-1 (e-ISBN)
  I. Blanchette, Victor S. II. Breakey, Vicky R. III. Revel-Vilk, Shoshana.
IV. Title: Pediatric thrombosis and hemostasis.
  [DNLM: 1. Hematologic Diseases. 2. Anticoagulants. 3. Child. 4. Hemostasis.
5. Infant. 6. Thrombosis. WS 300]
  RJ270
  618.92'157--dc23

2013009736

Bibliographic Indices. This publication is listed in bibliographic services.

Disclaimer. The statements, opinions and data contained in this publication are solely those of the individual authors and contributors and not of the publisher and the editor(s). The appearance of advertisements in the book is not a warranty, endorsement, or approval of the products or services advertised or of their effectiveness, quality or safety. The publisher and the editor(s) disclaim responsibility for any injury to persons or property resulting from any ideas, methods, instructions or products referred to in the content or advertisements.

Drug Dosage. The authors and the publisher have exerted every effort to ensure that drug selection and dosage set forth in this text are in accord with current recommendations and practice at the time of publication. However, in view of ongoing research, changes in government regulations, and the constant flow of information relating to drug therapy and drug reactions, the reader is urged to check the package insert for each drug for any change in indications and dosage and for added warnings and precautions. This is particularly important when the recommended agent is a new and/or infrequently employed drug.

All rights reserved. No part of this publication may be translated into other languages, reproduced or utilized in any form or by any means electronic or mechanical, including photocopying, recording, microcopying, or by any information storage and retrieval system, without permission in writing from the publisher.

© Copyright 2013 by S. Karger AG, P.O. Box, CH–4009 Basel (Switzerland)
www.karger.com
Printed in Germany on acid-free and non-aging paper (ISO 9706) by Bosch Druck, Ergolding
ISBN 978–3–318–02197–4
e-ISBN 978–3–318–02198–1

Contents

XIII   **Contributors**
XVII   **Preface**

Chapter 1
1   **Pediatric Thrombosis and Hemostasis: A Historical Perspective**
    V.R. Breakey, V.S. Blanchette

- 1   **Thrombosis in Childhood**
- 2   **Hemostatic Disorders in Children: The Evolution of Hemophilia Care**
- 3   **The Future of Pediatric Thrombosis and Hemostasis**
- 4   **Acknowledgment**
- 4   **References**
- 4   **Abbreviations**

Chapter 2
5   **Primary and Secondary Hemostasis, Regulators of Coagulation, and Fibrinolysis: Understanding the Basics**
    S. Revel-Vilk, M.L. Rand, S.J. Israels

- 5   **Introduction**
- 5   **Primary Hemostasis**
- 7   **Secondary Hemostasis**
- 9   **Regulators of Coagulation**
- 11   **Fibrinolysis**
- 13   **Conclusion**
- 13   **References**
- 13   **Abbreviations**

Chapter 3
14   **An Approach to the Bleeding Child**
    S. Revel-Vilk, M.L. Rand, S.J. Israels

- 14   **Introduction**
- 14   **History**
- 16   **Physical Examination**
- 18   **Laboratory Investigations**
- 21   **References**
- 22   **Abbreviations**

Chapter 4
Bleeding in the Neonate — 23

L. Avila, D. Barnard

- 23 **Developmental Hemostasis**
- 24 **Platelet Disorders: Neonatal Thrombocytopenia**
- 34 **Recommendations for Platelet Transfusions**
- 35 **Coagulation Factor Deficiencies**
- 37 **Combined Disorders**
- 38 **Diagnostic Algorithm: Approach to Bleeding in the Neonate**
- 41 **Acknowledgment**
- 41 **References**
- 41 **Abbreviations**

Chapter 5
Platelet Disorders in Children — 42

V. van Eimeren, W.H.A. Kahr

- 42 **Introduction**
- 43 **Diagnosis of Platelet Disorders**
- 46 **Thrombocytopenia**
- 51 **Platelet Function Defects**
- 57 **Conclusion**
- 57 **Acknowledgment**
- 57 **References**
- 58 **Abbreviations**

Chapter 6
Managing Hemophilia in Children and Adolescents — 59

J.D. Robertson, J.A. Curtin, V.S. Blanchette

- 59 **Introduction**
- 60 **General Management Principles**
- 64 **Inhibitors**
- 66 **Management of Bleeding Episodes**
- 69 **Specific Sites of Bleeding**
- 73 **Management of Surgery and Other Invasive Procedures**
- 73 **Chronic Complications of Hemophilia**
- 76 **Management of the Newborn with Suspected or Possible Hemophilia**
- 76 **Conclusion**
- 76 **Acknowledgment**
- 77 **References**
- 78 **Abbreviations**

Chapter 7

79 von Willebrand Disease in Children

V.R. Breakey, M. Carcao

- 79 Introduction
- 79 Pathophysiology of von Willebrand Disease
- 81 Clinical Presentation
- 81 Diagnosis
- 84 Management
- 88 Conclusion
- 89 Acknowledgment
- 89 References
- 89 Abbreviations

Chapter 8

90 Rare Congenital Factor Deficiencies in Childhood

F. Xavier, V.S. Blanchette

- 90 Introduction
- 90 Factor XI Deficiency
- 93 Factor VII Deficiency
- 95 Fibrinogen Disorders
- 97 Factor XIII Deficiency
- 99 Other Rare Inherited Coagulation Disorders
- 103 Conclusion
- 103 Acknowledgment
- 104 References
- 104 Abbreviations

Chapter 9

105 Acquired Bleeding Disorders in Children

R. Kumar, M. Steele

- 105 Introduction
- 105 Disseminated Intravascular Coagulation
- 109 Thrombotic Microangiopathic Disorders
- 109 Hemolytic Uremic Syndrome
- 111 Thrombotic Thrombocytopenic Purpura
- 114 Coagulopathy of Chronic Liver Disease
- 116 Bleeding in Chronic Renal Failure
- 118 Acquired Hemophilia
- 119 Acquired von Willebrand Syndrome
- 121 Hypoprothrombinemia-Lupus Anticoagulant Syndrome
- 121 Acquired Inhibitors after Bovine Thrombin Exposure
- 122 Conclusion
- 122 Acknowledgment
- 122 References
- 123 Abbreviations

Chapter 10

A Diagnostic Approach to a Child with Thrombosis — 124

M. Rizzi, C. Barnes

- 124 Introduction
- 125 History
- 126 Physical Examination
- 128 Diagnostic Imaging
- 131 Laboratory Investigations
- 132 Laboratory Thrombophilia
- 138 Anatomical Thrombophilia
- 139 Conclusion
- 139 Acknowledgment
- 139 References
- 140 Abbreviations

Chapter 11

Venous Thrombosis — 141

V.E. Price, L.R. Brandão, S. Williams

- 141 Introduction
- 141 Deep Vein Thrombosis
- 144 Catheter-Related Thrombosis
- 146 Pulmonary Embolism
- 148 Venous Thrombosis in Neonates
- 148 Venous Thrombosis in Cancer Patients
- 149 Inferior Vena Cava Filter
- 149 Venous Stents
- 149 Post-Thrombotic Syndrome
- 152 Conclusion
- 152 Acknowledgment
- 152 References
- 153 Abbreviations

Chapter 12

Arterial Thrombosis — 154

S. Revel-Vilk, M. Albisetti, M.P. Massicotte

- 154 Introduction
- 154 Arterial Catheter-Related Thrombosis
- 156 Umbilical Artery Catheter-Related Thrombosis
- 158 Aortic Thrombosis
- 160 Arterial Stents – Non-Cardiac, Non-CNS
- 160 Non-Catheter-Related Arterial Thrombosis
- 160 Complications of Arterial Thrombosis
- 161 Conclusion
- 161 Acknowledgment
- 162 References
- 162 Abbreviations

Chapter 13

163 **Thromboembolic Events at Specific Organ Sites**

V. Labarque, A.K.C. Chan, S. Williams

163 Introduction
163 Kidney-Related Thromboembolic Events
169 Liver-Related Thromboembolic Events
175 Mesenteric Vascular Thrombosis
176 Splenic Vein Thrombosis
177 Long-Term Complications
177 Conclusion
177 Acknowledgment
177 References
178 Abbreviations

Chapter 14

179 **Pediatric Stroke**

A. Andrade, R. Ichord, N. Dlamini, S. Williams, G. deVeber

179 Introduction
179 Arterial Ischemic Stroke
187 Cerebral Sinovenous Thrombosis
191 Transient Ischemic Attack
192 Conclusion
192 Acknowledgment
192 References
193 Abbreviations

Chapter 15

194 **Bleeding and Clotting in Children with Cardiac Disease**

Y. Diab, B.W. McCrindle, L.R. Brandão

194 Introduction
195 Mechanical Circulatory Support for Pediatric Cardiac Disease
197 Cardiac Conduits, Shunts and Stents
200 Prosthetic Valves
200 Bleeding in Children with Cardiac Disease
202 Thromboembolism in Children with Cardiac Disease
203 Thromboembolism in Children with Congenital Heart Disease
205 Thromboembolism in Children with Acquired Heart Disease
205 Specific Thromboembolic Events in Pediatric Cardiac Disease
210 Thromboprophylaxis in Pediatric Cardiac Disease
211 Conclusion
211 Acknowledgment
211 References
212 Abbreviations

Chapter 16
Antithrombotic Therapy in Children
214
T. Biss, P. Monagle

214	**Introduction**
214	**Unfractionated Heparin**
216	**Low-Molecular-Weight Heparin**
218	**Vitamin K Antagonists**
221	**New Anticoagulant Agents**
223	**Antiplatelet Therapy**
224	**Thrombolysis**
225	**Heparin-Induced Thrombocytopenia**
226	**Management of Anticoagulant Therapy during Surgery**
228	**Management of Antithrombotic Therapy in Children with Thrombocytopenia**
229	**Thromboprophylaxis**
230	**Acknowledgment**
230	**References**
231	**Abbreviations**

Appendix I
Reference Ranges for Common Tests of Bleeding and Clotting
232
V.R. Breakey

232	**Reference Ranges for Common Tests of Bleeding and Clotting**
232	**Variations of Reference Values Based on Age**
234	**References**
234	**Abbreviations**

Appendix II
Common Products Used to Manage Bleeding and Clotting
235
E. Simpson, M. Liebman

235	**Blood and Blood Product Information**
237	**Factor Concentrates**
240	**Other Agents for Achieving Hemostasis**
241	**Acknowledgment**
241	**References**
241	**Abbreviations**

242 Abbreviations

245 Subject Index

Contributors

Manuela Albisetti, MD
p. 154
Senior Pediatrics Registrar (FMH)
Director, Thrombosis and Hemophilia Care Center
Division of Hematology
University Children's Hospital
Steinwiesstrasse 75
CH-8032 Zürich (Switzerland)
manuela.albisetti@kispi.uzh.ch

Andrea Andrade, MD
p. 179
Fellow, Children's Stroke Program
Division of Neurology
The Hospital for Sick Children
555 University Avenue
Toronto, ON M5G 1X8 (Canada)
dra.andand@gmail.com

Laura Avila, MD, PhD(c)
p. 23
Fellow, Pediatric Thrombosis and Hemostasis Program
Division of Hematology/Oncology
The Hospital for Sick Children
555 University Avenue
Toronto, ON M5G 1X8 (Canada)
laura.avila@sickkids.ca

Dorothy Barnard, MD, PhD, FRCPC
p. 23
Professor (retired), Division of Pediatric Hematology/Oncology
Department of Pediatrics
IWK Health Center
Dalhousie University
5850/5980 University Avenue
P.O. Box 9700
Halifax, NS B3K 6R8 (Canada)
barndr@gmail.com

Chris Barnes, MBBS(Hons), FRACP, FRCPA
p. 124
Paediatric Haematologist
Department of Haematology
Royal Children's Hospital
The University of Melbourne
Flemington Road
Parkville, Vic. 3052 (Australia)
chris.barnes@rch.org.au

Tina Biss, BMedSci, BM BS(Hons), MD, MRCP(Lond), FRCPath
p. 214
Consultant Haematologist and Associate Clinical Researcher
The Newcastle Hospitals NHS Foundation Trust
Royal Victoria Infirmary
Queen Victoria Road
Newcastle upon Tyne NE1 4LP (UK)
tina.biss@ncl.ac.uk

Victor S. Blanchette, MA, MB BChir(Cantab), FRCP(C), FRCP
pp. 1, 59, 90
Professor of Pediatrics
University of Toronto
Medical Director, Pediatric Thrombosis and Hemostasis Program
Division of Hematology/Oncology
The Hospital for Sick Children
555 University Avenue
Toronto, ON M5G 1X8 (Canada)
victor.blanchette@sickkids.ca

Leonardo R. Brandão, MD, MSc
pp. 141, 194
Pediatric Hematologist
Division of Hematology/Oncology
The Hospital for Sick Children
555 University Avenue
Toronto, ON M5G 1X8 (Canada)
leonardo.brandao@sickkids.ca

Vicky R. Breakey, MD, MEd, FRCPC
pp. 1, 79, 232
Pediatric Hematologist/Oncologist
Assistant Professor, Division of Pediatric Hematology/Oncology
McMaster Children's Hospital
McMaster University
HSC 3N27A – 1280 Main Street West
Hamilton, ON L8S 4K1 (Canada)
breakev@mcmaster.ca

Manuel Carcao, MD, MSc, FRCPC
p. 79
Pediatric Hematologist/Oncologist
Co-Director, Hemophilia Clinic
Associate Professor, Division of Hematology/Oncology
The Hospital for Sick Children
555 University Avenue
Toronto, ON M5G 1X8 (Canada)
manuel.carcao@sickkids.ca

Anthony K.C. Chan, MBBS, FRCPC, FRCP(Glas), FRCPI, FRCPCH, FRCPath
p. 163
Professor of Pediatrics, Chief of Service
Division of Pediatric Hematology/Oncology
McMaster Children's Hospital
McMaster University
HSC 3N27A – 1280 Main Street West
Hamilton, ON L8S 4K1 (Canada)
akchan@mcmaster.ca

Julie A. Curtin, MBBS(Hons I), PhD, FRACP, FRCPA
p. 59
Paediatric Haematologist
Department of Haematology
The Children's Hospital at Westmead
Cnr Hawkesbury Road and Hainsworth Street
Locked Bag 4001
Westmead, N.S.W. 2145 (Australia)
julie.curtin@health.nsw.gov.au

Gabrielle deVeber, MD, FRCPC
p. 179
Director, Children's Stroke Program
Division of Neurology
The Hospital for Sick Children
555 University Avenue
Toronto, ON M5G 1X8 (Canada)
gabrielle.deveber@sickkids.ca

Yaser Diab, MD
p. 194
Attending Hematologist
Division of Hematology
Center for Cancer and Blood Disorders
Children's National Medical Center
111 Michigan Avenue NW
Washington, DC 20010 (USA)
ydiab@childrensnational.org

Nomazulu Dlamini, MBBS, MRCPCH, MSc(Lon)
p. 179
Consultant Paediatric Neurologist
Evelina Children's Hospital London
Newcomen Centre at St. Thomas'
Floor 1, Stairs D, South Wing
St. Thomas Hospital
Westminster Bridge Road
London SE1 7EH (UK)
nomazulu.dlamini@gstt.nhs.uk

Rebecca Ichord, MD
p. 179
Associate Professor
Department of Neurology
Perelman School of Medicine
University of Pennsylvania
Director, Pediatric Stroke Program
Department of Neurology, CTRB 10th Floor
Children's Hospital of Philadelphia
3501 Civic Center Boulevard
Philadelphia, PA 19104 (USA)
ichord@email.chop.edu

Sara J. Israels, MD, FRCPC
pp. 5, 14
Professor
Section of Pediatric Hematology/Oncology
Department of Pediatrics and Child Health
University of Manitoba
675 McDermot Avenue
Winnipeg, MB R3E 0V9 (Canada)
israels@cc.umanitoba.ca

Walter H.A. Kahr, MD, PhD, FRCPC
p. 42
Departments of Pediatrics and Biochemistry
University of Toronto
Hematologist, Division of Hematology/Oncology
Scientist, Program in Cell Biology
The Hospital for Sick Children
555 University Avenue
Toronto, ON M5G 1X8 (Canada)
walter.kahr@sickkids.ca

Riten Kumar, MD, MSc
p. 105
Fellow, Pediatric Thrombosis and Hemostasis Program
Division of Hematology/Oncology
The Hospital for Sick Children
555 University Avenue
Toronto, ON M5G 1X8 (Canada)
riten.kumar@sickkids.ca

Veerle Labarque, MD, PhD
p. 163
Assistant Professor, Department of Pediatrics
Pediatric Hemato-Oncology
University Hospitals Leuven
Herestraat 49
B–3000 Leuven (Belgium)
veerle.labarque@uzleuven.be

Mira Liebman, MDCM, FRCPC
p. 235
Resident, Department of Pathobiology and Laboratory Medicine
Mount Sinai Hospital
University of Toronto
600 University Avenue, 6th Floor 6-500
Toronto, ON M5G 1X5 (Canada)
mira.liebman@mail.mcgill.ca

M. Patricia Massicotte, MD, MHSc, FRCPC
p. 154
Professor of Pediatrics
University of Alberta, Peter Olley Chair
Pediatric Thrombosis
Director, KIDCLOT Program
Stollery Children's Hospital
3-539 ECHA 11405-87th Avenue NW
Edmonton, AB T6G 1C9 (Canada)
patti.massicotte@albertahealthservices.ca

Brian W. McCrindle, MD, MPH
p. 194
Professor of Pediatrics
University of Toronto
Labatt Family Heart Centre
The Hospital for Sick Children
555 University Avenue
Toronto, ON M5G 1X8 (Canada)
brian.mccrindle@sickkids.ca

Paul Monagle, MBBS, MD, MSc, FRACP, FRCPA, FCCP
p. 214
Stevenson Professor and Assistant Dean
Royal Children's Hospital Academic Centre, and Head, Department of Paediatrics, The University of Melbourne
Paediatric Haematologist, Department of Haematology
Royal Children's Hospital
Honorary Fellow, Critical Care and Neurosciences, and Group Leader, Haemotology Research
Murdoch Childrens Research Institute
50 Flemington Road
Melbourne, Vic. 3010 (Australia)
paul.monagle@rch.org.au

Victoria E. Price, MBChB, MMed (Pediatrics)
p. 141
Pediatric Hematologist/Oncologist
Division of Pediatric Hematology/Oncology
Department of Pediatrics
IWK Health Center
Dalhousie University
5850/5980 University Avenue
P.O. Box 9700
Halifax, NS B3K 6R8 (Canada)
vicky.price@iwk.nshealth.ca

Margaret L. Rand, PhD
pp. 5, 14
Professor of Laboratory Medicine and Pathobiology, Biochemistry, and Pediatrics
University of Toronto
Senior Associate Scientist, Physiology and Experimental Medicine Program
Division of Hematology/Oncology
The Hospital for Sick Children
555 University Avenue
Toronto, ON M5G 1X8 (Canada)
margaret.rand@sickkids.ca

Shoshana Revel-Vilk, MD, MSc
pp. 5, 14, 154
Director, Pediatric Hematology Center
Senior Lecturer of Pediatrics, Hadassah
Hebrew-University Medical School
Department of Pediatric Hematology/
Oncology
Hadassah Hebrew-University Hospital
P.O. Box 12000
IL–91120 Jerusalem (Israel)
shoshanav@hadassah.org.il

Mattia Rizzi, MD, PhD
p. 124
Fellow, Pediatric Thrombosis and
Hemostasis Program
Division of Hematology/Oncology
The Hospital for Sick Children
555 University Avenue
Toronto, ON M5G 1X8 (Canada)
mattia.rizzi@sickkids.ca

Jeremy D. Robertson, MBBS,
FRACP, FRCPA
p. 59
Paediatric Haematologist/
Haematopathologist
Director, Paediatric Haematology
Royal Children's Hospital
Queensland Children's Health Service
Herston, Qld. 4029 (Australia)
j.robertson@uq.edu.au

Ewurabena Simpson, MD, MPH,
FRCPC
p. 235
Pediatric Hematologist/Oncologist
Division of Hematology/Oncology
Children's Hospital of Eastern Ontario
401 Smyth Road
Ottawa, ON K1H 8L1 (Canada)
esimpson@cheo.on.ca

MacGregor Steele, MD, FRCPC
p. 105
Pediatric Hematologist, Division of
Pediatric Hematology, Suite C4-438
Alberta Children's Hospital
2888 Shaganappi Trail NW
Calgary, AB T3B 6A8 (Canada)
macgregor.steele@
albertahealthservices.ca

Viola van Eimeren, MD
p. 42
Pediatrician, Department of Pediatric
Hematology and Oncology
University Medical Center
Hamburg-Eppendorf
Martinistrasse 52
DE–20246 Hamburg (Germany)
violavaneimeren@gmail.com

Suzan Williams, MD, MSc,
FRCPC
p. 141, 163, 179
Pediatric Hematologist
Division of Hematology/Oncology
The Hospital for Sick Children
555 University Avenue
Toronto, ON M5G 1X8 (Canada)
suzan.williams@sickkids.ca

Frederico Xavier, MD
p. 90
Pediatric Hematologist, Indiana
Hemophilia and Thrombosis Center
8402 Harcourt Road, Suite 500
Indianapolis, IN 46260 (USA)
fxavier@IHTC.org

Preface

The Hospital for Sick Children (SickKids) in Toronto, Canada, has a history of excellence in pediatric thrombosis and hemostasis. Dr. Alvin Zipursky was recruited to lead a combined Division of Pediatric Hematology, Oncology and Stem Cell Transplantation in 1981 and brought with him vigor for growing the non-malignant hematology component of the program. In the years that followed, many experts in the field positioned themselves at SickKids for clinical training, practice and research. In 1983, Dr. Victor Blanchette joined the Division. With a particular interest in bleeding disorders, he was dedicated to the pursuit of collaborative research. He recognized the value of joining together with colleagues nationally and internationally to share ideas and conduct research studies. Dr. Blanchette also recognized the importance of training future generations of young, academically oriented pediatric hematologists/oncologists. In 2001, he worked with an industry sponsor (Baxter BioScience, Canada) to develop an endowed fellowship in pediatric thrombosis and hemostasis at SickKids. This stable financial support ensured that the Division's thrombosis and hemostasis program could fund one physician trainee per year. What has resulted is an impressive alumnus of 15 fellows from 12 countries (Argentina, Australia, Austria, Belgium, Canada, Germany, Ghana, Israel, South Africa, Thailand, UK and the USA). Many of these fellows now hold leadership positions in the Pediatric Hematology/Oncology Divisions in their academic institutions and continue to pursue an interest in the field of the inherited and acquired bleeding and clotting disorders in children. In addition, many others have come to observe, train and participate in research in thrombosis and hemostasis at SickKids.

In 2010, at a SickKids Fellows' reunion lunch at the World Federation of Hemophilia Congress in Buenos Aires, the idea for this handbook was developed. Although many of these former SickKids Thrombosis and Hemostasis fellows did not train together, strong alliances have formed due to their connections to the SickKids program. All present agreed that a handbook in pediatric thrombosis and hemostasis was lacking and would benefit those practicing in the field. It was agreed that the book should be evidence based and relevant internationally. Most importantly, it was felt that the book should be clinically sound and practical.

In addition to the print version of the text, we are pleased to provide an online version of the book (available at http://www.karger.com/sickkids). An online tool is available for readers to give feedback and to interact with the editorial team.

We sincerely hope that this handbook helps to fill a gap in the library of pediatric medicine. We envision its use by a wide spectrum of physicians, trainees and allied health professionals. We look forward to the opportunity to update the content both online and in hard copy as new evidence is published and practice changes over time.

Victor S. Blanchette, Toronto, Ont., Canada
Vicky R. Breakey, Hamilton, Ont., Canada
Shoshana Revel-Vilk, Jerusalem, Israel

Chapter 1

Pediatric Thrombosis and Hemostasis: A Historical Perspective

Vicky R. Breakey
Victor S. Blanchette

Throughout medical school and residency, trainees frequently hear the old adage 'kids are not just little adults'. Nowhere in pediatrics is this truer than in the physiology of coagulation. In fact, the coagulation system evolves in utero and continues to develop over the course of childhood. In the late 1980s, Maureen Andrew and her colleagues at McMaster University studied healthy newborns and subsequently preterm infants to better understand postnatal development of the human coagulation system and determine appropriate reference ranges [1, 2]. Additional work describing the maturation of the hemostatic system in children and adolescents was published by Andrew et al. [3] in 1992. These landmark studies confirmed significant and important differences in the physiology of coagulation and fibrinolysis in pediatric patients.

Thrombosis in Childhood

Unlike hemostatic disorders, thrombosis has long been considered a condition of adults. The first reported case of inherited coagulopathy described a Norwegian family and was published by Egeberg in 1965. Since then, mutations in numerous genes have been implicated in congenital thrombophilia. Some of the most severe presentations are homozygous mutations that manifest in infancy and childhood. Issues around who and when to test for inherited thrombophilias remain the source of much debate amongst experts in the field [4].

In addition to the clots that occur secondary to inherited mutations, acquired thromboembolic events also present in childhood. In the early 1990s, Dr. Andrew started the first surveillance program across Canada to determine the incidence and nature of thromboembolic diseases in childhood [5]. They found the incidence of DVT/PE to be 5.3/10,000 hospital admissions or 0.07/10,000 children. Follow-up data at a mean of 2.86 years gave additional insights, suggesting a heavy burden of mortality in this group of 16%. Death due to DVT/PE occurred in 2%, all of whom had central venous catheter-associated thrombosis. Morbidity was high with 8% having recurrent thrombosis, and 12% having post-phlebitic syndrome.

Following the initiation of the registry, Dr. Andrew led the development of two practical clinical treatment initiatives. The first was a telephone consultation service, called '1800-NO-CLOTS' which logged well over 4,000 international physician pediatric thrombosis consults in the first 8 years and continues to be active today. The second initiative was the development of institutional pathways for thrombosis treatment. The latter, entitled 'Thromboembolism and Stroke Protocols' was published in 1997 [6]. This practical pocketbook is now in its third edition. These initiatives were well received internationally and continue to be utilized by physicians around the world.

Despite the perceived rarity of thrombosis in childhood, increasing complex medical interventions, central venous catheters and cancer therapies, in particular, have led to a much higher burden of disease. Improved awareness has elevated clinical suspicion, thus increasing the diagnosis of thromboembolic events. Pediatric guidelines for the management of clots were first included in the 5th edition of the American College of Chest Physicians Chest Guidelines for Antithrombotic and Thrombolytic Therapy in 1995. The 9th edition of the guideline was published in 2012 [7]. This document has become the preeminent resource for the management of pediatric thrombosis; however, many recommendations are still based on adult data.

Hemostatic Disorders in Children: The Evolution of Hemophilia Care

Historically, congenital bleeding disorders like hemophilia were considered to be pediatric conditions as patients' life spans were limited due to bleeding. Over the course of the second half of the 20th century, hemophilia care saw considerable advancements, first with the discovery of cryoprecipitate in the 1960s and quickly thereafter with the development of easy to reconstitute and administer lyophilized FVIII and FIX plasma-derived clotting factor concentrates. Tragically, the tainted blood scandal of the 1980s resulted in the death of many young hemophilia patients who were infected with hepatitis virus and/or HIV. This devastating circumstance resulted in intense pressure to develop safe, virus-inactivated plasma-derived FVIII and FIX concentrates and subsequently to engineer synthetic, recombinant FVIII and FIX replacement products. Recombinant FVIII became available in 1988, followed by a recombinant FIX product in 1997. These synthetic products have become the mainstay of hemophilia treatment in much of the developed world.

With improved accessibility to factor replacement and decreased risk of transmission of infectious diseases, the opportunities for regular replacement therapy (prophylaxis) increased. The first FVIII prophylaxis was given in the late 1950s by Inga Marie Nilsson in Sweden [8]. Early studies of prophylaxis were optimistic, suggesting that infusing factor regularly could dramatically improve outcomes. The Swedish group devised the Malmo protocol, which aimed to keep factor levels at >1%, essentially converting severe hemophiliacs to the moderate phenotype with a substantial reduction in the frequency of spontaneous bleeding. Factor was given at a dose of 25–40 IU/kg for a minimum of 3 times weekly for FVIII deficiency, and twice weekly for FIX deficiency. Data showed that early institution of prophylaxis before bleeding is optimal for preventing joint disease. Investigators reported that anything less than full-dose prophylaxis, or prophylaxis started at an older age (>3 years), did not completely prevent significant hemophilic arthropathy in boys with severe hemophilia A [9]. Manco-Johnson et al. [10] were the first to prospectively study prophylaxis in severe hemophilia. The USA Joint Outcome Study randomized 63 boys (<30 months of age) with severe hemophilia to one of two treatment regimens, either primary prophylaxis using the Malmo regimen, or an on-demand regimen in which they received 40 IU/kg of factor with each joint bleed, followed by 25 IU/kg the next day and 2 days later. The primary outcome was preservation of normal joint structure in ankles, knees and elbows as seen with plain-film radiography and MRI at 6 years of age. The results of this prospective randomized controlled trial demonstrated that prophylaxis was significantly better than on-demand therapy for preventing hemarthroses and preserving joint structure and function in boys with hemophilia. With prophylaxis, severe hemophilia patients have far less joint disease. Their lifespan in developed countries approaches that of the general population.

Despite dramatic improvements in hemophilia care, there is still much work to be done. Research into the development and management of inhibitors is ongoing. Although there are excellent clinical outcomes in high-income countries, 80% of the world's hemophilia patients live in places where the cost of safe factor concentrates prohibits its routine usage. It should be noted that hemophilia is only one example of a multitude of hemostatic disorders that affect children. The more rare disorders receive less research funding and are in general less well studied.

The Future of Pediatric Thrombosis and Hemostasis

As we move forward, two essential things must be considered to further develop and advance the field of pediatric thrombosis and hemostasis. The first is continued research in this field. In this small patient population of uncommon disorders, physicians and researchers must continue to form alliances and collaborations. We must continue to pursue representation on committees of large organizations, such as the subcommittee for perinatal and pediatric issues in the ISTH and work together with those who provide adult hematology care. In addition, research collaborations at national and international levels will increase patient enrollment numbers and promote the success of prospective clinical studies. We must find creative ways to overcome additional barriers beyond small numbers of patients, which include practical limitations to the number and volume of blood samples needed and financial constraints on funding for pediatric research [11]. In providing improved evidence, we will promote the best care for our patients.

Secondly, we must support trainee education and sub-specialization. In pediatrics, we face an ongoing struggle to ensure that non-malignant hematology receives sufficient attention in intensive combined pediatric hematology/oncology training curricula. If hematology is taught well by enthusiastic teachers, more trainees will opt to focus in this area. An editorial in the *Journal of Thrombosis and Hemostasis* suggested a dramatic decline in the number of physicians interested in careers in the area of bleeding disorders [12]. There was a call for additional fellowship programs to support the education of a new generation of specialists in this area, and it was suggested that training should not be concentrated in one area alone, but should embrace both thrombosis and hemostasis, at least for young academic physicians entering the field [13]. Since that time, many additional fellowships have been started, most funded by industry sponsors. There is no data to show the number of trainees pursuing those fellowships, but human resources continue to be an important issue.

In summary, the history of the study and care of disorders of pediatric thrombosis and hemostasis is a tale of innovative thought, hard work and dedication. Our predecessors were talented and driven to build the science that supports our clinical practice. The story continues to evolve and much is left to be discovered. International research collaborations and focused efforts to mentor young academically oriented physicians will ensure that new gains continue to be made in the coming years.

Acknowledgment

The authors would like to express their appreciation for the thoughtful comments provided by Drs. Anthony K.C. Chan (Hamilton, Ont., Canada), Gabrielle DeVeber (Toronto, Ont., Canada), M. Patricia Massicotte (Edmonton, Alta., Canada) and Paul Monagle (Melbourne, Vic., Australia) who reviewed this chapter.

References

1 Andrew M, Paes B, Milner R, Johnston M, Mitchell L, Tollefsen DM, et al: Development of the human coagulation system in the full-term infant. Blood 1987;70:165–172.
2 Andrew M, Paes B, Milner R, Johnston M, Mitchell L, Tollefsen DM, et al: Development of the human coagulation system in the healthy premature infant. Blood 1988;72:1651–1657.
3 Andrew M, Vegh P, Johnston M, Bowker J, Ofosu F, Mitchell L: Maturation of the hemostatic system during childhood. Blood 1992;80:1998–2005.
4 Heleen van Ommen C, Middeldorp S: Thrombophilia in childhood: to test or not to test. Semin Thromb Hemost 2011;37:794–801.
5 Monagle P, Adams M, Mahoney M, Ali K, Barnard D, Bernstein M, et al: Outcome of pediatric thromboembolic disease: a report from the Canadian childhood thrombophilia registry. Pediatr Res 2000;47:763–766.
6 Andrew M, deVeber G: Pediatric Thromboembolism and Stroke Protocols, ed 1. Hamilton, BC Decker, 1997.
7 Monagle P, Chan AK, Goldenberg NA, Ichord RN, Journeycake JM, Nowak-Gottl U, et al: Antithrombotic therapy in neonates and children: antithrombotic therapy and prevention of thrombosis, ed 9: American College of Chest Physicians Evidence-Based Clinical Practice Guidelines. Chest 2012;141(suppl 2):e737S–e801S.
8 Nilsson IM, Blomback M, Ahlberg A: Our experience in Sweden with prophylaxis on haemophilia. Bibl Haematol 1970;34:111–124.
9 Nilsson IM: Experience with prophylaxis in Sweden. Semin Hematol 1993;30(suppl 2):16–19.
10 Manco-Johnson MJ, Abshire TC, Shapiro AD, Riske B, Hacker MR, Kilcoyne R, et al: Prophylaxis versus episodic treatment to prevent joint disease in boys with severe hemophilia. N Engl J Med 2007;357:535–544.
11 Manco-Johnson MJ: Pediatric thrombophilia and thrombosis: an historical perspective. Hematology Am Soc Hematol Educ Program 2008;2008:227.
12 Mannucci PM, Roberts HR: Uncertain times for research on hemophilia and allied disorders. J Thromb Haemost 2005;3:423.
13 Blanchette VS: Uncertain times for research on hemophilia and allied disorders. J Thromb Haemost 2006;4:682.

Abbreviations

DVT	Deep vein thrombosis
FVIII	Factor VIII
FIX	Factor IX
HIV	Human immunodeficiency virus
ISTH	International Society on Thrombosis and Haemostasis
MRI	Magnetic resonance imaging
PE	Pulmonary embolism

Chapter 2

Primary and Secondary Hemostasis, Regulators of Coagulation, and Fibrinolysis: Understanding the Basics

Shoshana Revel-Vilk
Margaret L. Rand
Sara J. Israels

Introduction

At the site of vessel wall injury, adhesion, activation and aggregation of platelets result in the formation of a platelet plug (primary hemostasis). Activation of the coagulation pathway results in the formation of covalently cross-linked fibrin that stabilizes the platelet plug (secondary hemostasis). Inhibitors of the coagulation cascade limit and confine the response (regulation of coagulation), and activation of the fibrinolytic pathway results in dissolution of the fibrin clot to maintain and/or restore blood vessel patency (fibrinolysis). The aim of this chapter is to summarize the complex process of hemostasis, highlighting points that are relevant to clinical practice (with referral to the relevant chapter, where applicable). Developmental hemostasis, i.e. the maturation of the hemostasis system from infancy to adulthood, is discussed in chapter 4.

Primary Hemostasis

Primary hemostasis is based on the formation of a platelet plug at a site of vascular injury. It has four sequential but overlapping phases: vasoconstriction, platelet adhesion, platelet activation and platelet aggregation [1, 2].

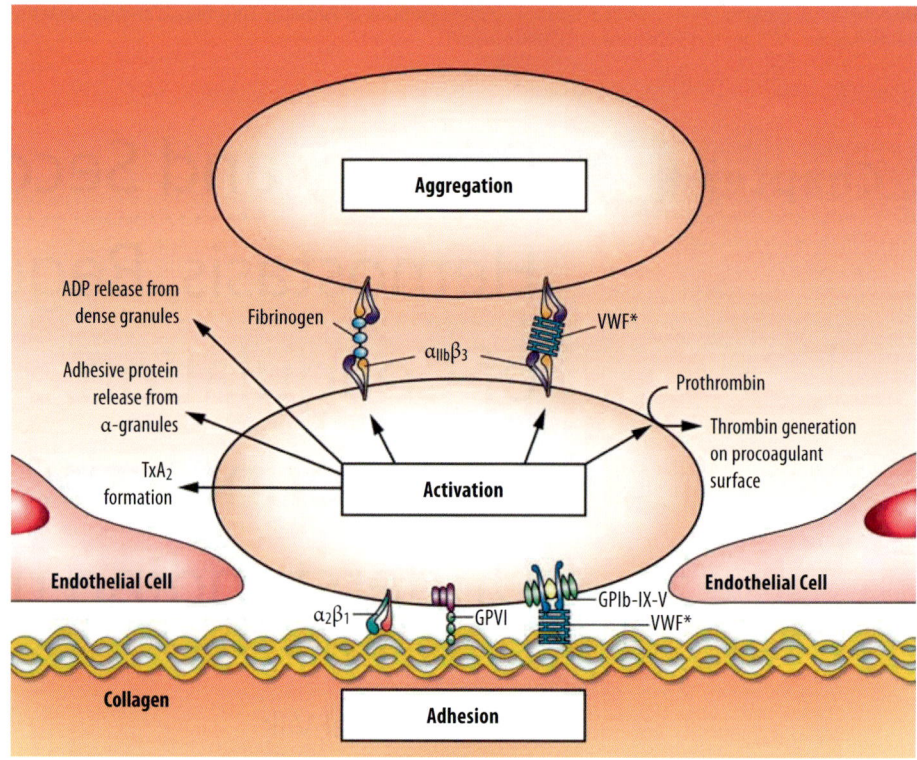

Figure 1. A simplified diagram of platelet adhesion, activation, and aggregation in response to blood vessel wall damage and exposure of subendothelium; the platelet plug that forms aids in the cessation of bleeding. Asterisk indicates interactions involving VWF that occur at high shear. Reproduced with permission from Israels and Rand [3].

Vasoconstriction

Immediate constriction of the vessel to temporarily decrease blood flow and pressure within the vessel occurs as a neurogenic response. Serotonin and TxA_2 released from the activated platelets further promote vasoconstriction.

Platelet Adhesion

In the bloodstream, red cells predominate in the axial stream, with platelets being marginated along the vessel wall by shear forces and collisions with red cells. As a result, platelets are well positioned to monitor the integrity of the vessel wall. When endothelial damage occurs, platelets are captured by exposed collagen fibrils, the most thrombogenic component of the subendothelial matrix (figure 1). Adhesion of platelets to collagen is influenced by shear stress. At low shear, binding occurs via the integrin $\alpha_2\beta_1$ (GPIa-IIa) and GPVI receptors, while at high shear, binding occurs via the GPIb-IX-V receptor and VWF bound to the collagen. Platelet adhesion at the site of vessel wall damage initiates activation events via intracellular signaling pathways.

Platelet Activation

Platelets adherent to the subendothelium undergo a dramatic shape change to an irregular sphere with multiple filipodia, spreading to increase their area of surface contact. During shape change, granules coalesce in the center of the platelet, fuse with the surface-connected canalicular system and release their contents to the exterior. Secretion of the aggregating agent ADP from dense granules amplifies platelet recruitment and activation (figure 1). Release of VWF and fibrinogen (adhesive proteins) from α-granules enhances platelet adhesion and aggregation. Release of the aggregating agent TxA$_2$, a second messenger synthesized via the COX-1 pathway, augments platelet activation and recruitment of additional platelets to the platelet plug (figure 1). ASA, the most commonly used antiplatelet drug, acts through irreversible inactivation of COX-1 (chapter 16).

Activated platelets undergo remodeling of the surface membrane resulting in exposure of phosphatidylserine on the cell surface. This negatively charged aminophospholipid provides a procoagulant surface for the assembly of the coagulation factors and generation of thrombin, the most potent platelet-aggregating agent (figure 1). Thrombin triggers further secretion of storage granule contents and formation of TxA$_2$, both of which act to enhance platelet activation.

Platelet Aggregation

Aggregation is an active process resulting from binding of the agonists ADP, TxA$_2$ and thrombin to their specific membrane receptors. ADP activates platelets via the P2Y$_1$ and P2Y$_{12}$ receptors; TxA$_2$, via the thromboxane-prostanoid receptor; and thrombin, via binding to GPIb-IX-V and cleaving PAR1 and PAR4 (protease-activated receptors 1 and 4). The antiplatelet drugs clopidogrel and prasugrel act through irreversible blocking of the P2Y$_{12}$ ADP receptor (chapter 16). Epinephrine stimulates aggregation via α$_2$-adrenerigic receptors, but only in the presence of other agonists. The binding of these agonists results in activation of intracellular signaling pathways, ultimately converting integrin α$_{IIb}$β$_3$ (GPIIb-IIIa) from a low-affinity resting state to a high-affinity activated state. Activated α$_{IIb}$β$_3$ binds to plasma fibrinogen and VWF, the latter at high shear (figure 1). Divalent fibrinogen and multivalent VWF function as bridges between α$_{IIb}$β$_3$ on adjacent activated platelets, resulting in aggregation and formation of the platelet plug.

An animation summarizing platelet plug formation in primary hemostasis can be viewed at the URL provided in [4]. Abnormalities of platelet adhesion, activation and/or aggregation are associated with increased mucocutaneous bleeding (chapter 5).

Secondary Hemostasis

Secondary hemostasis results in the formation, via the coagulation pathway, of covalently cross-linked fibrin that stabilizes the platelet plug [5]. The pathway is complex and involves many different proteins: zymogens (inactive precursors) of serine proteases (FII, FVII, FIX, FX, FXI, FXII); cofactors (TF, FVIII, FV); a transglutaminase zymogen (FXIII); and fibrinogen. A serine protease is an enzyme with the amino acid serine in its active site that hydrolyzes specific peptide bonds in proteins, and a transglutaminase is an enzyme that forms peptide bonds between the side chains of specific glutamine and lysine amino acid residues. Congenital and acquired deficiencies of FII, FV, FVII, FVIII, FIX, FX, FXI, FXIII and fibrinogen are associated with increased bleeding (chapters 6 and 8).

Serial activation of the serine protease zymogens and FVIII and FV, and feedback amplification loops result in the activation of FII (prothrombin) to FIIa (thrombin; figure 2) (note: activated coagulation factors are denoted by the suffix 'a'). The activation of the serine protease zymogens occurs on negatively charged phospholipid membrane surfaces of activated platelets, monocytes and endothelial cells. Thrombin is a multifunctional enzyme that catalyzes reactions that promote coagulation, particularly the conversion of fibrinogen to fibrin monomer, but also reactions that limit coagulation, including activation of the anticoagulant protein C.

The serine protease coagulation zymogens are synthesized in the liver. Vitamin K is an essential cofactor for γ-carboxylation of the N-terminal

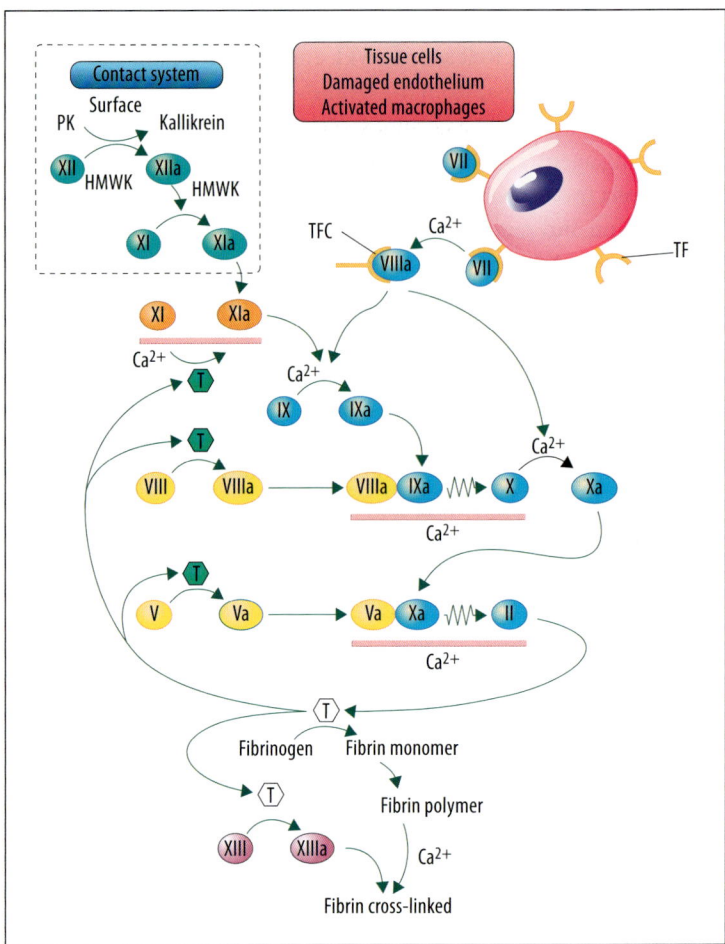

Figure 2. A serial activation of coagulation zymogens and feedback amplification loops starting from the exposure/release of TF and ending in the generation of thrombin (T). PK = Prekallikrein; TFC = TF complex. © Mechanisms in Medicine Inc.

glutamic acid residues of the vitamin K-dependent zymogens FII, FVII, FIX and FX; γ-carboxylation enhances the association of these factors with negatively charged phospholipid membrane surfaces. Vitamin K deficiency is associated with increased bleeding risk in newborns (chapter 4), and older children (chapter 9). Vitamin K antagonists are used for oral anticoagulation therapy (chapter 16). FVIII is synthesized in the liver and endothelial cells, and FV is synthesized in the liver and megakaryocytes (and stored in the α-granules of megakaryocytes and platelets). TF is an integral membrane GP that normally does not come into contact with flowing blood.

Coagulation proceeds by the formation of three enzyme complexes: the TF complex (TF/FVIIa), the tenase complex (FVIIIa/FIXa) and the prothrombinase complex (FVa/FXa). Each of these complexes involves a vitamin K-dependent protein (FVIIa, FIXa, FXa) and a membrane-bound cofactor (TF, FVIIIa, FVa). The coagulation pathway has three sequential overlapping phases: initiation, amplification and propagation.

Initiation of Coagulation

At the site of vessel wall injury, blood comes into contact with cells that express TF on their surfaces, and TF complexes (TF/FVIIa) are formed

[6]. Historically referred to as the extrinsic pathway because of the extravascular location of TF, this pathway is the primary initiator of hemostasis in vivo. The TF/FVIIa complex activates small amounts of FX and FIX. FXa forms a complex with FVa to convert small amounts of FII (prothrombin) to FIIa (thrombin). Therapeutically, recombinant FVIIa is used to initiate hemostasis in patients with hemophilia complicated by inhibitors (chapter 6), or Glanzmann thrombasthenia (chapter 5).

Amplification of Coagulation

Thrombin formed during initiation activates platelets, exposing the negatively charged membrane surface and releasing FV from the α-granules, and activates FXI, FVIII and FV on the activated platelet surface.

Propagation of Coagulation

On the activated platelet surface, FIXa, formed during the initiation phase and activated by platelet-bound FXIa, binds to FVIIIa, and with Ca^{2+}, in the tenase complex, activates FX to FXa. FXa then associates with FVa and Ca^{2+} in the prothrombinase complex, resulting in a burst of thrombin generation.

The thrombin formed during the propagation phase of coagulation is of sufficient concentration to promote fibrin clot formation. Thrombin cleaves fibrinopeptides A and B from fibrinogen to form fibrin monomer; fibrin monomers polymerize spontaneously to form an insoluble fibrin mesh. Thrombin also converts FXIII to FXIIIa that stabilizes the fragile clot by covalently cross-linking fibrin, making the fibrin polymer resistant to lysis.

The Contact System

The contact factors play a minor role in initiating coagulation in vivo (figure 2) [7]. However, they are important in the initiation of the coagulation cascade in vitro (referred to as the 'intrinsic pathway'), as measured by the aPTT. Surface contact activates FXII to FXIIa in the presence of prekallikrein and HMWK. FXIIa activates prekallikrein to kallikrein and FXI to FXIa. Kallikrein feeds back to activate additional FXII and cleaves HMWK to release bradykinin. In vivo, the activation of FXI is not dependent on the contact proteins, and thus deficiencies of FXII, prekallikrein or HMWK are not associated with abnormal bleeding. The aPTT is a functional screening test for the intrinsic pathway of coagulation (chapter 3) and is used for monitoring UFH therapy (chapter 16).

Regulators of Coagulation

Inhibitors of coagulation limit and confine the hemostatic response to vascular damage by a multistep cascade [8]. There are three major inhibitors of coagulation: TFPI, antithrombin, and the protein C system (figure 3).

Tissue Factor Pathway Inhibitor

TFPI binds and inhibits FXa, and then the FXa/TFPI complex binds and inhibits FVIIa bound to TF. It is the only efficient inhibitor of the TF/FVIIa complex, and thus it regulates the initiation phase of coagulation [9].

Antithrombin

Antithrombin, a serine protease inhibitor, slowly reacts with and irreversibly inhibits FXIa, FXa, FIXa, and FIIa (thrombin). The inhibition of more than one factor in the cascade amplifies its effect. Glycosaminoglycans such as heparan sulfate on the endothelial surface bind to antithrombin and act as cofactors that accelerate antithrombin's inhibitory effect (approximately 1,000-fold in the case of thrombin inhibition) (figure 3a). The anticoagulant effect of heparin is the result of its acceleration of serine protease inhibition by antithrombin (chapter 16). Decreased plasma levels of antithrombin are associated with an increased risk for thrombosis (chapter 10).

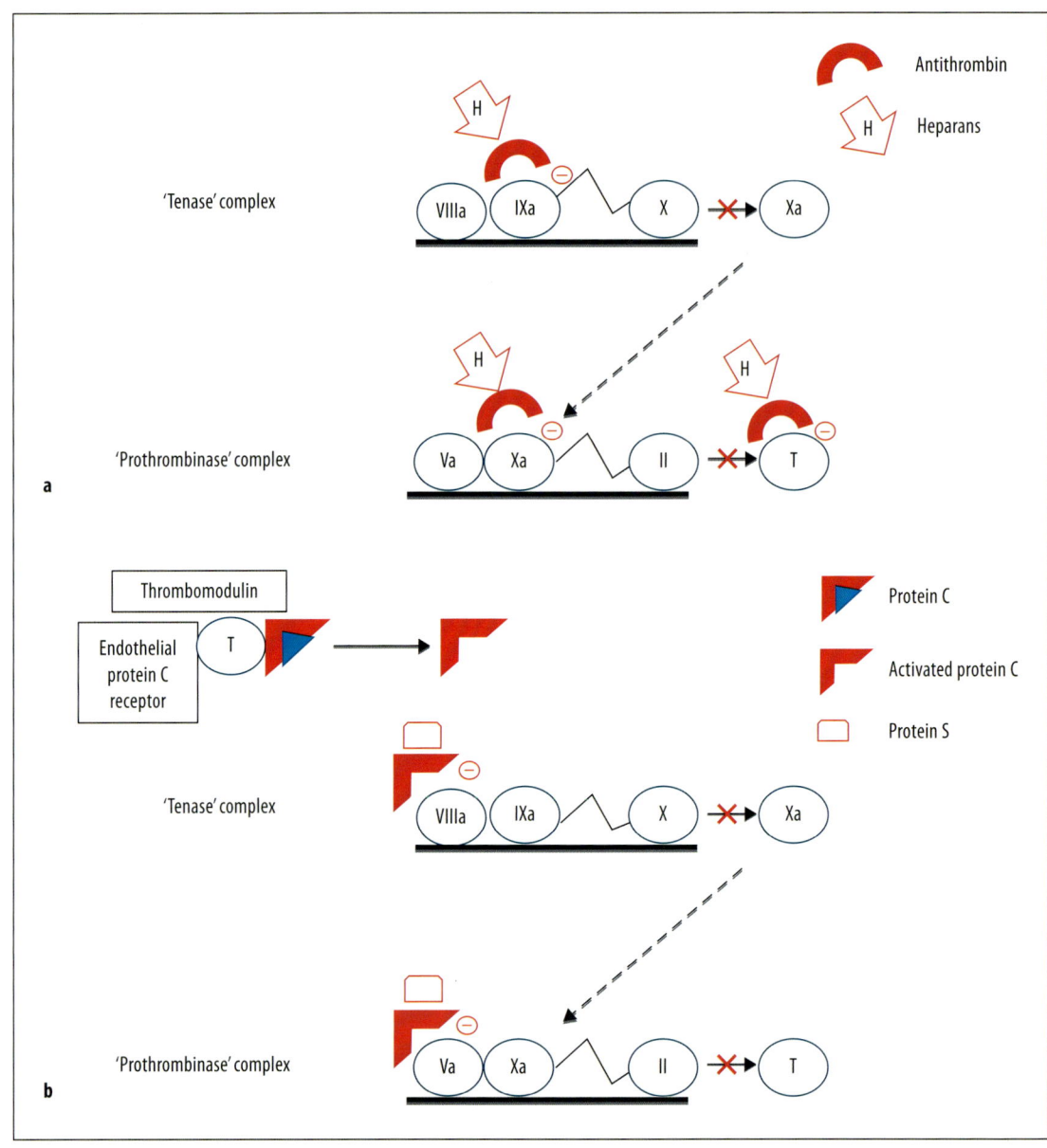

Figure 3. Inhibitors of coagulation. **a** Antithrombin (AT) pathway. **b** Protein C pathway.

Protein C System

Protein C, a vitamin K-dependent zymogen, is activated on the endothelial surface by thrombin bound to thrombomodulin. Thrombin bound to thrombomodulin gains the potential to activate protein C, but it loses its capacity to cleave fibrinogen. The endothelial protein C receptor is a cofactor that amplifies the activation of protein C by thrombin/thrombomodulin (figure 3b). aPC degrades cofactors FVIIIa and FVa. Amplification occurs because one molecule of thrombin can activate many molecules of protein C, and each molecule of aPC can cleave many molecules of FVIIIa or FVa. Protein S, a vitamin K-dependent cofactor for aPC, accelerates the cleavage of FVIIIa and FVa. Decreased plasma levels of protein C or protein S, or mutations causing aPC resistance (e.g. FV Leiden), are associated with increased risk for thrombosis (chapter 10).

Other Inhibitors

Several other proteins, including heparin cofactor II, protein C inhibitor, protein Z and Z-dependent protease inhibitor, contribute to the regulation of coagulation, but play less clinically significant roles.

Fibrinolysis

The major enzyme of the fibrinolytic pathway is plasmin [10, 11]. It is the product of plasminogen cleavage by specific plasminogen activators, t-PA and u-PA (figure 4). Plasmin cleaves fibrin into soluble fragments (FDPs). Proteases released by neutrophils and other cells can also degrade fibrin to end products that are removed by phagocytosis. Analogous to the coagulation system, the fibrinolytic system is regulated by both activators and inhibitors [12].

Plasminogen Activators

t-PA, a serine protease synthesized by endothelial cells, is the primary intravascular activator of plasminogen (figure 4a). The binding of plasminogen and t-PA to fibrin forms a ternary complex, which amplifies the activity of t-PA several hundred times and ensures that only fibrin-bound plasminogen is activated. When plasminogen is cleaved, plasmin remains bound to fibrin, where it is protected from inhibitors and is optimally positioned to degrade fibrin. Recombinant t-PA is currently an important drug used for therapeutic thrombolysis (chapter 16).

u-PA (figure 4b) is synthesized by monocytes/macrophages, fibroblasts and epithelial cells, and is found in urine, plasma and the extracellular matrix. u-PA is secreted as an inactive single-chain molecule. At sites of vascular injury, kallikrein, FXIIIa, thrombin or plasmin can cleave single-chain u-PA into a two-chain active form. Activated u-PA enhances fibrinolysis by further activation of plasminogen. The single-chain form also has enhanced activity when bound to receptors on leukocytes and platelets. In contrast to t-PA, u-PA can activate plasmin in the absence of fibrin. Urokinase can also be used for therapeutic thrombolysis (chapter 16).

Inhibitors of Plasminogen Activation

PAI-1, a serine protease inhibitor, is the primary inhibitor of t-PA and u-PA (figure 4a). It is synthesized in the liver, endothelial cells and megakaryocytes, and is stored in endothelial cells and platelet α-granules. Fibrinolytic enzymes bound to fibrin are protected from inhibition; unbound enzymes are not. PAI-1 forms stable complexes with unbound t-PA and u-PA that are cleared by the liver.

TAFI inhibits fibrinolysis by interfering with formation of the fibrin-plasminogen-t-PA complex. TAFI is activated to TAFIa by high concentrations of thrombin (thereby linking coagulation and fibrinolysis). Reduced thrombin generation results in decreased TAFIa and an increased rate of clot lysis; this mechanism may contribute to the premature lysis of clots in hemophilia (chapter 6). TAFIa is inactivated by plasmin; reduced plasmin formation results in increased TAFIa activity.

Inhibitors of Plasmin

$α_2$-AP (also called $α_2$-plasmin inhibitor), a serine protease inhibitor, is the primary inhibitor of plasmin. It is synthesized in the liver, circulates in plasma and is stored in platelet α-granules. $α_2$-AP neutralizes both fibrin-bound and free (unbound) plasmin by binding to its catalytic and

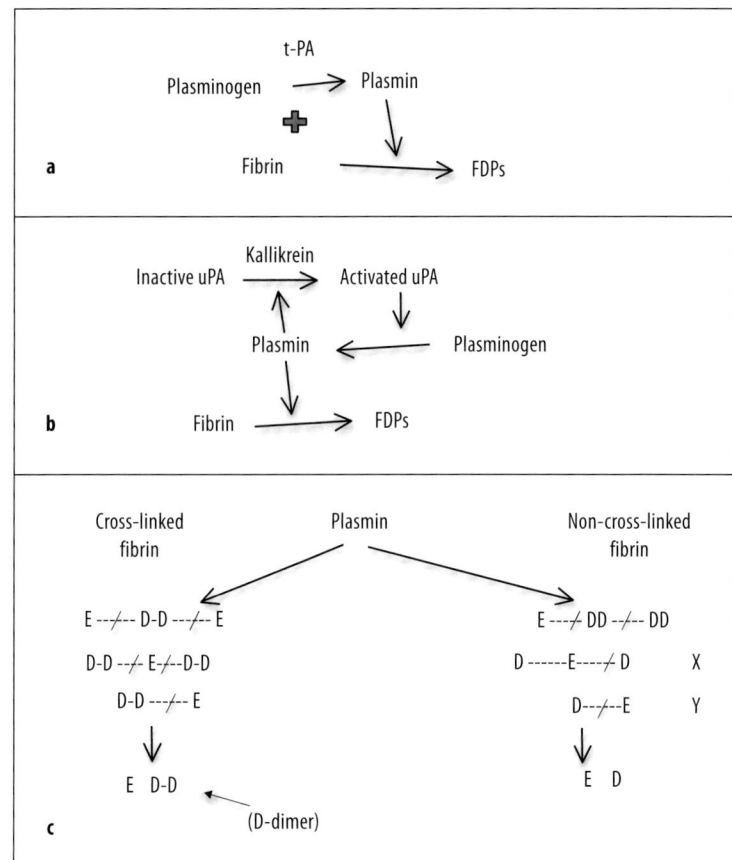

Figure 4. Schema of fibrinolysis. **a** t-PA binds to plasminogen and fibrin to form a complex: t-PA-plasminogen-fibrin complex. **b** Activated u-PA activates plasminogen in the absence of fibrin. Plasmin activates u-PA. **c** FDPs from cross-linked fibrin and non-cross-linked fibrin.

lysine-binding sites. The $α_2$-AP-plasmin complexes are cleared by the liver.

$α_2$-Macroglobulin, a nonspecific protease inhibitor, also inhibits plasmin. It is synthesized by endothelial cells and macrophages, and is stored in platelet α-granules. It functions as a salvage inhibitor in the event of major systemic activation of the fibrinolysis system.

Fibrin Degradation Products

The degradation of fibrin by plasmin produces lytic fragments of the fibrin polymer. The products differ depending on the substrate (figure 4c). Cross-linked fibrin is degraded to one fragment E and two cross-linked D-D fragments (D-dimers). Fibrinogen and non-cross-linked fibrin are degraded to fragment X. Further lysis of fragment X generates fragments Y and D. Fragment Y is further degraded to fragments D and E.

Elevated plasma levels of FDPs can be observed in the setting of thrombosis, inflammation, consumptive coagulopathy, liver disease or malignancy (see chapter 10). The presence of elevated D-dimers in plasma indicates lysis of cross-linked fibrin. D-dimer measurement can be used in conjunction with additional clinical assessment to exclude the diagnosis of venous thromboembolism (chapter 11).

Conclusion

Hemostasis is a complex process that relies on the equilibrium between procoagulant and anticoagulant factors that interact to ensure appropriate hemostatic plug formation at sites of vascular injury. Disruption of this equilibrium resulting from structural abnormalities or aberrant concentrations of the components can lead to either hemorrhage or thrombosis. Understanding how the balance in the hemostatic system is maintained, and how it can be disrupted, is key to the diagnosis and management of hemostatic and thrombotic disorders.

References

1. Israels SJ, Kahr WH, Blanchette VS, Luban NL, Rivard G, Rand ML: Platelet disorders in children: a diagnostic approach. Pediatr Blood Cancer 2011;56:975.
2. Rand ML, Israels SJ, McNicol A: Platelet structure and function; in Israels SJ (ed): Mechanisms in Hematology, ed 4. Core Health Services, 2010; www.mechanismsinhematology.ca.
3. Israels SJ, Rand ML: What we have learned from inherited platelet disorders. Pediatr Blood Cancer 2013;60(suppl 1):S2–S7.
4. http://www.youtube.com/watch?v=0pnpoEy0eYE.
5. Teitel JM: Coagulation cascade; in Israels SJ (ed): Mechanisms in Hematology, ed 4. Core Health Services, 2010; www.mechanismsinhematology.ca.
6. Mackman N: The role of tissue factor and factor VIIa in hemostasis. Anesth Analg 2009;108:1447.
7. Maas C, Oschatz C, Renne T: The plasma contact system 2.0. Semin Thromb Hemost 2011;37:375.
8. Houston DS: Regulators of coagulation; in Israels SJ (ed): Mechanisms in Hematology, ed 4. Core Health Services, 2010; www.mechanismsinhematology.ca.
9. Adams M: Tissue factor pathway inhibitor: new insights into an old inhibitor. Semin Thromb Hemost 2012;38:129.
10. Chan AKC, Chan HHW, Berry LS: Fibrinogen, factor XIII and fibrinolysis; in Israels SJ (ed): Mechanisms in Hematology, ed 4. Core Health Services, 2010; www.mechanismsinhematology.ca.
11. Parmar N, Albisetti M, Berry LR, Chan AK: The fibrinolytic system in newborns and children. Clin Lab 2006;52:115.
12. Schaller J, Gerber SS: The plasmin-antiplasmin system: structural and functional aspects. Cell Mol Life Sci 2011;68:785.

Abbreviations

α_2-AP	α_2-Antiplasmin
ADP	Adenosine 5′-diphosphate
aPC	Activated protein C
aPTT	Activated partial thromboplastin time
ASA	Acetylsalicylic acid
COX	Cyclooxygenase
FDPs	Fibrin degradation products
FII	Factor II (prothrombin)
FV	Factor V
FVII	Factor VII
FVIII	Factor VIII
FIX	Factor IX
FX	Factor X
FXI	Factor XI
FXII	Factor XII
FXIII	Factor XIII
GP	Glycoprotein
HMWK	High-molecular-weight kininogen
PAI-1	Plasminogen activator inhibitor type 1
PK	Prekallikrein
TAFI	Thrombin-activatable finbrinolysis inhibitor
TF	Tissue factor
TFPI	Tissue factor pathway inhibitor
TFC	TF complex
t-PA	Tissue-plasminogen activator
TxA$_2$	Thromboxane A$_2$
UFH	Unfractionated heparin
u-PA	Urokinase plasminogen activator
VWF	von Willebrand factor

Chapter 3 An Approach to the Bleeding Child

Shoshana Revel-Vilk
Margaret L. Rand
Sara J. Israels

Introduction

Bleeding in a child can be a diagnostic challenge because of the wide range of possible causes, but making a specific diagnosis is clinically important in order to provide appropriate therapy. An excessive bleeding response to commonly encountered challenges suggests the possibility of an underlying bleeding disorder. Symptoms such as bruising and epistaxis occur frequently in children without underlying bleeding disorders, and so determining which child requires further investigation can be difficult. Even when initial symptoms appear unimpressive, children with underlying bleeding disorders may be at increased risk for significant bleeding associated with surgical procedures or trauma.

Bleeding disorders can be inherited or acquired, and include coagulation factor deficiencies, platelet deficiencies and/or dysfunctions, and VWD [1, 2]. The evaluation of a child presenting with bleeding should include a comprehensive medical and bleeding history, a complete family history, a detailed physical examination and selected laboratory tests as outlined in algorithm 1.

History

Medical History

Clinical evaluation of a bleeding patient begins with a detailed history, with emphasis on the child's age, sex, past medical history, clinical presentation, and family history.

Age
Most cases of severe inherited hemostatic defects will be diagnosed in infancy because of significant mucocutaneous bleeding, postcircumcision bleeding, bleeding from the umbilical stump or ICH. However, moderate and mild inherited hemostatic defects may not present with clinical bleeding until an older age, or until the child is exposed to a hemostatic challenge. Thus, the possibility of an inherited hemostatic defect should

Table 1. Clinical abnormalities associated with inherited bleeding disorders

Coagulation defects	
FXIII deficiency	poor wound healing, severe scar formation
Platelet function defects	
Hermansky-Pudlak syndrome	oculocutaneous albinism
Chediak-Higashi syndrome	oculocutaneous albinism, infections, neutrophil peroxidase-positive inclusions
ARC syndrome	arthrogryposis, renal dysfunction, cholestasis
MYH9-related disorders	cataracts, sensorineural hearing defect, nephritis
Leukocyte adhesion deficiency type III	recurrent severe infections, delayed separation of the umbilical cord, neutrophilia
Thrombocytopenia	
Wiskott-Aldrich syndrome	eczema, immunodeficiency
Thrombocytopenia with absent radii, amegakaryocytic thrombocytopenia with radioulnar synostosis	skeletal defects
DiGeorge/velocardiofacial syndrome	cleft palate, cardiac defects, facial anomalies, learning disabilities
Paris-Trousseau/Jacobsen syndrome	cardiac defects, craniofacial anomalies, mental retardation
X-linked thrombocytopenia and dyserythropoiesis with or without anemia/X-linked thrombocytopenia-thalassemia	microcytosis of red blood cells, unbalanced hemoglobin chain synthesis resembling β-thalassemia minor

be considered in a child with clinically significant bleeding symptoms/signs, regardless of the age at presentation.

Acquired bleeding disorders can present at any age. For example, although ITP commonly presents between the ages of 2–10 years, presentation from the age of 3 months until adulthood can occur.

Sex

Some of the inherited hemostatic defects such as hemophilia A (FVIII deficiency), hemophilia B (FIX deficiency), Wiskott-Aldrich syndrome/X-linked thrombocytopenia, and X-linked thrombocytopenia with dyserythropoiesis are due to mutations on the X chromosome. A family history of bleeding limited to males suggests an X-linked disorder. All other inherited and acquired hemostatic defects occurs in both sexes, although there is an elevated rate of diagnosis of VWD, platelet defects and FXI deficiency in women because of menorrhagia [3].

General Medical History

Presentation of signs and symptoms other than bleeding can provide a clue to the diagnosis of inherited hemostatic disorders (table 1). A detailed medical history is essential for the diagnosis of acquired hemostatic disorders. A history of weakness, fever, weight loss, etc., can suggest malignancy. Liver disease affects synthesis of multiple coagulation factors. Cholestasis, fat malabsorption or antibiotic use can cause vitamin K deficiency. Sepsis is associated with consumptive coagulopathy and thrombocytopenia. Uremia can be associated with acquired platelet dysfunction. The use of medications can be associated with drug-induced thrombocytopenia, or platelet dysfunction (chapter 5).

Bleeding History

Type and pattern of bleeding are important indicators of possible diagnoses. Mucocutaneous bleeding such as petechiae, bruising, epistaxis, gastrointestinal bleeding and/or menorrhagia suggests disorders of platelets, VWD, or the vasculature. There may be prolonged bleeding following surgery and/or dental extractions. In contrast, spontaneous or excessive bleeding into soft tissues, muscles and joints, or delayed surgical bleeding suggests disorders of coagulation factors. It should be noted that coagulation factor disorders may also cause mucocutaneous bleeding, epistaxis, or gastrointestinal bleeding. ICH, postcircumcision bleeding or severe mucosal bleeding in early infancy requires immediate investigation for a coagulation factor deficiency. Bleeding from the umbilical cord stump within the first days of life is strongly suggestive of FXIII deficiency or afibrinogenemia.

The onset and acuity of bleeding can also aid in indicating a specific diagnosis. Acquired disorders may have an acute onset (e.g. ITP) compared with inherited disorders where symptoms are present for months or years. Challenges to the hemostatic system are often required to make a bleeding disorder clinically evident, so that mild/moderate bleeding disorders may not be appreciated until events such as trauma, surgery, or menarche occur.

The recognition of significant clinical bleeding is the first step in the diagnosis of bleeding disorders [4]. In children with severe bleeding disorders, the bleeding history is usually clear. However, children presenting with mild/moderate bleeding symptoms may have bleeding symptoms such as recurrent epistaxis or bruises that are also common among healthy children. The distinction between normal children and those with bleeding disorders can be difficult to make.

The use of standardized scores to quantitate bleeding symptoms is recommended. Recently, a PBQ (an adaptation of the standardized MCM DM-1 VWD questionnaire), was developed and validated (table 2) [5–7]. It provides a summative score for 13 bleeding symptoms: epistaxis, cutaneous bleeding, bleeding from minor wounds, oral cavity bleeding, gastrointestinal bleeding, bleeding post-tooth extraction, postsurgical bleeding, menorrhagia, postpartum hemorrhage, muscle hematoma, hemarthrosis, central nervous system bleeding and 'other', pediatric-specific bleeding symptoms (postcircumcision bleeding, umbilical stump bleeding, cephalohematoma, macroscopic hematuria, postvenipuncture bleeding, conjunctival hemorrhage). The mean bleeding score in healthy children was 0.5, and a bleeding score of ≥2 was defined as abnormal. The PBQ was validated prospectively as a screening tool for the diagnosis of VWD and studies validating it for the diagnosis of other bleeding disorders are ongoing.

Family History

In addition to the child's bleeding history, the family history may provide important clues about the potential inheritance of an underlying bleeding disorder. For example, an autosomal-dominant inheritance pattern would be in keeping with type 1 VWD and some platelet function disorders, and a sex-linked pattern, with FVIII or FIX deficiency. Consanguinity in a family increases the risk of autosomal-recessive disorders. Evaluation of the bleeding history in family members by a validated bleeding questionnaire could be useful for appreciating the significance of the family bleeding history.

Generally, there is little racial or ethnic predisposition to bleeding disorders. However, there are some bleeding disorders which are more prevalent in certain populations, e.g. FXI deficiency among Jews of Ashkenazi (European) origin and among the Basque population of south-western France and north-eastern Spain. Autosomal-recessive bleeding disorders can be more common in small, geographically or ethnically isolated communities sharing common genes.

Physical Examination

A careful physical examination for evaluation of clinical bleeding and associated abnormalities is an essential part in the diagnosis of hemostatic

Table 2. Pediatric bleeding questionnaire scoring key

Symptom	–1	0	1	2	3	4
Epistaxis	–	no or trivial (≤5 per year)	>5 per year or >10 min duration	consultation only	packing, cauterization or antifibrinolytics	blood transfusion, replacement therapy or desmopressin
Cutaneous	–	no or trivial (≤1 cm)	>1 cm and no trauma	consultation only	–	–
Minor wounds	–	no or trivial (≤5 per year)	>5 per year or >5 min duration	consultation only or steri-strips	surgical hemostasis or antifibrinolytics	blood transfusion, replacement therapy or desmopressin
Oral cavity	–	no	reported at least one	consultation only	surgical hemostasis or antifibrinolytics	blood transfusion, replacement therapy or desmopressin
Gastrointestinal tract	–	no	identified cause	consultation or spontaneous	surgical hemostasis, antifibrinolytics, blood transfusion, replacement therapy or desmopressin	–
Tooth extraction	no bleeding in at least 2 extractions	none done or no bleeding in 1	reported, no consultation	consultation only	resuturing, repacking or antifibrinolytics	blood transfusion, replacement therapy or desmopressin
Surgery	no bleeding in at least 2 surgeries	none done or no bleeding in 1	reported, no consultation	consultation only	surgical hemostasis or antifibrinolytics	blood transfusion, replacement therapy or desmopressin
Menorrhagia	–	no	reported or consultation only	antifibrinolytics or contraceptive pill use	D&C or iron therapy	blood transfusion, replacement therapy, desmopressin or hysterectomy
Postpartum	no bleeding in at least 2 deliveries	no deliveries or no bleeding in 1 delivery	reported or consultation only	D&C, iron therapy or antifibrinolytics	blood transfusion, replacement therapy or desmopressin	–
Muscle hematoma	–	never	post-trauma, no therapy	spontaneous, no therapy	spontaneous or traumatic, requiring desmopressin or replacement therapy	spontaneous or traumatic, requiring surgical intervention or blood transfusion
Hemarthrosis	–	never	post-trauma, no therapy	spontaneous, no therapy	spontaneous or traumatic, requiring desmopressin or replacement therapy	spontaneous or traumatic, requiring surgical intervention or blood transfusion
Central nervous system	–	never	–	–	subdural, any intervention	intracerebral, any intervention
Other: postcircumcision umbilical stump cephalohematoma macroscopic hematuria postvenipuncture conjunctival hemorrhage	–	no	reported	consultation only	surgical hemostasis, antifibrinolytics or iron therapy	blood transfusion, replacement therapy or desmopressin

An Approach to the Bleeding Child

disorders. Mucocutaneous bleeding suggests a disorder of primary hemostasis, i.e. VWD or platelet dysfunction/deficiency, or a vascular disorder. In males, deep hematomas, hemarthroses, or evidence of chronic joint abnormalities suggests hemophilia. Acquired bleeding disorders may present in the context of coexisting illness. Lymphadenopathy and/or organomegaly suggest an infiltrative process such as malignancy or a storage disease. Signs of liver failure suggest acquired coagulation factor deficiencies. Additional congenital anomalies may suggest the presence of a syndromic bleeding disorder (table 1).

A pattern of bruising that is not consistent with accidental injury should raise the concern about nonaccidental trauma.

Laboratory Investigations

Laboratory screening tests for suspected bleeding disorders provide additional diagnostic indicators that direct more specific investigations. Algorithm 1 provides an approach to evaluation of a child with bleeding symptoms.

Screening Tests

Initial tests to screen for bleeding disorders should include a CBC, blood film, PT and aPTT.

CBC (blood collected into EDTA) is performed to exclude thrombocytopenia. It should be noted, however, that automated cell counters (counters based on impedance rather than optical technology) may underestimate platelet counts and under- or overestimate mean platelet volume when platelet size is outside of the established reference interval. The CBC also provides information about additional cytopenias, and other WBC and RBC abnormalities.

Peripheral blood film (blood collected into EDTA) provides additional information regarding platelet number, size, clumping and granularity (the platelet count can be estimated by the number of platelets per ×100 field multiplied by 20×10^9/l). Pseudothrombocytopenia resulting from clumping of platelets collected in EDTA anticoagulant can be identified by examination of the blood film, and confirmed by re-collecting a specimen in citrate anticoagulant in which clumping will not occur. Examination of the peripheral blood film is essential in the evaluation of a child with a suspected platelet disorder (chapter 5). If true thrombocytopenia is diagnosed, the next step would be to differentiate between new onset acquired thrombocytopenia, chronic acquired thrombocytopenia and congenital thrombocytopenia (algorithm 1; chapter 5).

Evaluation of WBC morphology allows identification of malignant blasts, granulocyte inclusions, such as Döhle like bodies, or other WBC abnormalities. Evaluation of RBC morphology is important to exclude a microangiopathic process as evidenced by presence of fragmented red blood cells, microcytosis, macrocytosis and other RBC abnormalities.

PT/INR (blood collected into citrate) measures the extrinsic and common pathway in the coagulation cascade (tissue factor, FVII, FX, FV, FII, fibrinogen). Results should be compared with age-specific laboratory reference intervals (Appendix), and are reported in seconds and/or as a percentage of a normal control sample. The INR is the ratio of a patient's PT to a normal control sample, raised to the power of the ISI value for the analytical system used: (observed PT/control PT)^{ISI}, where ISI = international sensitivity index (sensitivity of thromboplastin). The INR was developed for guiding management in patients treated with oral VKA and was not meant to be used for evaluation of bleeding. However, as some laboratories now report only the INR, it has been included in algorithm 1. A prolonged PT/high INR (with normal aPTT) suggests FVII deficiency, or use of VKA such as warfarin.

▶

Algorithm 1. Evaluation of a child presenting with bleeding symptoms.

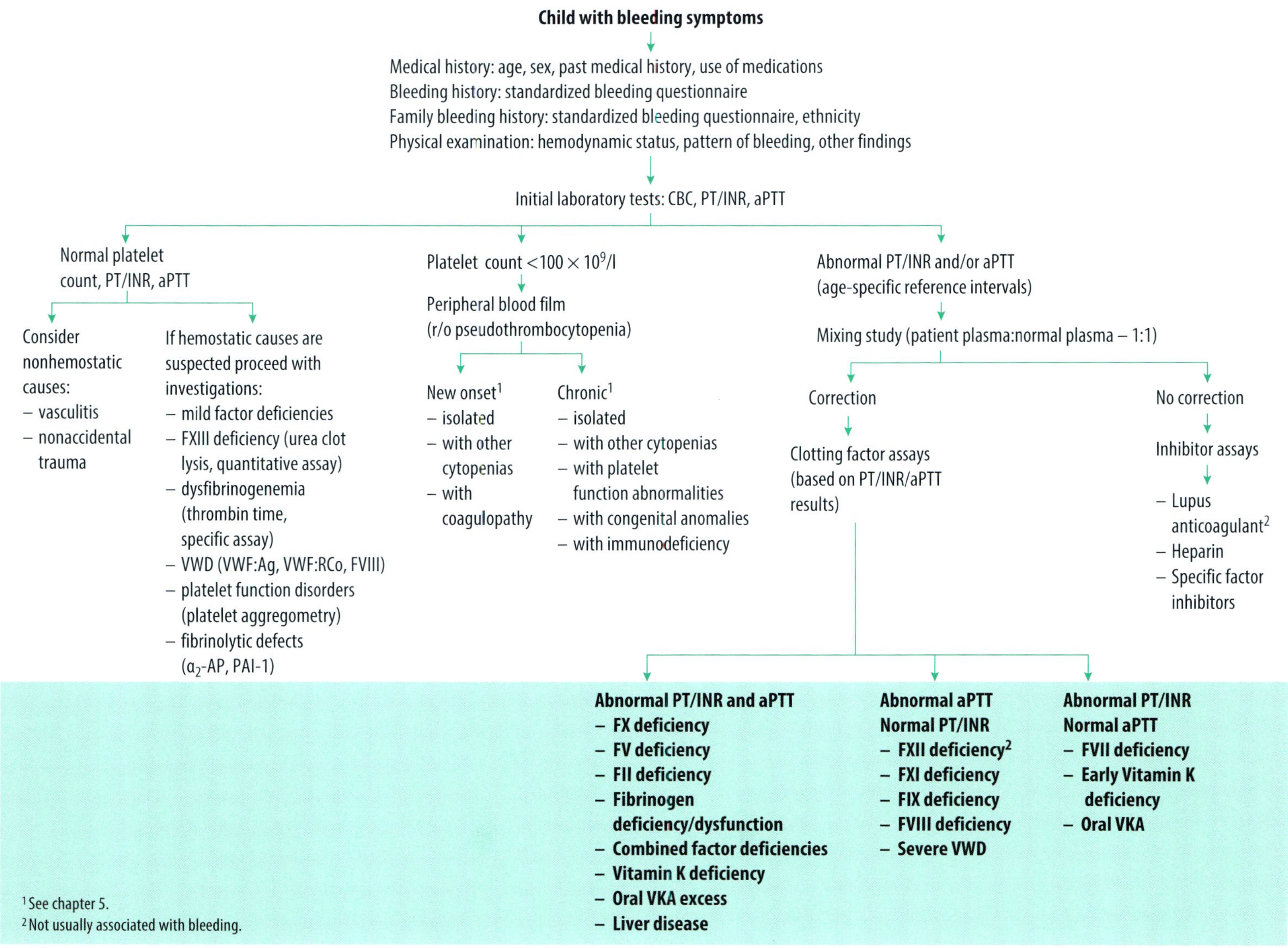

Child with bleeding symptoms

Medical history: age, sex, past medical history, use of medications
Bleeding history: standardized bleeding questionnaire
Family bleeding history: standardized bleeding questionnaire, ethnicity
Physical examination: hemodynamic status, pattern of bleeding, other findings

Initial laboratory tests: CBC, PT/INR, aPTT

Normal platelet count, PT/INR, aPTT

Consider nonhemostatic causes:
– vasculitis
– nonaccidental trauma

If hemostatic causes are suspected proceed with investigations:
– mild factor deficiencies
– FXIII deficiency (urea clot lysis, quantitative assay)
– dysfibrinogenemia (thrombin time, specific assay)
– VWD (VWF:Ag, VWF:RCo, FVIII)
– platelet function disorders (platelet aggregometry)
– fibrinolytic defects (α_2-AP, PAI-1)

Platelet count <100 × 10^9/l

Peripheral blood film (r/o pseudothrombocytopenia)

New onset[1]
– isolated
– with other cytopenias
– with coagulopathy

Chronic[1]
– isolated
– with other cytopenias
– with platelet function abnormalities
– with congenital anomalies
– with immunodeficiency

Abnormal PT/INR and/or aPTT (age-specific reference intervals)

Mixing study (patient plasma:normal plasma – 1:1)

Correction → Clotting factor assays (based on PT/INR/aPTT results)

No correction → Inhibitor assays
– Lupus anticoagulant[2]
– Heparin
– Specific factor inhibitors

Abnormal PT/INR and aPTT
– FX deficiency
– FV deficiency
– FII deficiency
– Fibrinogen deficiency/dysfunction
– Combined factor deficiencies
– Vitamin K deficiency
– Oral VKA excess
– Liver disease

Abnormal aPTT Normal PT/INR
– FXII deficiency[2]
– FXI deficiency
– FIX deficiency
– FVIII deficiency
– Severe VWD

Abnormal PT/INR Normal aPTT
– FVII deficiency
– Early Vitamin K deficiency
– Oral VKA

[1] See chapter 5.
[2] Not usually associated with bleeding.

An Approach to the Bleeding Child

aPTT (blood collected into citrate) measures the intrinsic and common pathways of coagulation (FXII, FXI, FIX, FVIII, FX, FV, FII, fibrinogen). The aPTT is less sensitive than the PT to deficiencies of the common pathway factors. Results should be compared with age-specific laboratory reference intervals (Appendix), and results are reported in seconds. An abnormally prolonged aPTT (with normal PT/INR) suggests FVIII or FIX deficiency (chapter 6) and FXI deficiency (chapter 8). Importantly, an aPTT within the reference range does not reliably exclude mild FVIII, FIX or FXI deficiency. Therefore, factor assays should be performed if specific deficiencies are suspected. FXII deficiency also causes a prolonged aPTT, but is not associated with clinical bleeding. A prolonged aPTT can occur in severe VWD, as a result of the associated FVIII deficiency (chapter 7).

The aPTT is also prolonged in the presence of inhibitors including heparin. Heparin contamination occurs most often in specimens drawn from arterial or central venous catheters. To avoid heparin contamination, an adequate volume of blood should be removed prior to sampling (chapter 16). Where that is not possible, heparin neutralization can be performed, usually by the addition of heparinase to the sample plasma.

Combined prolongation of PT/INR and aPTT can result from inherited deficiencies of individual factors in the common pathway: FX, FV, FII and fibrinogen, or from the rare inherited deficiency of the vitamin K-dependent coagulation factors (chapter 8). More commonly, combined abnormalities of aPTT and PT/INR are the result of acquired deficiencies of multiple coagulation factors (chapter 9).

A mixing study (patient plasma 1:1 normal plasma) (blood collected into citrate) is done when an abnormal PT and/or an aPTT is identified. The patient's plasma is mixed with normal plasma in a 1:1 ratio, and the screening tests are repeated. This test differentiates between factor deficiency (mixing corrects the PT or aPTT) and the presence of an inhibitor (mixing does not correct the PT or aPTT). The most common inhibitor that results in noncorrection of the aPTT with mixing is a lupus anticoagulant. This is often an incidental finding in children and is not associated with clinical bleeding. Specialized assays will confirm its presence. Specific factor inhibitors also interfere with correction of screening tests by mixing with normal plasma. Confirmation requires specific inhibitor assays (chapter 9).

PT and aPTT reagents used for testing have variable sensitivities to coagulation factors and insensitive reagents may result in false negative (i.e. normal) results for mild deficiencies. If there is a strong suspicion of a coagulation factor deficiency, specific factor assays should be performed.

TT and fibrinogen measurement (blood collected into citrate): TT measures the thrombin-induced conversion of fibrinogen to fibrin. A prolonged TT suggests a quantitative or qualitative abnormality of fibrinogen or the presence of heparin in the sample. A quantitative measurement of fibrinogen should also be performed.

PT, aPTT, and TT do not screen for factor XIII deficiency.

Urea clot lysis test (blood collected into citrate) measures the solubility of the clot with the addition of urea. An abnormal test suggests severe FXIII deficiency or hypofibrinogenemia. Clot solubility is increased only at very low levels of FXIII levels (<3%) and therefore does not detect mild/moderate deficiencies. A quantitative assay of FXIII should be used to confirm the result of this screening test (chapter 8).

Bleeding time (using a device appropriate for size of child): a lancet device is used to make a standardized cut on the volar surface of the forearm, and the time it takes for bleeding to stop is measured. The bleeding time test was widely used as a screening test for primary hemostasis disorders, but is less often used now because of difficulties in standardization.

Platelet function analyzer, PFA-100® (blood collected into citrate) is an instrument in which primary, platelet-related hemostasis is simulated.

A small sample of anticoagulated whole blood (0.8 ml) is aspirated via a narrow-diameter capillary through a microscopic aperture cut into a membrane coated with the platelet agonists collagen and epinephrine or collagen and adenosine 5′-diphosphate. The high shear rate generated under the standardized flow conditions and presence of the chemical stimuli result in platelet adhesion, activation and aggregation at the aperture, building a stable platelet plug. The time required to obtain full occlusion of the aperture is reported as the closure time. The closure time is prolonged by low levels of VWF, thrombocytopenia, decreased hematocrit, and by some platelet function abnormalities (e.g. severe disorders such as Bernard-Soulier syndrome and Glanzmann thrombasthenia). Due to issues of both sensitivity and specificity, use of the PFA-100® as a routine screening test is still debated. However, the small blood volume needed for this test compared with the much larger volume required for platelet function testing by aggregometry (10 ml or more) is an advantage, especially for screening very young children for VWD or severe platelet function disorders.

Testing for Defects in Primary Hemostasis

VWF antigen and activity (ristocetin cofactor assay) (blood collected into citrate): these tests measure the level and the activity of VWF for the diagnosis of VWD. Specialized laboratory evaluations of VWF to determine VWD subtype are discussed in chapter 7.

Platelet function testing (blood collected into citrate): the most common method of assessing platelet function is light transmission aggregometry, in which the increase in light transmission through a rapidly stirred sample of citrated platelet-rich plasma as recorded as platelets aggregate (chapter 5). As a fresh blood sample is needed for aggregation testing, the patient may have to be referred to a center with a specialized laboratory [8]. Specialized testing including measurement of granule secretion, dense granule enumeration by whole mount electron microscopy, flow cytometric assessment of surface receptors and evaluation of platelet ultrastructure by transmission electron microscopy are discussed in chapter 5.

Fibrinolysis Inhibitors

Abnormalities of *fibrinolysis inhibitors (blood collected into citrate)*, such as $α_2$-AP and PAI-1, can cause rare bleeding disorders because of increased fibrinolysis [9].

Genetic Testing

The genetic mutations associated with inherited hemostatic disorders are gradually being revealed. If available, mutational analysis aids in accurate diagnosis and improves genetic counseling and prenatal diagnosis. Recommendations for genetic testing for specific disorders are provided in the relevant chapters.

References

1 Carcao MD, Blanchette VS: Work-up of a bleeding child; in Lee C, Berntorp E, Hoots K (eds): Textbook of Hemophilia, ed 2. London, Blackwell, 2010, p 118.
2 Revel-Vilk S: Clinical and laboratory assessment of the bleeding pediatric patient. Semin Thromb Hemost 2011;37:756.
3 James AH, Kouides PA, Abdul-Kadir R, Dietrich JE, Edlund M, Federici AB, Halimeh S, Kamphuisen PW, Lee CA, Martinez-Perez O, McLintock C, Peyvandi F, Philipp C, Wilkinson J, Winikoff R: Evaluation and management of acute menorrhagia in women with and without underlying bleeding disorders: consensus from an international expert panel. Eur J Obstet Gynecol Reprod Biol 2011;158:124.
4 Rodeghiero F, Kadir RA, Tosetto A, James PD: Relevance of quantitative assessment of bleeding in haemorrhagic disorders. Haemophilia 2008;14(suppl 3):68.
5 Bowman M, Riddel J, Rand ML, Tosetto A, Silva M, James PD: Evaluation of the diagnostic utility for von Willebrand disease of a pediatric bleeding questionnaire. J Thromb Haemost 2009;7:1418.
6 Biss TT, Blanchette VS, Clark DS, Bowman M, Wakefield CD, Silva M, Lillicrap D, James PD, Rand ML: Quantitation of bleeding symptoms in children with von Willebrand disease: use of a standardized pediatric bleeding questionnaire. J Thromb Haemost 2010;8:950.
7 Biss TT, Blanchette VS, Clark DS, Wakefield CD, James PD, Rand ML: Use of a quantitative pediatric bleeding questionnaire to assess mucocutaneous bleeding symptoms in children with a platelet function disorder. J Thromb Haemost 2010;8:1416.

8 Harrison P, Mackie I, Mumford A, Briggs C, Liesner R, Winter M, Machin S: Guidelines for the laboratory investigation of heritable disorders of platelet function. Br J Haematol 2011;155:30.
9 Hayward CP: Diagnosis and management of mild bleeding disorders. Hematology Am Soc Hematol Educ Program 2005;2005:423.

Abbreviations

α_2-AP	α_2-Antiplasmin
aPTT	Activated partial thromboplastin time
CBC	Complete blood count
FII	Factor II (prothrombin)
FV	Factor V
FVII	Factor VII
FVIII	Factor VIII
FIX	Factor IX
FX	Factor X
FXI	Factor XI
FXII	Factor XII
FXIII	Factor XIII
ICH	Intracranial hemorrhage
INR	International normalized ratio
ITP	Immune thrombocytopenia
PAI-1	Plasminogen activator inhibitor type 1
PBQ	Pediatric Bleeding Questionnaire
PFA-100®	Platelet function analyzer-100
PT	Prothrombin time
RBC	Red blood cell
TT	Thrombin time
VKA	Vitamin K antagonist
VWD	von Willebrand disease
VWF	von Willebrand factor
VWF:Ag	VWF antigen
VWF:RCO	VWF activity (ristocetin cofactor assay)
WBC	White blood cell

Chapter 4 Bleeding in the Neonate

Laura Avila
Dorothy Barnard

Developmental Hemostasis

The term 'developmental hemostasis' has been used since the 1980s to describe age-dependent changes in the hemostatic system [1]. Hemostasis is a dynamic system that develops over time, beginning during intrauterine life and evolving throughout the neonatal period.

Size and ultrastructure of platelets of both full-term and premature neonates are similar to those of adults, with MPV ranging between 7 and 9 fl. Functionally, platelets in neonates are relatively hyporesponsive, showing impaired aggregation and secretion in vitro. Higher levels and enhanced function of VWF may help compensate for this impairment. Platelet reactivity increases with GA. The duration of this platelet hyporeactivity remains unclear.

Coagulation proteins do not cross the placenta. They are synthesized by the fetus and reach measurable levels at 10 weeks GA. Functional levels of these proteins gradually increase during gestation and after birth, attaining near adult values at approximately 6 months of age. Lower concentrations of coagulation proteins in healthy premature infants are compensated for by accelerated maturation, so that levels also reach adult ranges within 6 months of age in these infants.

These physiological age-related changes in the coagulation system provide effective protection to the healthy neonate. Thus, despite lower functional levels of most prothrombotic and antithrombotic factors in comparison to adults, healthy neonates are not particularly prone either to bleeding or to developing thrombotic disorders.

Plasma levels of coagulation FV, FVIII, FXIII and VWF are close to, or even higher than, adult values at birth. Whereas the functional activity of fibrinogen is reduced in neonates in comparison to older children, fibrinogen levels are increased due to the presence of a fetal variant. Plasma levels of FII, FVII, FIX and FX (the vitamin K-dependent coagulation proteins) and of FXI, FXII, prekallikrein and HMWK (the contact pathway coagulation proteins) at birth are

Table 1. Definitions

Term	Definition
Neonatal period	first 28 days of extrauterine life
Low birth weight infant	birth weight <2,500 g
Very low birth weight infant	birth weight <1,500 g
Extremely low birth weight infant	birth weight <1,000 g
Preterm newborn	infant born before week 37 GA
Term newborn	infant born between weeks 37 and 42 GA
Small for gestational age infant	infant with birth weights below the 10th percentile for GA
Large for gestational age infant	infant with a birth weight above the 90th percentile for GA

approximately half of adult values, as shown in the Appendix (reference values for newborns). Furthermore, the capacity of newborns to generate thrombin is decreased and delayed compared to that of adults. Similarly, the rate of thrombin inhibition is slower in neonates; whereas levels of antithrombin and heparin cofactor II are lower at birth, levels of α_2-macroglobulin are higher. The latter plays a more relevant role as a thrombin inhibitor in neonates than in adults, and likely helps compensate for the low levels of antithrombin in newborns. Other coagulation inhibitors such as protein C and S are also low at birth (approximately one third of normal adult values, please refer to the Appendix), and mature during the first 6 months of life. Nonetheless, the levels of free and active protein S are close to adult levels due to the absence of its binding protein, C4b.

The overall fibrinolytic activity of neonatal plasma is low; neonatal plasminogen concentration is not only lower compared to adult values, but the plasminogen has a different glycosylation pattern, which may be responsible for its less efficient conversion to plasmin.

Understanding these age-related differences in coagulation proteins is essential when evaluating a newborn infant with abnormal bleeding or a thrombus (clot). For example, the aPTT is prolonged in healthy neonates, mirroring the differences in coagulation proteins described above, particularly with respect to low concentrations of contact factors. However, this physiologic prolongation of aPTT is not associated with a higher risk of bleeding events in neonates. Tables describing reference ranges of routine coagulation laboratory tests, coagulation factor levels and natural coagulation inhibitor levels in healthy full-term can be found in the Appendix.

Bleeding disorders in the neonate will be described in the following sections, classified according to three categories: platelet disorders, coagulation factor deficiencies and combined disorders. Some definitions used throughout this chapter are listed in table 1.

Platelet Disorders: Neonatal Thrombocytopenia

Thrombocytopenia in neonates has classically been defined as an absolute platelet count below 150×10^9/l, irrespective of the GA. However, this traditional definition remains controversial, as recent data suggest that preterm infants often have platelet counts in the range of 100–150×10^9/l [2, 3]. Irrespective of the definition used, a repeated platelet count lower than 100×10^9/l, confirmed in a venous blood sample and

Table 2. Causes of neonatal thrombocytopenia by age of onset and clinical status

Onset	Disorder	Severity	Clinical findings
Fetal and early-onset thrombocytopenia (<72 h postnatal age)	chronic fetal hypoxia (e.g. pregnancy-induced hypertension, fetal growth restriction)	mild to moderate	suggestive prenatal history, small for gestational age
	alloimmune thrombocytopenia	severe	well-appearing
	autoimmune thrombocytopenia	moderate	well-appearing
	genetic syndromes	moderate	dysmorphic features, congenital anomalies
	viral infections	variable	ill-appearing
	perinatal asphyxia	moderate	ill-appearing
	inherited thrombocytopenia	variable	well-appearing, dysmorphic features in some cases
Late-onset thrombocytopenia (>72 h of age)	NEC	moderate to severe	ill-appearing
	fungal infections/sepsis	severe	ill-appearing
	drugs	moderate to severe	variable appearance at presentation
Variable onset	DIC	severe	ill-appearing
	bacterial infections/sepsis	variable	ill-appearing
	Kasabach-Merritt phenomenon	severe	vascular tumors
	thrombosis (e.g. portal vein, renal vein)	moderate	variable appearance at presentation
	metabolic diseases	variable	ill-appearing

Modified from refs. [4, 5].

by examination of a peripheral blood smear by an experienced individual, deserves further investigation.

Thrombocytopenia, as traditionally defined (i.e. <150 × 10^9/l), has a relatively low incidence in the general neonatal population, occurring in 0.5–2% of unselected newborns as detected by cord blood sampling, and is severe (i.e. platelets <50 × 10^9/l) in only 30% of those cases. Conversely, thrombocytopenia is the most common abnormal hemostatic finding in the neonatal intensive care unit and occurs in as many as 50% of neonates during the course of their hospital stay. It is especially common in premature and extremely low birth weight infants. Severe thrombocytopenia has been reported in 2% of patients admitted to neonatal intensive care units.

A practical approach to identifying the etiology of neonatal thrombocytopenia includes consideration of the time of onset as well as the clinical status of the neonate. Early thrombocytopenia is defined as thrombocytopenia presenting within the first 72 h of postnatal life and late thrombocytopenia as presenting thereafter. According to this approach, the most frequent causes of neonatal thrombocytopenia are summarized in table 2.

Fetal and Early-Onset Thrombocytopenias
Chronic Fetal Hypoxia

This condition, which may develop as part of maternal hypertensive disorders, maternal diabetes, and fetal growth restriction, is the most common cause of early-onset thrombocytopenia. Thrombocytopenia in the context of chronic fetal hypoxia tends to be mild to moderate. If all major hypertensive disorders of pregnancy are considered (pre-eclampsia, pre-existing hypertension and gestational hypertension), chronic fetal hypoxia affects approximately 10% of newborns. Although the pathogenesis of neonatal thrombocytopenia in the context of maternal hypertension is not clear, it is thought to be associated with decreased platelet production.

Not surprisingly, due to the intricate relationship between maternal environment and fetal growth, thrombocytopenia is also seen in small-for-gestational-age infants. The mechanism of thrombocytopenia in small-for-gestational-age infants is thought to involve reduced platelet production. Low megakaryocytic mass and failure to adequately increase thrombopoietin levels have been reported.

Clinical Findings

Most infants are asymptomatic and thrombocytopenia is identified incidentally on a routine complete blood count. In general, thrombocytopenia associated with either maternal hypertension or fetal growth restriction is less severe and tends to improve spontaneously within 7–10 days after birth without requiring therapy (e.g. platelet transfusions) [4].

Fetal and Neonatal Alloimmune Thrombocytopenia

FNAIT is the most common cause of severe thrombocytopenia in an otherwise healthy neonate; however, it is important to note that up to one third of FNAIT patients have an additional condition that could account for a low platelet count.

FNAIT results from maternal immunization against paternally inherited fetal platelet alloantigens, which are not present on maternal platelets. Fetal platelets express alloantigens early in the second trimester of gestation and cross the placenta. Exposure of an antigen-negative mother to fetal platelets bearing a 'foreign' platelet antigen of paternal origin leads, in some cases, to maternal alloimmunization and production of alloantibodies directed against the 'foreign' platelet alloantigen [6]. Transport of maternal alloantibodies across the placenta into the fetal circulation occurs via fetal Fc receptors expressed in the placenta. The maternal alloantibodies opsonize fetal platelets leading to their accelerated removal from the circulation by phagocytic cells in the fetal reticulo-endothelial system. In addition, reduced platelet production due to targeting of fetal megakaryocytes by maternal alloantibodies has been described.

HPA, derived from glycoproteins located in the platelet membrane, are the offending antigens in essentially all cases of FNAIT. Twenty-seven different HPAs have been implicated to date. HPA-1a, is expressed on the platelets of 98% of Caucasians and is by far the most common antigen involved in this race (80–90% of all FNAIT cases), followed by HPA-5b. HPA-4 antigen is the most frequent cause of severe FNAIT in Asians.

The frequency of FNAIT in a Caucasian population has been estimated to be 1 in 1,000–2,000 live births. Severe FNAIT due to HPA-1a incompatibility occurs in 1 in 2,500 pregnancies. Of note, 20% of affected cases present during the first pregnancy. The majority of patients present with cutaneous bleeding (petechiae, ecchymoses). The most feared complication of FNAIT is ICH, which occurs in 10–20% of clinically detected cases; at least 50% of ICH cases occur in utero. FNAIT is reportedly the most common cause of severe ICH in term newborns. Whereas antenatal intra-ventricular hemorrhage is the most frequent type of ICH, an intraparenchymal bleed is suggestive of FNAIT.

Diagnosis

Diagnosing FNAIT serves two purposes: (1) to assist with the management of the index case, and (2) to help plan future pregnancies. The main component of laboratory diagnosis is based on the detection of anti-platelet antibodies in the maternal serum. Monoclonal antibody-specific immobilization of platelet antigens is the gold standard laboratory test but is labor intensive. Increasingly, a solid-phase ELISA test is used. To determine the implicated platelet antigen, platelet phenotyping and/or genotyping of both parents (by PCR, fluorescence or ELISA-based techniques) are required.

Management

Platelet transfusion is indicated in an attempt to maintain a platelet count above $30 \times 10^9/l$ in well-appearing neonates without other risk factors because platelet function may be impaired among these patients, above $50 \times 10^9/l$ in patients with clinically significant bleeding, and above $100 \times 10^9/l$ in infants with ICH (see recommendation for platelet transfusions section). Since FNAIT is self-limited, and recovery of the platelet count usually occurs within 1–4 weeks, prophylactic platelet transfusion aims to prevent severe bleeding such as ICH. Transfusion of safe (i.e. tested for infectious diseases), irradiated and washed maternal platelets or HPA-1a-5b-negative random donor platelets, which are compatible in more than 90% of cases of Caucasian background are suitable choices. However, these products are rarely available in the acute setting. When not available, random donor platelets should be transfused as they produce acceptable increments in platelet counts in some cases. Because of the strong possibility of no response, or a very limited response, to random donor platelets, it is recommended that a 30-min to 1-hour post-transfusion platelet count be obtained following an infusion of random donor platelets in a newborn infant with suspected FNAIT. Concomitant IVIG (1 g/kg daily for 1–3 days) is recommended in cases who fail to respond to the initial infusion of random donor platelets. Although effective in some cases, IVIG takes time to produce a clinically relevant increase in platelet counts. In cases with organ- or life-threatening bleeding refractory to random donor platelets and IVIG every effort should be made to obtain compatible antigen-negative platelets from the mother or a volunteer blood donor. Methylprednisolone 30 mg/kg i.v. administered over 1 h is reserved for affected infants with life-threatening bleeding unresponsive to frontline therapy (i.e. IVIG, platelet transfusions). Use and dosing of recombinant FVIIa in this clinical setting remains controversial. If used, doses of 30 µg/kg every 3–4 h for a total of 6–7 doses, depending on clinical response, is a possible starting regimen for consideration by the clinical team caring for the affected infant.

Imaging

Imaging studies (ultrasound, MRI or CT) to rule out ICH in neonates with severe thrombocytopenia is recommended, since the presence of ICH guides the threshold for platelet transfusion (see above) and is the most relevant predictor of clinically relevant FNAIT for future pregnancies.

Future Pregnancies

The recurrence rate of FNAIT is approximately 90%; furthermore, thrombocytopenia usually worsens in subsequent pregnancies [6]. The predictive value of high maternal HPA-1a antibody titers for severity of disease in the fetus is controversial, since severely affected neonates may be born to mothers with low titers. In contrast, a history of a previous child affected with ICH remains the best predictor of earlier and more severe thrombocytopenia due to FNAIT during subsequent pregnancies. Cases of a FNAIT affected fetus whose siblings sustained ICH are considered high-risk. Treatment of the mother with repeated infusions of IVIG and/or corticosteroid therapy during the pregnancy is recommended in cases where the fetus is known to be antigen-positive [7].

Genetic Counseling

The risk of recurrence depends on the paternal zygosity for the pathologic platelet alloantigen. If the father is heterozygous, PCR testing via amniocentesis for fetal platelet genotyping should be considered. Mothers who have delivered an infant with proven FNAIT should be referred to a specialist obstetric unit for counseling and management.

Neonatal Autoimmune Thrombocytopenia

Thrombocytopenia can occur in neonates born to mothers affected by autoimmune thrombocytopenia. Maternal ITP is the most common condition, but autoimmune thrombocytopenia can also be secondary to other diseases such as SLE or autoimmune thyroid disease. Similar to FNAIT, transplacental transport of maternal platelet autoantibodies is implicated in the pathogenesis of neonatal autoimmune thrombocytopenia. However, in neonatal autoimmune thrombocytopenia, the thrombocytopenia tends to be mild to moderate. Approximately 10% of neonates born to mothers with ITP are severely thrombocytopenic (platelet count <50 × 10^9/l); less than 5% will have platelet counts below 20 × 10^9/l. Whereas a clinical history of a thrombocytopenic sibling in the neonatal period is the best predictor of severe neonatal autoimmune thrombocytopenia in future pregnancies, the predictive value of the maternal platelet count remains controversial.

Clinical Findings

Minor bleeding, including cutaneous bleeding and cephalohematoma, is the most common manifestation and may occur in 3% of those affected. As opposed to FNAIT, ICH is rare in neonatal autoimmune thrombocytopenia and the frequency is estimated to be at or below 1%.

Management

Infants born to mothers with a history of ITP should have their platelet count repeatedly checked during the first few days of life, since the nadir of thrombocytopenia is usually reached after birth and typically during the first 2–5 days of life. Resolution follows 7 days to a few weeks later. If the platelet count is below 30 × 10^9/l during the first week of life, below 20 × 10^9/l after that or if there is life-threatening bleeding, IVIG should be administered. The recommended initial dose is 1 g/kg daily administered intravenously over 6–8 h for a total of 1–3 days. In cases with organ (e.g. ICH) or life-threatening bleeding or if IVIG is not available, corticosteroid therapy (methylprednisolone 30 mg/kg i.v. × 3 days or prednisone 3–4 mg/kg/day in divided doses orally × 3–4 days with no tapering) is recommended. Head imaging studies are recommended in cases of severe thrombocytopenia or if clinically indicated.

Genetic Syndromes

Thrombocytopenia has been reported in many syndromes, including Turner syndrome, trisomy 13, trisomy 18, and triploidy. In addition to a lower platelet count, larger platelets have been reported in neonates with Down syndrome (constitutional trisomy 21). Thrombocytopenia may also be associated with the transient myeloproliferative disorder that can occur in 10% of newborns with Down syndrome.

Clinical Findings

Clinical findings vary by syndrome. In any thrombocytopenic infant with dysmorphic features and/or congenital anomalies it is prudent to consider chromosomal syndromes that may affect platelet production and/or bone marrow function.

Management

See 'Recommendations for Platelet Transfusions' below.

Perinatal Asphyxia
See 'Combined Disorders'.

Inherited Thrombocytopenias

The following is a brief description of the causes of inherited thrombocytopenia, classified according to platelet size (figure 1). Further details can be found in chapter 5.

Inherited Thrombocytopenia with Small Size Platelets

Syndromes Associated with WAS Protein Gene Mutations. Mutations in the gene that encode the WAS protein on the short arm of the X

Small platelets
- Wiskott-Aldrich syndrome
- X-linked thrombocytopenia

Normal-sized platelets
- Thrombocyopenia with absent radii
- Amegakaryocytic thrombocytopenia with radioulnar synostosis
- Congenital amegakaryocytic thrombocytopenia
- Familial platelet disorder with predisposition for development of acute myeloid leukemia

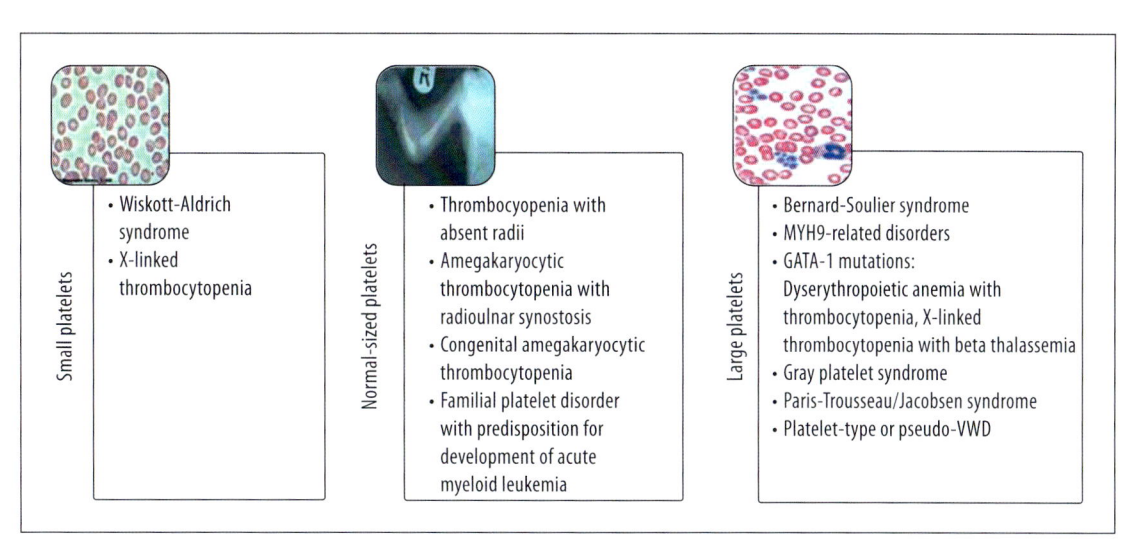

Large platelets
- Bernard-Soulier syndrome
- MYH9-related disorders
- GATA-1 mutations: Dyserythropoietic anemia with thrombocytopenia, X-linked thrombocytopenia with beta thalassemia
- Gray platelet syndrome
- Paris-Trousseau/Jacobsen syndrome
- Platelet-type or pseudo-VWD

Figure 1. Inherited thrombocytopenias according to platelet size. Adapted from Balduini et al. [8].

chromosome are responsible for a wide spectrum of clinical phenotypes, characteristically encompassing classic WAS and X-linked thrombocytopenia. Clinical manifestations associated with the WAS protein gene mutation are rare, occurring in 4–10 in a million individuals. Classic WAS features include: thrombocytopenia in the neonatal period; susceptibility to infections due to combined immunodeficiency in early infancy; extensive eczema in infancy and childhood; and a tendency to develop malignancies (such as B cell lymphomas, leukemias) and autoimmune diseases (such as hemolytic anemia, neutropenia, arthritis, vasculitis and inflammatory bowel disease) later in life.

Thrombocytopenia, often severe, is characterized by the presence of small platelets (3.8–5 fl, half the mean volume of normal platelets). Signs of cutaneous bleeding and bloody diarrhea often present in the neonatal period; bleeding from the umbilical stump and circumcision is also relatively common. X-linked thrombocytopenia is a milder variant, with less frequent and less severe clinical manifestations, particularly eczema and infections.

Conventional supportive treatment usually includes IVIG and antimicrobial prophylaxis. With regard to thrombocytopenia, platelet transfusion is only indicated in case of active bleeding. Platelets should be irradiated before transfusion because of the association of immunodeficiency with WAS. Splenectomy usually increases platelet counts and may be indicated in older children. However, it should be avoided if at all possible because of the risk of postsplenectomy overwhelming sepsis, particularly in WAS cases. The only definitive therapy for WAS is a hematopoietic stem cell transplantation.

Inherited Thrombocytopenia with Normal Size Platelets

Thrombocytopenia with Absent Radii. The inheritance pattern of this complex genetic disorder remains unclear. Deletion in chromosome 1q21.1 is a necessary component, but not sufficient for the phenotype to develop. TAR is characterized by congenital or early thrombocytopenia and bilateral absence of the radii. The thumbs can be hypoplastic but are always present. Thrombocytopenia, due to abnormal megakaryocytopoiesis, is usually present at birth or develops early in infancy. Bleeding manifestations can be severe in neonates; however, platelet counts can fluctuate and spontaneous improvement in the platelet count occurs after the first year of life. Interestingly, almost half of these patients have associated cow's milk allergy, and thrombocytopenia can be triggered by exposure to these dairy products. Platelet transfusions should be given in the event of bleeding episodes.

Amegakaryocytic Thrombocytopenia with Radioulnar Synostosis. Homeobox 11 gene mutation has been identified as responsible for this rare syndrome. Early neonatal amegakaryocytic thrombocytopenia and bilateral proximal fusion of the radius and ulna characterize this autosomal-dominant disorder. It is also associated with sensorineural hearing loss and the development of aplastic anemia in childhood.

Congenital Amegakaryocytic Thrombocytopenia. CAMT is an autosomal-recessive disorder that presents with severe thrombocytopenia and bleeding manifestations at birth with progression to bone marrow failure and pancytopenia during childhood. CAMT is secondary to a variety of mutations in the thrombopoietin receptor, with subsequent failure to respond to its stimuli. Levels of thrombopoietin in plasma are characteristically elevated. Newborns with CAMT can have severe bleeding episodes during the first weeks of life. Two types of CAMT have been described clinically: type I presents with early severe pancytopenia and platelet counts usually below 20×10^9/l, and type II is characterized by milder manifestations, with transient increases in platelet counts during the first year of life and pancytopenia occurring later in childhood. No physical abnormalities are usually present, and their presence strongly suggests a different diagnosis. Management includes supportive therapy with platelet transfusion if clinical bleeding occurs; adjunctive therapies (i.e. antifibrinolytic agents) can be utilized for minor bleeding events. Hematopoietic stem cell transplantation remains the only curative therapy available at present.

Inherited Thrombocytopenia with Large Size Platelets

Myosin, Heavy Chain 9, Nonmuscle (MYH9)-Related Disorders. May-Hegglin anomaly, Sebastian platelet syndrome, Epstein syndrome and Fechtner syndrome are a group of rare and predominantly autosomal dominant macrothrombocytopenias encompassed in the MYH9 related disorders. The finding of pathognomonic Döhle body-like neutrophil cytoplasmic inclusions in conventionally stained (i.e. May-Grünwald-Giemsa or Wright) peripheral blood smears or by immunofluorescence confirms the diagnosis of an MYH9 related disorder. These aggregates contain myosin IIA, ribosomes and MYH9 mRNA, the latter being responsible for the appearance of the inclusions. However, mRNA is degraded with time and therefore, the inclusions may be difficult to detect in standard stains. In contrast, immunofluorescence staining is a sensitive (100%) and specific (95%) technique for detection of these inclusions. Apart from the presence of macrothrombocytopenia (MPV >12 fl) at birth, sensorineural deafness, cataracts and nephritis can occur and are usually detected later in life. Platelet counts are variable. Cutaneous bleeding manifestations such as easy bruising can be present during the neonatal period, though bleeding is not usually a major problem in these patients; further, newborns do not seem to be at higher risk for ICH. The nonhematologic manifestations usually develop later in life. Platelet transfusions are indicated to control bleeding complications.

Bernard-Soulier Syndrome. BSS is a rare autosomal-recessive disorder secondary to quantitative or qualitative abnormalities in the platelet GP Ib complex that cause abnormal VWF-mediated adhesion to the exposed vascular endothelium. Affected patients usually have moderate macrothrombocytopenia. Bleeding symptoms and signs such as epistaxis, cutaneous, and gingival bleeding start early in childhood, particularly after hemostatic challenges or trauma. Although it usually presents later, a few cases have been reported in the neonatal period. In a recent systematic review of BSS in pregnancy, it was reported that 6 of 24 newborns in whom platelet count was available developed FNAIT due to maternal sensitization against GP Ib complex [9]. Two of those cases suffered severe bleeding events (ICH and severe fetal gastrointestinal bleeding resulting in intrauterine death), 1 newborn was asymptomatic and 3 presented with minor cutaneous bleeding manifestations.

Diagnosis of BSS can be established by the presence of macrothrombocytopenia, abnormal ristocetin-induced platelet agglutination and low or absent GP Ib complex (CD 42a–d) by flow cytometry. Management of bleeding in children with BSS is discussed in detail in chapter 5.

Gray Platelet Syndrome. The hallmark of this rare disorder is thrombocytopenia associated with abnormal large platelets that display markedly decreased or absent alpha granules. Mutations in the neurobeachin-like 2 gene have recently been identified as a cause of this syndrome, which probably involves defective protein storage or packaging during biogenesis of the platelet alpha-granules. Although GPS can present soon after birth (usually with easy bruising), the mean onset is in early childhood. The severity of bleeding symptoms and the degree of thrombocytopenia vary but tend to be mild to moderate. Severe hemorrhage is most commonly associated with menometrorrhagia later in life. The typical appearance of platelets in conventionally stained peripheral blood smears (i.e. pale gray and larger than normal) is highly suggestive of this syndrome; electron microscopy confirms the diagnosis. Management of bleeding in GPS is addressed in chapter 5.

Inherited Thrombocytopenias Related to GATA-1 Mutations. Dyserythropoietic anemia with thrombocytopenia (or X-linked macrothrombocytopenia), X-linked thrombocytopenia with beta-thalassemia, Down syndrome-associated transient myeloproliferative disorder, Down syndrome-associated acute megakaryoblastic leukemia, and congenital erythropoietic anemia are rare conditions caused by mutations in the GATA-1 gene. Defective megakaryocyte maturation with severe thrombocytopenia and bleeding since birth has been reported in cases of dyserythropoietic anemia with thrombocytopenia. Moderate thrombocytopenia due to dysmegakaryocytopoiesis, platelet dysfunction, reticulocytosis, and globin synthesis imbalance resembling beta-thalassemia have been described among patients with X-linked thrombocytopenia with beta-thalassemia.

Down syndrome-associated transient myeloproliferative disorder occurs in 10% of newborns with trisomy 21. The median age at diagnosis is 3 days of life and 40% of cases have platelet counts below 100×10^9/l. Common findings are hepatosplenomegaly, pleural or pericardial effusions, ascites and liver fibrosis secondary to megakaryocytic infiltration, vesiculopapular skin lesions, anemia, leukocytosis and thrombocytopenia. Transient myeloproliferative disorder resolves within 3 months in the majority of cases; however, early mortality occurs in 10–20%, and 20% of affected patients develop acute myeloid leukemia later in life.

Thrombocytopenia Paris-Trousseau Type and Jacobsen Syndrome. Clinical findings in these two syndromes, which are both related to terminal 11q deletions, typically overlap. Cognitive impairment, dysmorphic features, growth retardation and cardiac abnormalities are commonly seen in both entities. Most patients affected by thrombocytopenia Paris-Trousseau type are diagnosed during the first month of life and present with severe thrombocytopenia and a mild bleeding phenotype. Dysmegakaryocytopoiesis with micromegakaryocytes is common. Thrombocytopenia, also due to dysmegakaryocytopoiesis, has been reported in 47% of patients with Jacobsen syndrome. Bleeding should be treated with platelet transfusions.

Platelet-Type VWD. Platelet-type VWD is an autosomal-dominant disorder caused by mutations in the gene encoding the alpha subunit of the platelet GP Ib complex. The abnormal GP Ib alpha receptor exhibits enhanced affinity with spontaneous binding to its ligand, VWF. As a consequence of this increased interaction, platelets and high molecular weight VWF multimers are cleared from circulation. Platelet-type VWD is rare, with only 55 cases reported to date, and features mild macrothrombocytopenia and a mild to moderate bleeding phenotype. Diagnosis is based on heightened platelet agglutination in the presence of low amounts of ristocetin, and/or flow cytometry. Patients with this disorder require platelet transfusion in the case of active bleeding.

Inherited Bone Marrow Failure Syndromes with Thrombocytopenia

CAMT, TAR and amegakaryocytic thrombocytopenia with radioulnar synostosis are described above.

Fanconi Anemia. Cytogenetic instability, progressive pancytopenia, and high risk to develop malignancies such as acute myeloblastic leukemia, characterize this autosomal recessive or, rarely, X-linked form of inherited bone marrow failure. Its phenotypic expression is highly variable: short stature, skin hyperpigmentation, abnormal thumbs and radii, microcephaly or hydrocephaly, microphthalmia and developmental delay are commonly found congenital abnormalities. Hematological manifestations of Fanconi anemia usually present later in childhood. However, cases of neonatal onset have been reported and it may present as isolated thrombocytopenia.

Late-Onset Thrombocytopenias (>72 h)

Necrotizing Enterocolitis

This disease of unclear pathophysiology almost exclusively affects very low birth weight infants, having a prevalence of 5–10%. It is characterized by the presence of an excessive inflammatory process and, therefore, systemic manifestations including hematological abnormalities are common. Thrombocytopenia has been reported to correlate with disease severity and mortality, and to indicate a poor prognosis. Moderate-to-severe thrombocytopenia (platelet count $<100 \times 10^9/l$) affects up to 90% of neonates with NEC at diagnosis and usually recovers after 7–10 days. Coagulopathy is seen in up to a third of affected patients. Peripheral platelet destruction appears to be the main mechanism, although decreased production may contribute. Platelet activating factor, implicated in the pathogenesis of NEC, may affect thrombopoiesis in unclear ways. The majority of infants are noted to have an incidental thrombocytopenia on a complete blood cell count performed as an investigation of NEC. Platelet concentrates should be administered following current neonatal transfusion guidelines (see below). In vivo survival of transfused platelets is expected to be short in patients with NEC.

Fungal Infections

Candidiasis is responsible for 5–10% of sepsis occurring after 72 h of life among very low birth weight infants infants, harboring higher risk of death than gram-positive organisms. Fungal and Gram-negative sepses have been associated with more frequent and more severe thrombocytopenia than Gram-positive infections. Mixed mechanisms of thrombocytopenia have been suggested (see bacterial infection/sepsis below). Less common fungi, *Pantoea agglomerans* and *Malassezia furfur* have been reported in neonates with thrombocytopenia and other associated conditions. The severity of the underlying conditions reported in many of these patients may account, at least in part, for the observed low platelet count.

Drug-Induced Thrombocytopenias

Drugs administered to either the mother or the neonate can cause neonatal thrombocytopenia. Cases related to administration of vancomycin, amphotericin B and valproic acid, have been described. The frequency of thrombocytopenia in neonates receiving linezolide has been estimated to be 2%. Indomethacin-associated thrombocytopenia has been reported in 10% of very low birth weight infants, though studies comparing surgical ligation and indomethacin in the treatment of ductus did not show significant difference between groups.

Drugs administered to the mother may induce IgG antibodies directed against drug epitopes that can lead to thrombocytopenia in the mother and also cross the placenta thus affecting the fetus. Cases of neonatal thrombocytopenia secondary to maternal exposure to quinine and to valproic acid have been reported.

Heparin administration can lead to heparin-induced thrombocytopenia in 0.2–5% of adult patients. Despite thrombocytopenia, affected patients are at higher risk of thrombotic complications. A recent review found no cases of heparin-induced thrombocytopenia among 325 neonates included in well-designed cohort studies. Thus, other causes of thrombocytopenia are more likely and should be investigated in neonates exposed to heparin.

Variable-Onset Neonatal Thrombocytopenias

Disseminated Intravascular Coagulation, Bacterial Infections and Kasabach-Merritt Phenomenon
See combined disorders below.

Viral Infections
Neonatal TORCH (toxoplasmosis, rubella, cytomegalovirus, herpes simplex virus-2) infections can present with thrombocytopenia. Mixed mechanisms may be responsible for thrombocytopenia, including impaired platelet production due to suppression of proliferation and cytotoxic effects on megakaryocytes and their precursors, and accelerated platelet removal. Cytomegalovirus is one of the most common causes of congenital infection. The classical findings include jaundice, hepatosplenomegaly, and petechiae and occur in 10–15% of affected patients. Platelet counts less than $50 \times 10^9/l$ are found in half of these cases.

Severe thrombocytopenia secondary to parvovirus B19 has been reported. Enterovirus infections have also been associated with neonatal thrombocytopenia in the context of hepatitis. HIV-associated thrombocytopenia is uncommon in affected neonates, although almost 50% of newborns exposed to HIV during pregnancy, though not necessarily infected, manifest low platelet counts after birth (ranging between 50 and $150 \times 10^9/l$). In HIV-infected infants, thrombocytopenia should improve approximately 1 week after starting adequate antiretroviral therapy.

Thrombosis
The peak incidence of thrombosis in children occurs during the neonatal period. Renal vein thrombosis, the most prevalent non-catheter-related thrombotic event in neonates, presents with a triad of thrombocytopenia, palpable abdominal mass and hematuria, though the complete triad is present in less than a quarter of patients. Almost 50% of neonates with renal vein thrombosis have thrombocytopenia at presentation. The large majority of cases are detected within the first 3 days of life. Platelet counts below $100 \times 10^9/l$ have also been reported in almost 20% of neonates with PVT. Almost half of these patients, however, had additional conditions (sepsis, NEC) that would account for the presence of thrombocytopenia. Management of neonatal venous thrombosis is covered in chapters 11 and 13.

Metabolic Diseases
A few inborn errors of metabolism, such as propionic acidemia, mevalonic aciduria, storage diseases (Gaucher disease), Pearson syndrome, and neonatal hemochromatosis have been reported to be associated with isolated cases of neonatal thrombocytopenias. Further description of each of these diseases is beyond the scope of this chapter.

Table 3. Recommendations for transfusion in neonates based on clinical condition and platelet count

Indication	Clinical condition	Threshold for platelet transfusion
Prophylaxis	high risk of bleeding (ECMO, perioperative time period)	$100 \times 10^9/l$
	intermediate risk of bleeding (unstable patient, invasive procedure)	$50 \times 10^9/l$
	low risk (stable neonates)	$20 \times 10^9/l$
Active bleeding	any	$50-100 \times 10^9/l$

Table 4. Recommendations for platelet transfusion in neonates, based on clinical condition and platelet mass

Clinical condition	Platelet mass*
On ECMO, immediately pre- or postsurgery	<800
Unstable (high risk of bleeding)	<400
Stable	<160

* Platelet mass is calculated by multiplying the platelet count (in platelets $\times 10^9/l$) by the MPV (in fl). For example, a platelet count of $50 \times 10^9/l$ and an MPV of 9 fl would equate to a platelet mass of 450. From Christensen [3], with permission.

Recommendations for Platelet Transfusions

Transfusion of platelet concentrates is the only therapy available for management of many causes of neonatal thrombocytopenia. However, careful consideration should be given to administration of platelets, as associated risks include transfusion reactions and transmission of viral or bacterial infections.

Guidelines for prophylactic platelet transfusions (i.e. the patient is not bleeding) are based almost entirely on expert opinion. The correlation between absolute platelet counts and risk of hemorrhage is not strong. Thus, despite severe thrombocytopenia being a risk factor for intraventricular hemorrhage, most premature newborns that develop severe intraventricular hemorrhage do not have preexisting thrombocytopenia. Both the clinical condition of the neonate and the platelet counts need to be taken into consideration when recommending thresholds for platelet transfusions (table 3).

Experts recommend a lower threshold for platelet transfusion ($30 \times 10^9/l$) in small, stable, premature neonates, particularly during the period when the risk of periventricular hemorrhage is high (i.e. first 3–4 days of life) and in cases of neonates with coagulopathy. The threshold for platelet transfusion in patients with FNAIT is also $30 \times 10^9/l$, since platelet function may be impaired in these patients [10].

However, the strategy described in table 3 does not consider abnormalities in platelet function. For this reason, a new approach to platelet transfusion has been suggested, based on platelet mass (table 4). Platelet mass can be easily be estimated multiplying platelet count (in platelets x $10^9/l$) by MPV (in fl). Because small platelets are less effective than large platelets in forming a platelet plug, platelet mass may be a better indicator of platelet function than absolute platelet count. This novel approach has proven to reduce the number of prophylactic platelet transfusions by 30%, without increasing the number of bleeding events, though the findings require further validation.

Platelets for neonatal transfusions should be single donor, Rh compatible and ABO type-specific. ABO compatibility of the plasma present in the platelet product is an important consideration when ABO type-specific products are not available. Group O platelets administered to group A or B neonates can cause hemolysis because of the passive transfer of anti-A or anti-B present in the plasma and, thus, platelets should be volume reduced. Platelets should be irradiated if administered to neonates with congenital immunodeficiency or malignancy and in cases of transfusions from family members, particularly when maternal platelets are transfused to newborns with FNAIT. Some centers irradiate all platelet transfusions administered to neonates in order to prevent transfusion-associated graft-vs.-host disease in potentially not-yet-diagnosed cases of cellular immunodeficiency. Cytomegalovirus seronegative or leukoreduced (to obtain a white cell count $<5 \times 10^6$/U) products are recommended, especially for low birth weight infants. The recommended volume of transfusion ranges between 10–20 ml/kg (corresponding to 6.5×10^{10} platelets of 50–60 ml or one random donor platelet unit). In the United States, platelets are dosed according to adult equivalent units (EU). For children <5 kg, 1 EU is recommended (corresponding to 5.5×10^{10} platelets in 25–50 ml of plasma). Dosing can vary, depending on the product available in the local blood bank.

Coagulation Factor Deficiencies

Inherited Deficiencies

Hemophilia A and B

These two X-linked disorders are increasingly diagnosed at earlier ages, either secondary to prenatal diagnosis (known carriers or family history) or due to early bleeding events. Hemophilia is the most common inherited bleeding disorder manifesting in neonates.

Delivery of the Infant with Possible/ Confirmed Hemophilia

The optimal mode of delivery is a matter of debate. The risk of ICH in neonates with hemophilia at delivery has been estimated at 3.5%. Whereas it is clear that instrumental delivery increases this risk, it is less clear how spontaneous vaginal delivery and cesarean section compare in this regard. The British Guidelines recommend a case-by-case approach, taking into account obstetric indications and fetal hemophilia status or gender to decide the mode of delivery (spontaneous vaginal delivery or programmed cesarean section). Invasive monitoring, scalp blood sampling, and instrumental delivery should be avoided.

Management of Infants Born to Known Carriers

A cord blood sample should be obtained to measure FVIII or FIX levels. Since FVIII levels are not low at birth, diagnosis is relatively simple in suspected cases of hemophilia A. Levels of FIX in newborns, on the other hand, are 35–70% that of adults, rendering the diagnosis of milder forms of hemophilia B more difficult. Intramuscular VK administration should be avoided until the diagnosis is clear and VK can be given orally in confirmed cases (see dose recommendations in VKDB section). Bleeding events occurring during the neonatal period should be managed with administration of recombinant or plasma-derived virus inactivated FVIII or FIX products. Where these treatment options are available, the use of cryoprecipitate (for hemophilia A cases) and FP (for hemophilia B cases) is not recommend since these blood products carry a risk, albeit small, of transmitting viral infections such as HIV and HCV. The half-life of the factor is expected to be shorter in infants for several reasons, including larger plasma volume, larger volume of distribution and higher liver to body ratio with increased weight-adjusted clearance. Therefore, close monitoring of factor levels is warranted. Short-term primary prophylaxis may be indicated in cases of traumatic or instrumental delivery. Performing a head ultrasound is recommended prior to the discharge of a neonate with moderate or severe hemophilia.

Index Cases Presenting with Bleeding Events

The diagnosis of hemophilia during the neonatal period is based on the presence of hemorrhagic manifestations in one third of the cases. Among such manifestations, circumcision, ICH, and heel stick bleeding are the most commonly reported initial sites of bleeding. Hemophilia should be suspected on the bases of an aPTT that is prolonged beyond age-appropriate normal ranges, and confirmation of diagnosis with factor level determination should follow.

Further details, including differential diagnosis and management of bleeding in children with hemophilia, is reviewed in detail in chapter 6.

Von Willebrand Disease

Type I, the most common type of VWD, is not usually recognized in the neonatal period due to increased VWF levels at this age. Type III, the most severe form where VWF is <1%, is an autosomal-recessive disorder that may manifest in newborns, but has rarely been reported. Type IIB, which is of interest in the newborn period due to its association with thrombocytopenia is reviewed in chapter 5.

Acquired Deficiencies
Vitamin K Deficiency Bleeding

VK serves as cofactor for the gamma-carboxylation of procoagulant proteins (FII, FVII, FIX and FX) and of natural anticoagulants (proteins C, S and Z). This post-translational modification allows calcium-mediated binding of these proteins to negatively charged phospholipids, which is key to their hemostatic activity. Formerly known as 'hemorrhagic disease of the newborn', VKDB encompasses three syndromes classified according to the time of onset: early, classic, and late VKDB. These syndromes have in common a reduction of VK-dependent factors (II, VII, IX and X) below the hemostatic level, which is correctable after VK administration.

Clinical Findings

Early VKDB occurs in the first day of life and is seen in neonates born to mothers receiving medication that interferes with VK activity, such as antituberculosis drugs, some antibiotics and VK antagonists. Anticonvulsants have also been traditionally implicated; however evidence is limited. Early VKDB is often severe and associated with cephalohematoma, ICH, and intra-abdominal bleeding. Classic VKDB presents between the 2nd and 7th day of life, and is secondary to inadequate or delayed feeding. Clinical manifestations are milder; mucocutaneous and gastrointestinal bleeding are more common, but ICH can occur. It can be prevented with administration of VK prophylaxis (see below). Late VKDB is defined as presenting between the first and the 12th week of extrauterine life, but it usually manifests between the 2nd and 8th week. The incidence of late VKDB has been estimated at 4.4–7.2 per 100,000 births [11]. It is more common in males and conveys a substantial risk of ICH (approximately 50%) and high mortality, estimated at 20%. Late VKDB is seen in exclusively breastfed infants and in children with underlying disorders associated with abnormal VK absorption. Breastfed infants are at risk of VKDB due to inadequate intake, since breast milk has a lower concentration of VK compared to commercial formulas, and due to lower VK production by their intestinal flora.

Diagnosis

Diagnosis of VKDB is based on the presence of prolonged INR (>3.5) or PT (>4 times the control value in seconds) with a normal platelet count and fibrinogen level. Rapid normalization (within 30–120 min) of the abnormal laboratory findings following VK administration confirms the diagnosis.

Management

Early VKDB can be treated with daily oral administration of 10 mg of VK to pregnant women at risk during the 2 weeks prior to delivery and has been advocated to prevent this disease. Classic and late VKDB can be effectively prevented with intramuscular administration of 0.5–1 mg of VK at birth. Oral administration can be used in some cases, such as neonates with hemophilia. However, to ensure protection with oral VK, administration should be repeated with either 25–50 µg daily or 1 mg weekly for 3 months. The recommended dose for premature infants is 0.3 mg/kg i.m. (preferred route) or 0.2 mg/dose i.v.. Treatment of symptomatic VKDB consists of intravenously or subcutaneously administered VK; the intramuscular route should be avoided due to the risk of bleeding. Plasma concentrates containing the VK-dependent coagulation factors may be indicated in severe or life-threatening bleeding.

Combined Disorders

Bacterial Infections and Sepsis

Sepsis is a systemic inflammatory response syndrome that occurs in the presence of, or as a result of, a suspected or proven infection. Thrombocytopenia can be found in the course of sepsis, with or without the presence of DIC. Bacterial sepsis has been associated to low platelet counts in approximately 20–60% of cases. The risk and severity of thrombocytopenia is reportedly higher with Gram-negative and fungal infections compared to Gram-positive infections. The duration of thrombocytopenia is variable, but is generally short (<5 days); increased MPV is a common finding due to the release of new platelets. Thrombocytopenia is thought to be multifactorial, and causes include enhanced peripheral clearance (secondary to endothelial damage with platelet activation, direct effect of toxins, and DIC) and decreased platelet production.

Disseminated intravascular Coagulation

DIC is an acquired disorder characterized by massive inflammatory response with microvascular endothelial damage and systemic activation of coagulation that can lead to organ dysfunction. In neonates, it can be secondary to several underlying conditions, such as sepsis, respiratory distress, severe asphyxia, NEC, liver dysfunction, and vascular tumors [12]. Laboratory findings include thrombocytopenia resulting from platelet consumption, microangiopathic hemolytic anemia, prolonged PT/INR and aPTT, elevated D-dimers, and a low fibrinogen level. The interpretation of all coagulation-related laboratory results requires comparison with age-appropriate reference values. The treatment of DIC primarily involves treatment of the underlying condition and supportive care. Further details can be found in chapter 9 on acquired bleeding disorders.

Asphyxia

Perinatal asphyxia is associated with moderate neonatal thrombocytopenia. Studies have shown that platelet counts are lower in newborns sustaining preadmission or intrapartum injury of some duration in comparison to newborns suffering acute asphyxia, thus suggesting that low platelet counts may be a marker to date the insulting event. The potential role of fibrinolytic system activation in cases of injury of some duration has been raised. In fact, asphyxiated newborns have reportedly lower fibrinogen levels and higher D-dimers in cord blood. Animal studies suggest decreased platelet survival in hypoxemic conditions, which could be related to activation of fibrinolysis or to antibody-mediated removal. In some cases, asphyxia can lead to DIC, thus accentuating coagulation abnormalities. Endothelial damage is another possible mechanism of hemostatic derangement.

Induced hypothermia (whole-body or head) is a therapeutic approach that aims to improve the neurological outcome of patients with hypoxic-ischemic events. It has been suggested that induced hypothermia increases the incidence of thrombocytopenia, but does not increase the risk of coagulopathy in newborns with perinatal asphyxia.

Kasabach-Merritt Phenomenon

The KMP is characterized by the presence of microangiopathic hemolytic anemia, consumptive coagulopathy and severe thrombocytopenia in the presence of an enlarging vascular tumor. KMP-associated mortality may be as high as 30% and is often related to bleeding complications [13]. Kaposiform hemangioendotheliomas and tufted angiomas are the vascular tumors underlying the KMP. These two rare vascular tumors are most commonly present at birth and show predilection for the upper body (trunk and extremities). The lesions are usually unifocal, warm and firm.

The pathophysiology of thrombocytopenia in KMP is primarily a result of platelet trapping, probably due to enhanced adhesion to the abnormal endothelium, which leads to platelet activation and subsequent activation of the coagulation and fibrinolytic system. Increased shear rate within the tumor may contribute to further platelet activation.

Laboratory features are severe thrombocytopenia ($<20 \times 10^9$/l), marked hypofibrinogenemia, high levels of fibrinogen degradation products and some degree of microangiopathic hemolytic anemia.

The acute management of KMP includes hemostatic support as required. FP, platelets and cryoprecipitate should be administered, accordingly, in cases of active intra-lesional or systemic bleeding, or if invasive procedures are planned. Platelets, including those transfused, display short survival (1–24 h) and close follow-up of platelet counts is advisable in the setting of acute bleeding.

First-line specific management of KMP involves the use of prednisone (5 mg/kg/day). Other therapeutic options should be discussed with specialists. Re-assessment is recommended after 2 weeks of treatment. In infants who respond to initial corticosteroid therapy, prednisone should be reduced by 10% per week starting after the second week until reaching a dose of 2 mg/kg/day. Weaning of corticosteroids should be slower after this point in time. Surgical excision of most lesions is not recommended because of hemorrhagic risks; embolization should be considered in cases with organ or life-threatening lesions (e.g. multiple hepatic lesions leading to cardiorespiratory compromise) or cases refractory to front-line therapies.

Neonatal Liver Failure

Coagulopathy due to hepatic dysfunction is one of the essential components of the diagnosis of this rare disorder. The presence of hemostatic abnormalities is largely explained by the crucial role of the liver in the synthesis and post-translational modification of the majority of the proteins that belong to secondary and tertiary hemostasis (i.e. coagulation factors, natural anticoagulants and proteins of fibrinolysis). Hemochromatosis and viral infections are the most common causes of liver failure among newborns. An algorithm for the initial diagnosis is shown (algorithm 1).

Diagnostic Algorithm: Approach to Bleeding in the Neonate

To finalize, we present a general approach to the diagnosis of bleeding disorders, which combines standard and broadly available laboratory tests and the most common disorders found in neonates (algorithm 2). See chapter 3 for further details on the approach to the bleeding child.

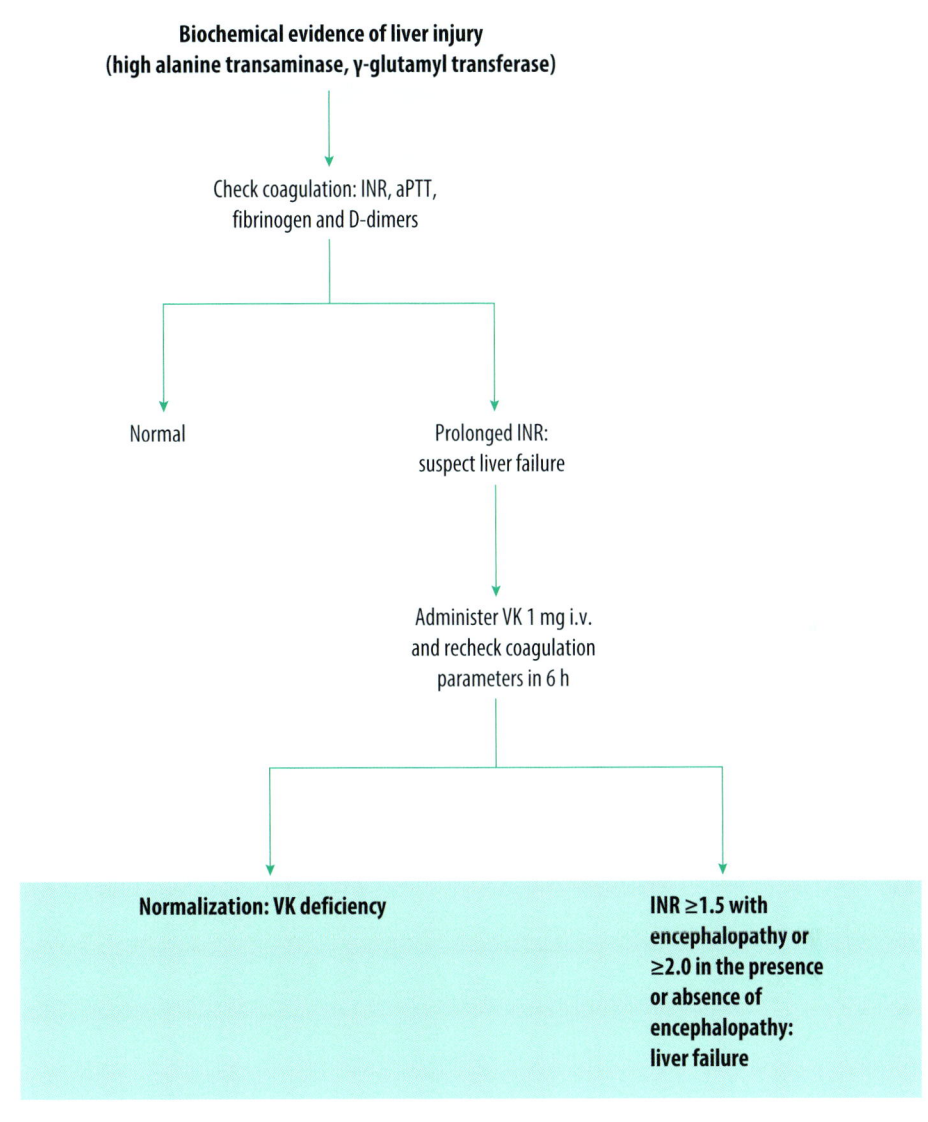

Biochemical evidence of liver injury
(high alanine transaminase, γ-glutamyl transferase)

↓

Check coagulation: INR, aPTT, fibrinogen and D-dimers

↓ Normal

↓ Prolonged INR: suspect liver failure

↓

Administer VK 1 mg i.v. and recheck coagulation parameters in 6 h

↓

Normalization: VK deficiency

INR ≥1.5 with encephalopathy or ≥2.0 in the presence or absence of encephalopathy: liver failure

Algorithm 1. Diagnosis of liver disease in neonates. From Shanmugam et al. [14], with permission.

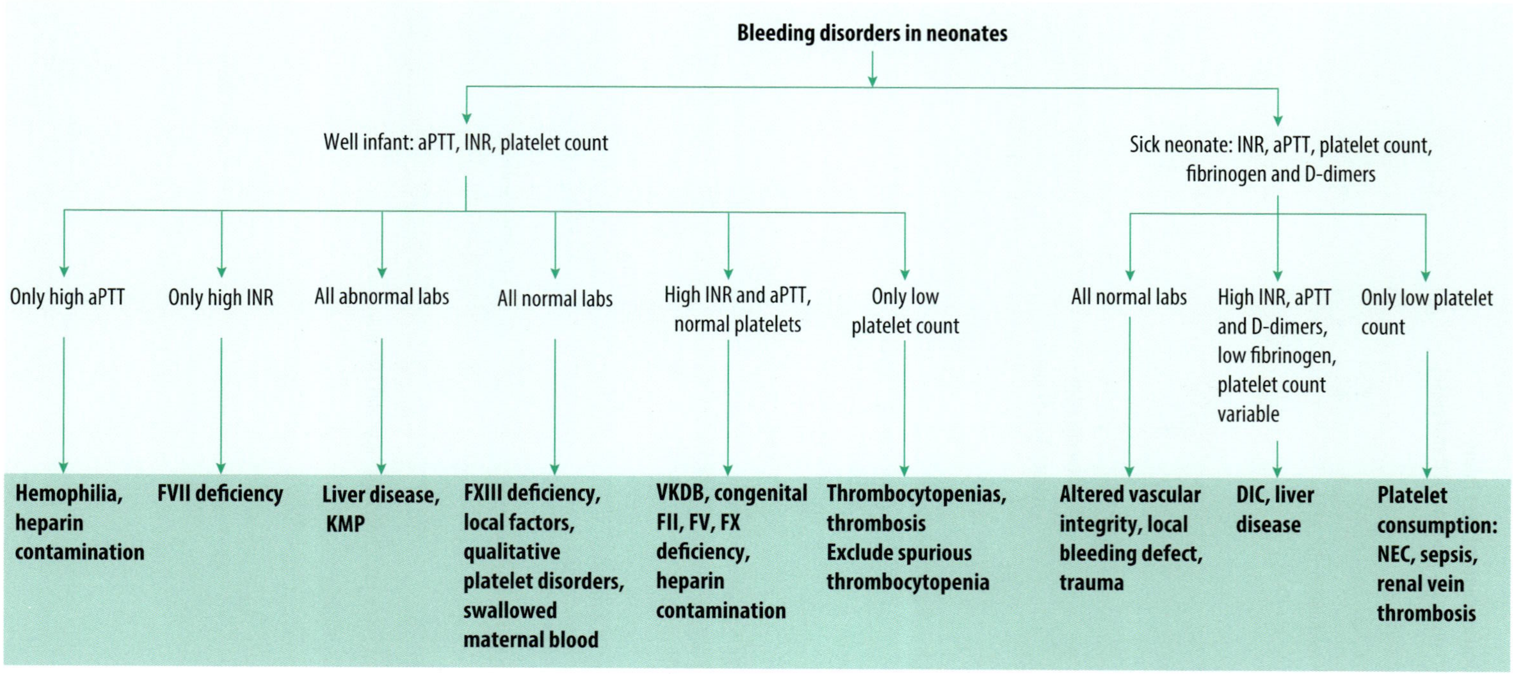

Algorithm 2. Diagnosis of bleeding disorders in neonates. From Goodnight et al. [15], with permission. The blood volumes required to perform laboratory tests should be taken into account, particularly in relation to premature infants. Although the amount of blood needed for these assays varies from laboratory to laboratory, most laboratories require 0.5 ml to perform a complete blood count, and 1 ml to run standard coagulation tests (including INR, aPTT, fibrinogen and D-dimers). The anticoagulant recommended for the standard coagulation tests is 3.2% tri-sodium citrate. In these containers, a 9:1 ratio of blood to anticoagulant is critical for valid coagulation test results.

Acknowledgment

The authors would like to express their appreciation for the thoughtful comments provided by Drs. Yaser Diab (Washington, D.C., USA), Johann Hitzler (Toronto, Ont., Canada), Heather Hume (Montreal, Que., Canada), Wendy Lau (Toronto, Ont., Canada), Naomi Luban (Washington, D.C., USA), Elena Pope (Toronto, Ont., Canada), and Claudio Solana (Buenos Aires, Argentina) who reviewed this chapter.

References

1 Monagle P, Ignjatovic V, Savoia H: Hemostasis in neonates and children: pitfalls and dilemmas. Blood Rev 2010;24:63–68.
2 Chakravorty S, Roberts I: How I manage neonatal thrombocytopenia. Br J Haematol 2012;156:155–162.
3 Christensen RD: Platelet transfusion in the neonatal intensive care unit: benefits, risks, alternatives. Neonatology 2011;100:311–318.
4 Roberts I, Stanworth S, Murray NA: Thrombocytopenia in the neonate. Blood Rev 2008;22:173–186.
5 Sola MC: Evaluation and treatment of severe and prolonged thrombocytopenia in neonates. Clin Perinatol 2004;31:1–14.
6 Bussel JB, Primiani A: Fetal and neonatal alloimmune thrombocytopenia: progress and ongoing debates. Blood Rev 2008;22: 33–52.
7 Pacheco LD, et al: Fetal and neonatal alloimmune thrombocytopenia: a management algorithm based on risk stratification. Obstet Gynecol 2011;118:1157–1163.
8 Balduini CL, et al: Inherited thrombocytopenias: a proposed diagnostic algorithm from the Italian Gruppo di Studio delle Piastrine. Haematologica 2003;88:582–592.
9 Peitsidis P, et al: Bernard Soulier syndrome in pregnancy: a systematic review. Haemophilia 2010;16:584–591.
10 Gibson BE, et al: Transfusion guidelines for neonates and older children. Br J Haematol 2004;124:433–453.
11 Van Winckel M, et al: Vitamin K, an update for the paediatrician. Eur J Pediatr 2009;168:127–134.
12 Veldman A, et al: Disseminated intravascular coagulation in term and preterm neonates. Semin Thromb Hemost 2010;36:419–428.
13 Ryan C, et al: Kasabach-Merritt phenomenon: a single centre experience. Eur J Haematol 2010;84:97–104.
14 Shanmugam NP, et al: Neonatal liver failure: aetiologies and management – state of the art. Eur J Pediatr 2011;170:573–581.
15 Goodnight SH, et al: In Goodnight SH, Hathaway WE (eds): Disorders of Hemostasis and Thrombosis: A Clinical Guide, ed 2. New York, McGraw-Hill, 2001, vol xiv, p 622.

Abbreviations

aPTT	Activated partial thromboplastin time
BSS	Bernard-Soulier syndrome
CAMT	Congenital amegakaryocytic thrombocytopenia
CT	Computed tomography
DIC	Disseminated intravascular coagulation
ECMO	Extracorporeal membrane oxygenation
ELISA	Enzyme-linked immunosorbent assay
EU	Equivalent unit
FII	Factor II (prothrombin)
FV	Factor V
FVII	Factor VII
FVIII	Factor VIII
FIX	Factor IX
FX	Factor X
FXI	Factor XI
FXII	Factor XII
FXIII	Factor XIII
FNAIT	Fetal and neonatal alloimmune thrombocytopenia
FP (FFP)	Frozen plasma (Fresh frozen plasma)
GA	Gestational age
GP	Platelet glycoprotein
GPS	Gray platelet syndrome
HCV	Hepatitis C virus
HIV	Human immunodeficiency syndrome
HMWK	High-molecular-weight kininogen
HPA	Human platelet alloantigens
ICH	Intracranial hemorrhage
INR	International normalized ratio
ITP	Immune thrombocytopenia
IVIG	Intravenous immunoglobulin
KMP	Kasabach-Merritt phenomenon
MPV	Mean platelet volume
MRI	Magnetic resonance imaging
mRNA	Messenger RNA
MYH9	Myosin heavy chain 9
NEC	Necrotizing enterocolitis
PT	Prothrombin time
PVT	Portal vein thrombosis
PCR	Polymerase chain reaction
SLE	Systemic lupus erythematosus
TAR	Thrombocytopenia with absent radii
VK	Vitamin K
VKDB	Vitamin K deficiency bleeding
VWD	von Willebrand disease
VWF	von Willebrand factor
WAS	Wiskott-Aldrich syndrome

Chapter 5 Platelet Disorders in Children

Viola van Eimeren
Walter H.A. Kahr

Introduction

This chapter reviews the causes and management of thrombocytopenia and PFDs in childhood. The section on thrombocytopenia will focus on ITP – the most common cause of a low platelet count in children – with an emphasis on diagnosis and treatment. The identification and management of congenital platelet defects with or without thrombocytopenia are described in the subsequent section. Congenital thrombocytopenia disorders are also described in chapter 4. Acquired platelet function abnormalities due to illness or medications will not be discussed in detail.

Platelets are essential cells in the arrest of bleeding and establishment of hemostasis (see chapter 2). They are rapidly recruited to areas of vessel injury and contribute to hemostasis by forming the primary hemostatic plug. In this process, they undergo a highly regulated set of functional responses that include: adhesion (platelet-vessel wall interaction), activation, secretion of granular contents (autocrine and paracrine stimulation), aggregation (platelet-platelet interaction), exposure of a catalytic surface for local thrombin generation and the release of factors from granules that promote endothelial cell repair and restore vessel architecture. Platelets must have normal function and be present in adequate numbers to allow these complex functions to occur [1].

In a well child, the most common sign of a platelet disorder is mild to moderate mucocutaneous bleeding. Hemorrhage is most frequently observed after trauma or surgery. Only severe platelet disorders present with spontaneous bleeding. Bleeding in patients with platelet disorders occurs with a rapid onset (at the time of trauma) rather than after a delay. Physical examination should focus on establishing the type and severity of bleeding. It is also important to exclude an underlying genetic syndrome (e.g. TAR) or collagen-vascular disorder (e.g. Ehlers-Danlos syndrome; chapter 3 and 4).

Table 1. Causes of acquired platelet dysfunction and/or thrombocytopenia

Antibody induced	ITP, TTP, HIT
Consumptive coagulopathy	disseminated intravascular coagulopathy, cardiopulmonary bypass, extracorporeal membrane oxygenation, Kasabach-Merritt syndrome
Drugs	NSAIDs (aspirin, ibuprofen, diclofenac, etc.), antiepileptics (valproic acid), psychiatric drugs (selective serotonin reuptake inhibitors), chemotherapy, etc.
Herbs	ginkgo, garlic, ginger, feverfew, ginseng, etc.
Systemic disease	renal failure, sepsis, myelodysplastic syndromes, leukemia, cardiac disease (e.g. valvular disease), liver disease, hypersplenism, HUS

Diagnosis of Platelet Disorders

Mild epistaxis or bruising is common in the general population, while platelet disorders are, in comparison, rare. To facilitate the correct diagnosis, the medical history, physical examination and laboratory investigations are crucial. The PBQ [2, 3] is a useful tool to assess bleeding severity in children with inherited platelet disorders (see chapter 3). A thorough family history detects dominant traits and reveals potential consanguineous relationships in the immediate or remote family. The medication history rules out acquired platelet disorders, which are significantly more common than inherited defects. Table 1 lists causes of acquired platelet dysfunction/thrombocytopenia in children [4, 5].

Diagnostic algorithms for patients with suspected platelet disorders (platelet function abnormalities and thrombocytopenia) guide physicians towards a diagnosis (algorithm 1) [6, 7]. Initial laboratory tests that aid in diagnosis include a CBC and white blood cell differential, inspection of the peripheral blood film, screening coagulation tests such as aPTT and PT (INR), and VWF screening tests (see chapter 3). With the history, physical examination and laboratory evaluation a preliminary differential diagnosis can be developed. Specialized testing such as platelet LTA, flow cytometry, immunofluorescence and electron microscopy, and genetic testing can be used to confirm a specific diagnosis.

Platelet Count and Morphology

The correct assessment of platelet size and number is an important initial step. Automated cell counters can underestimate platelet counts when platelet size is outside of the established reference range. Similarly, the MPV may be under- or overestimated, as the largest and smallest platelets are excluded from the analysis. If platelet clumping is seen on the blood film, a platelet count from a blood sample collected in 3.2% sodium citrate should be analyzed to rule out pseudothrombocytopenia. A peripheral blood film stained with Wright's or May-Grünwald-Giemsa and examined using a light microscope not only serves in yielding accurate platelet counts and size, but may reveal additional important information regarding other blood cells. For example, Döhle-like inclusions in neutrophils are indicative for MYH9-related disorders, and large pale platelets are characteristic of the GPS. Disorders related to mutations in the *GATA-1* gene exhibit an abnormal red blood cell morphology. Whole mount electron microscopy

▶

Algorithm 1. Algorithm and differential diagnosis for suspected platelet disorders. Modified from Israels et al. [6]. Further testing for specific diagnoses may include electron and immunofluorescence microscopy, lumiaggregometry, flow cytometry, genotyping, platelet protein analysis and bone marrow studies. Scott syndrome is not included. Thrombocytopenia is classified according to congenital (bold + italics) and acquired defects. ATRUS = Amegakaryocytic thrombocytopenia with radioulnar synostosis; FPD/AML = familial platelet disorder and predisposition to acute myelogenous leukemia; THC2 = autosomal dominant thrombocytopenia.

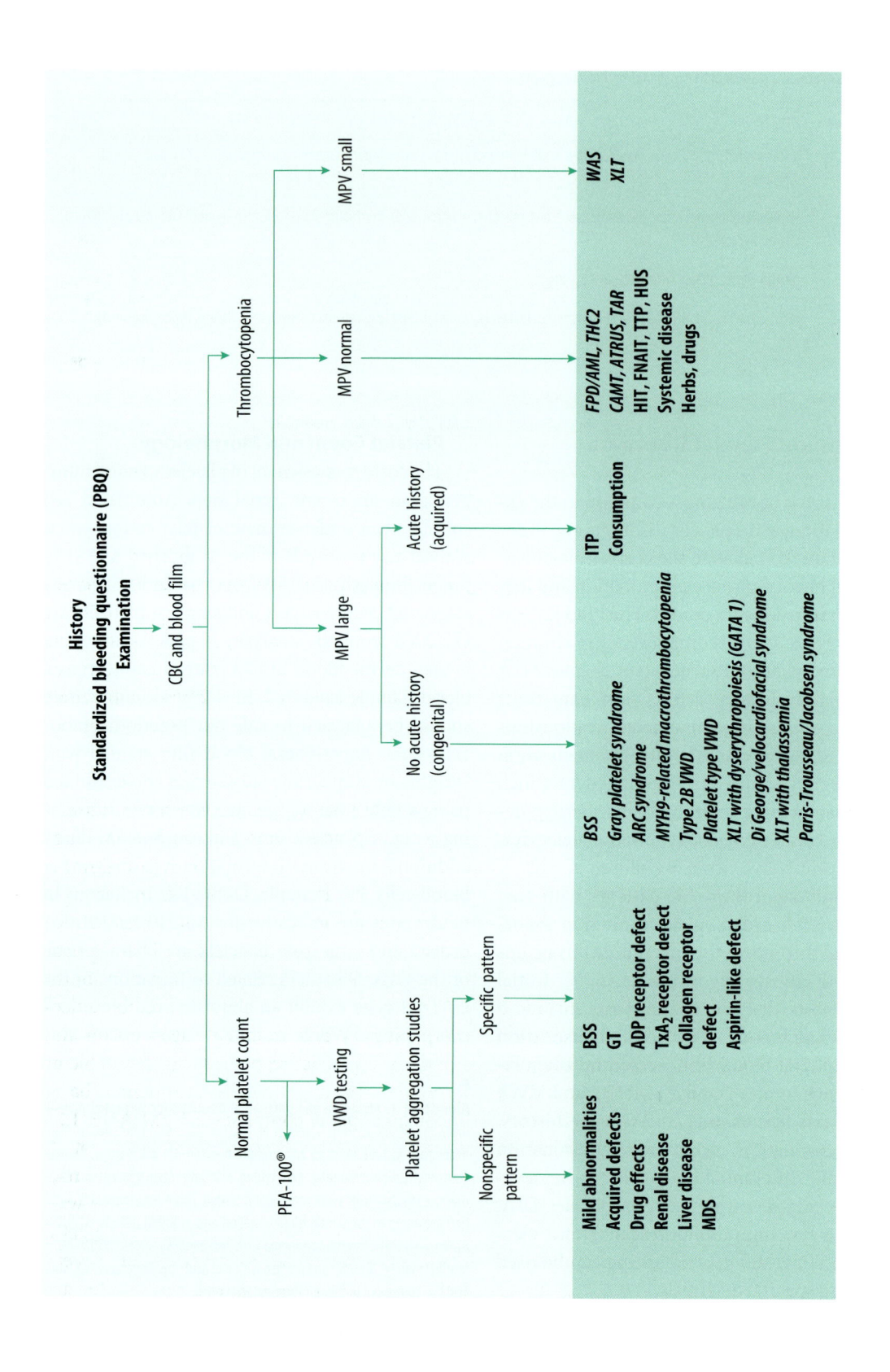

History
Standardized bleeding questionnaire (PBQ)
Examination
CBC and blood film

- Normal platelet count
  - PFA-100®
    - VWD testing
    - Platelet aggregation studies
      - Nonspecific pattern
        - Mild abnormalities
        - Acquired defects
        - Drug effects
        - Renal disease
        - Liver disease
        - MDS
      - Specific pattern
        - BSS
        - GT
        - ADP receptor defect
        - TxA$_2$ receptor defect
        - Collagen receptor defect
        - Aspirin-like defect

- Thrombocytopenia
  - MPV large
    - No acute history (congenital)
      - *BSS*
      - *Gray platelet syndrome*
      - *ARC syndrome*
      - *MYH9-related macrothrombocytopenia*
      - *Type 2B VWD*
      - *Platelet type VWD*
      - *XLT with dyserythropoiesis (GATA 1)*
      - *Di George/velocardiofacial syndrome*
      - *XLT with thalassemia*
      - *Paris-Trousseau/Jacobsen syndrome*
    - Acute history (acquired)
      - ITP
      - Consumption
  - MPV normal
    - *FPD/AML, THC2*
    - *CAMT, ATRUS, TAR*
    - HIT, FNAIT, TTP, HUS
    - Systemic disease
    - Herbs, drugs
  - MPV small
    - *WAS*
    - *XLT*

44 van Eimeren · Kahr

Table 2. Aggregation findings for platelet function disorders

Disorder	Characteristic findings on LTA
BSS or VWD	markedly reduced platelet agglutination with ristocetin
Type 2B VWD or platelet type VWD	increased agglutination with low concentrations of ristocetin
GT	absent response to all agonists (aggregation cannot occur because fibrinogen cannot bind) except ristocetin (agglutination)
Secretion defect or δ-granule defect	reduced secondary wave of aggregation (ADP, epinephrine, collagen) suggesting a failure of δ-granule release or a deficiency of platelet δ-granules
ASA (or defects in the COX pathway)	absent aggregation to arachidonic acid; decreased or absent aggregation with collagen; normal response to U46619
ADP receptor defect	abnormal aggregation response to ADP (slight and rapidly reversible)

of platelets quantifies dense granules (δ-granules), whereas TEM evaluates the platelet ultrastructure and α-granule content. Immunofluorescence microscopy with antibodies directed against myosin IIA can detect abnormal distributions of myosin IIA in neutrophils even when Döhle-like inclusions are not obvious on blood films in patients with MYH9-related disease.

Platelet Aggregometry

Platelet adhesion, aggregation and secretion are assessed using in vitro platelet aggregometry. To minimize preanalytical variables such as platelet activation or hemolysis, blood should be collected by an experienced phlebotomist using a standardized atraumatic protocol as described by Harrison et al. [7]. Blood is collected in 3.2% sodium citrate and should be kept at room temperature (20–25°C not 4°C) and ideally analyzed between 30 min and 2 h of blood collection (not more than 4h). Antiplatelet drugs (NSAIDs including ASA, clopidogrel, prasugrel, cangrelor), anticoagulants (heparinoids, vitamin K antagonists, direct thrombin inhibitors), as well as many other drugs such as caffeine and nicotine should be avoided (for a complete list see table 1 in Harrison et al. [7]). Platelet aggregometry measures the ability of platelets to aggregate after stimulation with specific agonists as detailed below, where light transmission changes in PRP or electrical impedance in 50% diluted whole blood can be measured. Characteristic aggregation tracings can be indicative of specific platelet disorders (table 2).

Light Transmission Aggregometry

LTA is the most common method of assessing platelet function but also requires the largest blood volumes (10–15 ml blood) to allow for sufficient PRP. It measures the change in light transmittance over time of rapidly stirred PRP after addition of platelet agonists. The aggregation tracing is observed for 5–10 min to monitor the lag phase, shape change (negative deflection), primary and secondary aggregation and any delayed platelet responses, e.g. reversible or spontaneous aggregation. A recommended baseline agonist panel comprises 2.5 μM ADP, 1.25 μg/ml collagen, 5 μM epinephrine (may not always give a full aggregation response due to natural variations in adrenoreceptor numbers with no related platelet defect), 1.2 mg/ml ristocetin and 1.0 mM arachidonic acid (all final concentrations in PRP). If the agglutination to ristocetin is normal, then retesting should additionally be performed with low dose (0.5–0.7 mg/ml) ristocetin to check for hyperfunction or gain of function (associated with type 2B and platelet type VWD). If results with 1.2 mg/ml ristocetin are absent, then retesting can be performed with addition of an external source of VWF to confirm either a VWF or GPIb defect. If arachidonic acid aggregation is abnormal, then further testing should be performed with 1.0 μM U46619 (a stable TxA_2 mimetic) to distinguish COX-1 inhibition (absent arachidonic acid response but normal to U46619) from a thromboxane receptor defect (absent arachidonic acid and U46619 response) [7].

Whole Blood Aggregometry

Whole blood aggregometry requires smaller blood volumes than LTA because it eliminates the need for PRP. It measures aggregation in saline-diluted whole blood as the change in electrical impedance between electrodes. The Multiplate® (multiple platelet function) analyzer is a recently developed 4-channel impedance aggregometer using standardized reagents. Due to its small sample volume (0.3 ml of blood or 0.175 ml using a special mini-test cell), it may be very useful for pediatric applications.

Lumiaggregometry Studies

Lumiaggregometry studies are useful in the identification of dense granule disorders. The lumiaggregometer measures platelet aggregation and secretion of dense granule ATP simultaneously. Released ATP oxidizes a firefly-derived luciferin-luciferase reagent to generate proportional chemiluminescence. Lumiaggregometry may be performed using whole blood or PRP. If secretion is abnormal, quantification of platelet-dense granules by whole mount electron microscopy can distinguish a defect in the dense granule secretion process from a decrease/absence in the number of dense granules.

Flow Cytometry (Citrated Blood)

This method involves incubating platelets with fluorochrome-conjugated antibodies directed against platelet proteins such as GPIb-IX-V (low to absent in BSS) or GPIIb-IIIa (low to absent in GT) where the platelet surface membrane proteins are quantified by flow cytometry. Testing can be carried out in whole blood, PRP or washed platelets and requires very small sample volumes (0.5 ml), making it useful in children and neonates. Flow cytometry may facilitate the diagnosis of BSS, GT, WAS and Scott syndrome.

Thrombocytopenia

Acquired causes of thrombocytopenia are significantly more common than congenital disorders. Neonatal acquired thrombocytopenia is most often the result of perinatal factors or due to allo- or autoimmune thrombocytopenia (see chapter 4). The platelet count history of the individual and family may be helpful in distinguishing between congenital and acquired causes. Causes of congenital thrombocytopenia are rare and diverse, and may also be accompanied by platelet function abnormalities [8, 9]. Inherited thrombocytopenias persist beyond the neonatal period and can be categorized clinically according to platelet size (algorithm 1). For further details on these disorders, see table 4 and chapter 4.

Immune Thrombocytopenia

Nomenclature, definitions and recommendations in the following section are based on the guidelines of the international Vicenza Consensus Conference [10], and two published international ITP guidelines [11, 12].

ITP is caused by an inappropriate immune response. Often there is a history of prodromal viral illness. Proposed pathogenic mechanisms include the development of antibodies to viral or bacterial antigens that cross-react with epitopes on platelet receptors, or autoreactive antibodies that have escaped immune selection. Splenic destruction of antibody-coated platelets, as well as the inhibition of megakaryopoiesis (in some cases), contribute to the low platelet count.

Primary ITP is defined as 'an autoimmune disorder characterized by isolated thrombocytopenia (peripheral blood platelet count <100 × 10^9/l) in the absence of other causes or disorders that may be associated with thrombocytopenia' [10]. Primary ITP is the single most common cause of thrombocytopenia in childhood with an incidence of 4/100,000 children per year. ITP is classified by duration: newly diagnosed (up to 3 months from diagnosis), persistent (3–12 months' duration) and chronic (≥12 months' duration).

Causes of secondary ITP (all forms of immune-mediated thrombocytopenia except primary ITP) include:
1. Autoimmune diseases: APLS, autoimmune thrombocytopenia and anemia (Evans syndrome), autoimmune lymphoproliferative syndrome, common variable immunodeficiency, SLE
2. Infectious diseases: cytomegalovirus, *Helicobacter pylori*, HCV, HIV, varicella zoster, Epstein-Barr virus
3. Drug effects: HIT (rare in young children), quinine

Clinical Presentation
Patients typically present with petechiae or purpura that develop acutely, accompanied by platelet counts <20 × 10^9/l. Patients/parents often report a prodromal illness or other immune stimulant such as allergic reaction, insect bite or immunization (there is a reported association with measles-mumps-rubella vaccine). ITP occurs more frequently in the fall and winter, and least frequently in the summer. Childhood ITP affects males and females equally; in adolescent girls, the disease is more likely to become chronic.

In contrast to severe thrombocytopenia associated with bone marrow failure syndromes, serious bleeding is rare in ITP, possibly due to more efficient function of the few remaining platelets. Only 3% of children with ITP have clinically significant symptoms such as severe epistaxis or GI bleeding. Severe bleeding is more likely in children with platelet counts <10 × 10^9/l. The incidence of ICH in children with ITP is approximately 0.1–0.5%. Risk factors for ICH in children with severe thrombocytopenia include head trauma and concomitant use of medications that inhibit platelet function. The term 'severe ITP' is reserved for patients with 'presence of bleeding symptoms at presentation sufficient to mandate treatment, or occurrence of new bleeding symptoms requiring additional therapeutic intervention with a different platelet-enhancing agent or an increased dose' [10].

Diagnosis
ITP remains a diagnosis of exclusion. The classic presentation is that of a previously healthy child who has acute onset of petechiae, bruising and/or bleeding with an otherwise normal physical examination. Laboratory investigations show isolated thrombocytopenia with normal to large platelet size and an otherwise unremarkable peripheral blood film. Other causes of thrombocytopenia must be ruled out. It is not necessary to perform a bone marrow aspirate in newly diagnosed patients who fulfill these criteria. Findings that are not typical for ITP and that should prompt additional testing include: weight loss or failure to thrive; bone or joint pain; family history of low platelets or easy bruising, thrombocytopenia present from birth; fever, recurrent infections, risk factors for HIV infection; skeletal or soft-tissue morphologic abnormalities, dysmorphic/syndromic features; lymphadenopathy; jaundice. In addition, abnormalities of additional cell lines also warrant further investigations, including consideration of a bone marrow examination. ITP that is refractory to therapy or recurs following an initial remission may also require further investigation. Caution should be

Table 3. Suggested laboratory assessment for suspected ITP with typical features

Initial investigation	
Complete blood count and differential WBC count, reticulocyte count, stained peripheral blood smear	multilineage involvement, leukemia or aplastic/myelodysplasia, hemolytic anemia, platelet size, cell inclusions
Blood type, Rh, direct antiglobulin/Coombs test	possible anti-D antibody treatment, autoimmune hemolytic disease
Quantitative serum immunoglobulin levels (IgG, IgA, IgM)	upfront only if treatment with intravenous immunoglobulin is considered, otherwise after 3–6 months if no improvement (rule out: common variable immune deficiency, WAS)
Recommended evaluations for children with no improvement after 3–6 months	
Bone marrow evaluation	recommended if ITP persists and suboptimal response to therapy
Identify potential infection	HIV/HCV/*H. pylori* if clinical suspicion or high local prevalence
Antinuclear antibody, C3, C4, anti-double-stranded DNA antibody testing	for clinical suspicion of SLE
APLA, including anticardiolipin antibody and lupus anticoagulant	to rule out APLS

taken with infants with Down syndrome in whom thrombocytopenia may herald the development of megakaryoblastic leukemia. Suggested laboratory investigations for suspected childhood ITP with typical features are shown in table 3.

Management

Two thirds of children with typical ITP achieve complete or partial remission of thrombocytopenia with no major bleeding complication within the first year after diagnosis, regardless of therapy.

Medications that interfere with platelet function should be discontinued (e.g. NSAIDs such as ASA and ibuprofen; antiepileptics, particularly valproic acid; selective serotonin reuptake inhibitors).

The child should not participate in high-impact sport activities that have a high risk of trauma or head injury, such as martial arts, American football, ice hockey and competitive soccer, until the platelet count is stable at ≥50 × 10^9/l. Swimming is allowed but diving is not. Other activities need not be restricted, and the child should be encouraged to continue with schooling. A medical alert bracelet may be appropriate.

Oral hygiene is crucial in order to prevent gingival bleeding, inflammation and severe periodontal diseases. Close cooperation between a patient's dentist and hematologist is warranted, especially in the case of dental/periodontal procedures. Tooth extractions and mandibular blocks should be avoided until the platelet count is greater than 30 × 10^9/l; for other dental work (cleaning, filling) the platelet count may be lower but >10 × 10^9/l [13]. Removal of wisdom teeth is a major challenge and should probably be done with a platelet count of ≥50 × 10^9/l. Effective local hemostatic measures may include suturing and the use of topical hemostatic agents. In addition, antifibrinolytic therapy before and after oral procedures may limit excessive hemorrhage (treatment specifics are given below).

In children with ITP who have already received their first dose of MMR vaccine, vaccine titers can be checked. If the child does not have adequate immunity, then the child should be reimmunized with MMR vaccine at the recommended age; otherwise, no further MMR vaccine should be given. Children with a history of ITP who are unimmunized should receive their scheduled first MMR vaccine [12].

It is recommended that children with no bleeding or mild bleeding (skin manifestations only, such as petechiae and bruising) be managed with observation alone, regardless of platelet count. The decision to observe requires a detailed discussion with the patient/family and guidance about prevention and monitoring of bleeding. A CBC and blood film should be repeated periodically to exclude the evolution of a serious bone marrow or other hematologic disorder. Treatment may be considered in patients for whom there is a question of compliance or if the family is geographically isolated. In addition, quality of life issues may warrant treatment, especially in older children with chronic ITP.

Clinically significant bleeding (any type of bleed exceeding skin manifestations only, such as mucosal hemorrhage) should prompt treatment initiation in all children with ITP. The treatment goal for acute ITP should be a rapid achievement of safe hemostatic levels of circulating platelets while awaiting a spontaneous remission. Hospital admission should be reserved for patients who have clinically significant bleeding or problematic psychosocial circumstances.

First-Line Treatment

For newly diagnosed children requiring treatment, IVIG or corticosteroids can be used. A single dose of IVIG (0.8 g/kg, rounded to the nearest vial) can be given with a follow-up platelet count checked 24–48 h after administration. A second dose can be given if there is no response. Side effects of IVIG include postinfusion headache, vomiting, allergic reactions, aseptic meningitis and renal failure. Anemia may develop due to hemolysis and/or there may be an acquired immune-mediated neutropenia. In children with acute ITP and platelet counts <20 × 10^9/l, IVIG raises the circulating platelet count >20 × 10^9/l in more than 80% of children and does so more rapidly than oral corticosteroids. The disadvantage is that it must be given intravenously and in a monitored setting.

Steroids are also useful in the acute setting. A 4-day course of higher dose steroids (prednisone 4 mg/kg/day divided twice daily, maximum dose 180 mg) is effective in 70–80% of patients and raises platelet counts to levels similar to those produced by IVIG within 72 h [14]. This approach results in fewer side effects than a lower dose of steroids given over a few weeks. Side effects most commonly include transient mood changes and gastritis, but other steroid effects are sometimes seen.

Intravenous anti-D (50–75 μg/kg, rounded to nearest vial) can be used in Rh-positive, nonsplenectomized children. Anti-D should not be given to patients with hemoglobin levels below 100 g/l or coexisting immune-mediated anemia (i.e. cases with a baseline moderate to strongly positive direct antiglobulin test). Rarely, anti-D may cause severe intravascular hemolysis and disseminated intravascular coagulation. Patients at increased risk are those with active viral infections (e.g. Epstein-Barr virus), malignant conditions or old age. Although less expensive than IVIG, a recent black box warning recommends that patients who receive anti-D should be observed in hospital for at least 8 h after admission for evidence of acute intravascular hemolysis (dipstick urinalysis positive for hemoglobin). This has curtailed its use in some centers.

An increase in the platelet count in response to the initial treatment supports a diagnosis of ITP and the immune nature of the thrombocytopenia.

Persistent/Chronic Immune Thrombocytopenia

Rituximab can be considered in patients who have significant thrombocytopenia and ongoing bleeding despite treatment with IVIG, corticosteroids or anti-D. Administration of rituximab, an anti-CD20 antibody, results in depletion of circulating B cells. It has been used with success in children with chronic refractory ITP. It may serve as an alternative to splenectomy or be given in cases where splenectomy has failed. Response with increasing platelet counts occurs over the period of a few weeks to a few months. The rate of durable responses (>50 × 10^9/l platelet count) in the largest pediatric series is approximately 30% [15]. With the exception of rare cases of serum sickness, rituximab is generally well tolerated. Additional potential side effects include hypotension and anaphylaxis. A very rare but severe sequel of the drug is progressive multifocal leukoencephalopathy. Rituximab-associated hypogammaglobulinemia is not significant in ITP patients without underlying immunodeficiency. The standard approach is to give 375 mg/m^2 weekly for 4 weeks.

Splenectomy may be considered for patients with a lack of response or an intolerance to medical therapies. It should also be considered in patients for whom thrombocytopenia or the medications are having a significant impact on the quality of life. However, it is suggested to delay a decision about splenectomy for at least 12 months (3 years in some centers) following diagnosis to allow time for spontaneous resolution, unless the ITP is associated with severe bleeding. The risk of death from ITP in childhood is extremely low (0.5%) but postsplenectomy overwhelming sepsis occurs in up to 3% despite antibiotic prophylaxis [16, 17]. Patients should be immunized against encapsulated bacteria (*Streptococcus pneumoniae*, *Haemophilus influenzae* type b and *Neisseria meningitidis*), at least 2–3 weeks prior to the procedure. If necessary, IVIG or steroids in known responders may be used to boost the platelet count before splenectomy to 30–50 × 10^9/l [18], as generally suggested for surgery in adults [13]. Preoperative platelet transfusions are rarely warranted, and their routine use should be discouraged. There is a suggestion that if platelets seem necessary to cover the surgery, these should be given once the splenic artery has been clamped [13]. Following splenectomy, antibiotic prophylaxis with oral penicillin or erythromycin is recommended to reduce the incidence of overwhelming postsplenectomy infection. An increased risk of sepsis probably persists for life, and it is therefore prudent to recommend antibiotic prophylaxis in compliant patients to be continued lifelong, but as a minimum, 2–3 years following the procedure.

Thrombopoietin receptor agonists have been licensed for use in adults with severe chronic ITP. Studies in children and adolescents are under way, but no recommendations for the use of these agents can be made at this time. In addition, high-dose dexamethasone and immunosuppressive agents have been used in a small number of children who failed to respond to more conventional therapy. Data for any single agent or combination of agents remain insufficient for specific recommendations.

Emergency Treatment/Surgery

An urgent increase in platelet count may be required for some thrombocytopenic patients needing surgical procedures, or in the event of life and organ-threatening hemorrhage. Concurrent administration of platelet transfusions, steroids and IVIG can be effective in resolving bleeding and restoring adequate platelet counts with minimal side effects. We recommend infusion of a larger than usual dose (2- to 3-fold) of platelets followed by i.v. methylprednisolone 30 mg/kg (maximum dose 1 g) followed by IVIG (1 g/kg). Emergency splenectomy may be considered, but the dangers of unplanned surgery, possible lack of immunization and the risk of surgical bleeding need to be evaluated carefully.

There is no evidence in ITP for a specific target platelet count for operative intervention or after trauma. Generally, in thrombocytopenic patients the bleeding risk is negligible when platelet counts are ≥50 × 10^9/l, but increases significantly when platelet counts are <20 × 10^9/l. Procedures considered high risk for bleeding include neurosurgery, vascular surgery, surgery of mucous membranes, spinal/peridural anesthesia and solid organ biopsy. In addition, patients with concomitant coagulation deficits are at higher risk of hemorrhage, and therefore screening for and correction of these deficits are required before surgery.

Platelet Function Defects

Congenital PFDs, especially secretion defects and nonspecific aggregation abnormalities, are very common and may be as prevalent as VWD, which is considered to be the most common inherited bleeding disorder (for details on VWD, see chapter 7). Nevertheless, the prevalence among the general population has not been established. Due to a challenging diagnostic evaluation and the requirement for specialized laboratory testing, a high percentage of patients remain undiagnosed. Table 4 lists the numerous, mostly rare, causes of PFDs, categorized according to the underlying pathophysiology. Various treatment choices/hemostatic agents are presented, and management of bleeding episodes is described according to clinical circumstances, as there are few disorder-specific therapies [19, 20].

Glycoprotein Disorders

These defects can be categorized according to receptor function into defects in platelet adhesion, defects of aggregation and defects of agonist receptors/signaling pathways. For this group of disorders, LTA is a useful tool to identify the specific functional defects (detailed in table 2), followed by flow cytometry to determine receptor numbers on the platelet surface.

Glanzmann Thrombasthenia [21]
In GT, an autosomal-recessively inherited disorder, quantitative or qualitative defects of the $\alpha IIb\beta_3$ integrin (GPIIb/IIIa) receptor result in abnormal platelet aggregation. In healthy individuals the activated receptor binds to fibrinogen or VWF, which cross-link platelets into aggregates. $\alpha IIb\beta_3$ integrin also provides a link between fibrin and the intracellular cytoskeletal proteins that mediate clot retraction, a process that fails to occur in patients with severe GT.

Patients with GT commonly present with severe mucocutaneous bleeding. Most GT patients present before the age of 5 years, often during the neonatal period, with purpura or petechiae or in early childhood with excessive bruising, epistaxis, gingival bleeds or bleeding after trauma or surgery. Dental extractions and exfoliation of the deciduous teeth may be associated with excessive bleeding. Iron deficiency anemia is common in children with GT due to blood loss. Major bleeding complications during the neonatal period, such as ICH, are rare. With the exception of menorrhagia/postpartum hemorrhage, severity of bleeding diminishes with age. Heterozygotes are asymptomatic, but have approximately half of the normal complement of $\alpha IIb\beta_3$ receptors on their platelets.

Platelet count and morphology in patients with GT are normal; however, platelet function is severely compromised due to defects in platelet aggregation. The PFA-100® closure times are significantly prolonged, typically >300 s (i.e. nonclosure) with both collagen/epinephrine and collagen/ADP cartridges (chapter 3). The PFA-100® can be a useful screening test to rule out a diagnosis of GT. Platelet aggregation studies will reveal absent aggregation with all agonists, except ristocetin-induced agglutination (GPIb-IX-V receptor mediated). $\alpha IIb\beta_3$ deficiency is quantified using flow cytometry or Western blotting. In neonates, flow cytometry is easily performed on small volumes of blood (LTA is difficult in neonates because of blood volumes required for testing). Gene analysis will lead to detection of mutations of the *ITGA2B* and *ITGB3* genes.

Bernard-Soulier Syndrome [22]
BSS results from defects of the GPIb-IX-V complex, the receptor for VWF on the platelet surface. BSS manifests as defective platelet adhesion. BSS is usually transmitted as a recessive trait. Heterozygotes in these families usually have normal platelet counts and no or mild bleeding

Table 4. Platelet function disorders

Disease	Clinical findings	Laboratory features
Glycoprotein defects		
Defects of platelet aggregation		
GT (GPIIb-IIIa defect)	autosomal recessive, severe bleeding diathesis from childhood	platelet count and morphology normal, PFA-100® closure times markedly prolonged, absence of aggregation with all agonists except ristocetin agglutination, flow cytometry identifies $αIIbβ_3$ deficiency
Defects in platelet adhesion		
BSS (GPIb-IX-V defect)	autosomal recessive, severe bleeding diathesis from childhood	macrothrombocytopenia (platelet count may fluctuate), PFA-100® closure times markedly prolonged, no agglutination with ristocetin, flow cytometry reveals GPIb-IX-V deficiency
DiGeorge/velocardiofacial syndrome (22q11.2 deletion, involving GPIb)	cleft palate, cardiac abnormalities, typical facies, learning disabilities, parathyroid and thymus abnormalities, mild to significant bleeding	normal/variable platelet function tests
Platelet type VWD (GPIb defect) synonym: pseudo-VWD	mild to moderate bleeding	gain of function mutation in GPIb of the GPIb-IX-V receptor (in type 2B VWD, the GPIb binding site on VWF is altered in the gain of function), macrothrombocytopenia, platelet clumps on blood film, increased platelet agglutination to low-dose ristocetin, high-molecular-weight VWF multimers reduced
Defects of agonist receptors and signaling pathways		
Collagen receptor defect (GPVI)	autosomal recessive, mild bleeding diathesis	reduced aggregation response to collagen
ADP receptor (P_2Y_{12}) defect	autosomal recessive, mild bleeding after trauma/surgery	abnormal aggregation response to ADP (slight and rapidly reversible)
Thromboxane A_2 (TP) receptor defect	autosomal recessive, mild bleeding diathesis	abnormal aggregation response to arachidonic acid and U46619 (stable analog of TXA_2)
Granule disorders		
α-Granule defects		
GPS	autosomal recessive, mild to moderate bleeding related to hemostatic stress, myelofibrosis	thrombocytopenia, large and pale gray platelets by light microscopy, absent/reduced α-granules by TEM
ARC syndrome	flexion contractures, hypotonia, cholestatic jaundice, renal tubular acidosis, failure to thrive, lethal during first year of life, various bleeding complications	pale gray platelets on peripheral smear, absent α-granules by TEM, P-selectin is absent
Quebec platelet disorder	autosomal dominant, delayed onset bleeding after surgery/trauma, not responsive to platelet transfusion but very responsive to antifibrinolytics	abnormal excess platelet urokinase plasminogen activator causing plasmin-mediated proteolysis of platelet α-granule proteins and fibrinolysis of blood clots due to platelet secretion; abnormal urokinase detected in platelet lysates using ELISA/Western blots; variable thrombocytopenia
Paris-Trousseau/Jacobsen syndrome	autosomal-dominant, mild bleeding tendency, developmental delay, cardiac, urogenital, skeletal, central nervous system, gastrointestinal and craniofacial anomalies	macrothrombocytopenia; giant α-granules (TEM) which cannot release their contents normally upon stimulation in a low percentage of platelets; two morphologically distinct populations of megakaryocytes in the bone marrow
δ-Granule defects/secretion defects		
Idiopathic δ-granule disorder	no systemic findings, mild bleeding diathesis	decreased/absent δ-granules on whole mount electron microscopy with defective ATP release measured by lumiaggregometry
Hermansky-Pudlak syndrome	autosomal recessive, oculocutaneous albinism, immunity defects, mild bleeding diathesis; pulmonary fibrosis, granulomatous colitis and neutropenia possible (subtype specific); most common genetic disorder in Puerto Rico	decreased/absent δ-granules on whole mount electron microscopy with defective ATP release measured by lumiaggregometry

Table 4. Continued

Disease	Clinical findings	Laboratory features
Chediak-Higashi syndrome	autosomal recessive, variable oculocutaneous albinism, recurrent life-threatening infections, death within first decade, mild bleeding diathesis	decreased δ-granules on whole mount electron microscopy, giant peroxidase-positive cytoplasmatic granules in neutrophils (abnormal lysosomes unable to digest phagocytosed bacteria), lymphohistiocytosis
αδ-Granule disorders	autosomal dominant or recessive, mild bleeding diathesis	pale gray platelets on blood film, absent α-granules on TEM, decreased δ-granules on whole mount electron microscopy
Platelet cytoskeletal defects WAS XLT	triad: eczema, microthrombocytopenia, immune deficiency; propensity to develop lymphomas and auto-immunity, x-linked (males affected), clinically significant bleeding often present from infancy, including ICH	small platelets accompanied by thrombocytopenia, decreased T-cell subsets, natural killer cell function, antibody production after vaccines and immunoglobulin levels, decreased α- and dense granules by whole mount electron microscopy/TEM; mutations in WAS protein
MYH9-related disorder (formerly Sebastian, May-Hegglin, Fechtner and Epstein syndromes)	autosomal dominant and de novo mutations, association with variable bleeding tendency, variable association with sensorineural deafness, cataracts and nephritis	macrothrombocytopenia, Döhle-like inclusions in neutrophils on blood film, myosin IIA clumps in neutrophils detected with immunofluorescence microscopy
Disorder of phospholipid exposure Scott syndrome	very rare, autosomal-recessive, bleeding with invasive procedures	defect of phospholipid exposure and microvesiculation, defective thrombin/fibrin formation, absent annexin A5 binding to activated platelets using flow cytometry

problems. However, there are dominant heterozygous forms of BSS with mild to moderate mucocutaneous symptoms. Hemizygous mutations can also cause BSS when associated with the DiGeorge/velocardiofacial syndrome, and may cause significant bleeding in these patients, even in the absence of a detectable platelet function abnormality but related to thrombocytopenia.

BSS generally presents in infancy with severe symptoms of abnormal primary hemostasis. However, age at onset and severity of bleeding symptoms may vary considerably between individuals. Bleeding may be more severe than expected for the degree of thrombocytopenia.

BSS should be considered when a patient presents with macrothrombocytopenia and severe bleeding problems. However, platelet counts can fluctuate over time in the same individual and may be very low, marginally low or normal. In homozygotes, the diagnosis is supported by markedly prolonged PFA-100® closure times, typically >300 s with both cartridges. A lack of platelet agglutination with high-dose ristocetin using LTA is confirmatory in the presence of normal plasma VWF levels. Flow cytometry measuring platelet surface GPIb-IX-V offers a quantitative method of confirming the diagnosis. Mutation testing of the *GPIBA*, *GPIBB*, and *GP9* genes can be performed.

Granule Disorders

Platelets contain two unique types of cytoplasmic storage granules: the α-granules and the dense (δ-)granules. α-Granules contain numerous proteins including coagulation factors (fibrinogen, VWF) growth factors, angiogenic factors, immune modulators, cytokines, bacteriostatic proteins and many others. δ-Granules contain pro-aggregatory factors such as ADP, calcium, polyphosphate, and 5-hydroxytryptamine (serotonin). During activation, the granules are centralized, and fuse with the open canalicular system and plasma membrane to release their contents to the exterior.

Granule disorders encompass α-granule defects (such as GPS, ARC syndrome, Quebec platelet disorder, Paris-Trousseau/Jacobsen syndrome) and δ-granule defects/secretion defects (Hermansky-Pudlak syndrome, Chediak-Higashi syndrome, nonsyndromic secretion defects). Nonsyndromic secretion defects are by far the most often encountered abnormalities within this group. In few patients, the usually mild to moderate bleeding tendency may be part of a more complex – and possibly severe – condition affecting other organ systems. Significant bleeding may result following surgery or trauma. Absence of α-granules can be visualized by thin-section TEM. δ-Granule quantification can be assessed by whole mount electron microscopy. Reduction of ATP release from δ-granules as found in secretion defects can be measured by lumiaggregometry. Characteristic findings of granule disorders are outlined in table 4.

Treatment and Hemostatic Agents

Supportive Care

Individuals with PFD should be managed by qualified specialists with expertise in bleeding disorders and registered with a bleeding disorder clinic, if possible. The patient/parent should be educated and issued written information about the condition. A medical alert bracelet should also be issued. Platelet inhibitor medication should be avoided. Advice on maintaining good dental hygiene is appropriate. Individuals with severe PFD (GT, BSS, severe forms of WAS) should not engage in contact sports.

Patients with severe inherited PFD are likely to be exposed to blood products in their life span. They should be immunized against hepatitis A and B and have annual monitoring of their liver function.

Local Measures

If bleeding is only mild to moderate, local measures such as suturing, compression, nasal packing, use of gelatin sponge or gauze dipped in tranexamic acid or topical recombinant human thrombin applied to superficial wounds or nasal mucosa may suffice. Recothrom® is preferred, where available, over a product that contains bovine proteins such as Tisseel® because it decreases the risk of antibody development.

Antifibrinolytic Agents

Tranexamic acid (Cyklokapron®) and ε-amino caproic acid (Amicar®), are lysine analogues that inhibit clot lysis by binding to plasminogen and are useful for control of mild/moderate bleeding manifestations, particularly at mucosal sites, such as epistaxis or menorrhagia. For elective interventions, they are usually commenced the day before and continued for 5–7 days thereafter.

Tranexamic acid is preferred because it is more potent (8-fold). It may be given either orally at a dose of 25 mg/kg (usual adult dose is 1.0–1.5 g) 3–4 times daily for 5–7 days, or i.v. at a dose of 10 mg/kg (adult dose 0.5–1 g) 2–3 times daily in cases of more serious bleeding. For patients with renal failure, dose adjustments of tranexamic acid are necessary (electronic medicines compendium, UK):

- serum creatinine 120–249 μmol/l twice daily: 10 mg/kg i.v. or 15 mg/kg oral
- serum creatinine 250–500 μmol/l once daily: 10 mg/kg i.v. or 15 mg/kg oral
- serum creatinine >500 μmol/l every 48 h: 10 mg/kg i.v.

Tranexamic acid may also be useful as a mouthwash for local oropharyngeal bleeding or bleeding from inflamed tonsils (10 ml of a 5% solution 4 times daily, which if swallowed, is equivalent to a dose of 500 mg) [19].

ε-Aminocaproic acid is given at a dose of 100 mg/kg infused over 15 min, followed by a maintenance dose of 10 mg/kg/h or 5 g bolus every 4 h. Oral pediatric dosing for ε-aminocaproic acid is 100–200 mg/kg initial dose with a maximum dose of 10 g, followed by 50–100 mg/kg/dose with a maximum dose of 5 g every 6 h, usually given for 5–7 days. Antifibrinolytic agents are contraindicated when there is urinary bleeding, due to the risk of obstruction from clot formation. Common side effects include nausea and diarrhea; long-term use has been associated with visual changes.

Desmopressin

DDAVP may be the agent of choice for mild/moderate bleeding problems where fibrinolytic inhibitors alone are ineffective. For surgery, it is given as a single dose immediately prior to the intervention and if bleeding persists, possibly again after 12 h. Although of limited benefit in patients with platelet receptor defects, patients with secretion defects may respond. A DDAVP challenge may be considered in cases where there is prolongation in the closure time using the PFA-100®, where a response is considered as normalization of the closure time when tested before, at 1 h, and 4 h after DDAVP administration. The mechanism of the DDAVP response in PFDs is not understood but may be the result of DDAVP-dependent increased levels of circulating VWF and FVIII. Side effects of DDAVP include flushing and hypotension. It causes fluid retention, and patients should be advised to restrict fluid intake for 24 h following administration. Intravenous fluids should be given with caution because fluid retention can result in severe hyponatremia and seizures, particularly in young children. As a result, it is not recommended in children <2 years of age [19, 20]. If given for more than a single dose, fluid balance and plasma electrolytes must be monitored carefully.

DDAVP administration is as follows:
1. Intravenous infusion over 30 min: the usual dose regimen is 0.3 µg/kg (up to a maximum of 20 µg) of a 4 µg/ml solution diluted to 30–50 ml in 0.9% saline. Peak levels of circulating VWF and FVIII are reached after 30–60 min.
2. Subcutaneous injection at a dose of 0.3 µg/kg. A more concentrated product is available containing 15 µg/ml. Peak levels of circulating VWF and FVIII are reached after 90–120 min.
3. Intranasal spray is available in a concentrated form (150 µg per dose) to be administered at 150 µg for a child over 30 kg in weight and 300 µg for an adult. Peak levels of circulating VWF and FVIII are reached after 90–120 min.

Platelet Transfusions

Platelet transfusions provide normal functioning platelets to the circulation in patients with PFDs, partially correcting the inherent platelet dysfunction (pediatric dose is 10–15 ml/kg per transfusion). Transfusion is the treatment of choice during major life-threatening bleeding episodes for moderate to severe PFDs and thrombocytopenia. It should also be used when other agents have failed. However, a careful risk-benefit assessment should be carried out due to the risks of transfusion-transmitted infections, allergic reactions and the risk of developing alloantibodies either to HLA antigens or absent GPs (in BSS and GT). Some centers recommend that patients with severe PFD should be typed for HLA to facilitate HLA-selected platelet units for transfusion. However, there is no good evidence to support the use of either ABO or HLA best-matched single donor apheresis platelets in preference to WBC-depleted pooled random donor platelets to avoid alloimmunization in GT and BSS cases, especially when platelet transfusion is required urgently. HLA and platelet-specific alloantibodies may limit response to platelet transfusion. Antibodies should be looked for in patients that have previously received transfusions and do not respond clinically to adequate doses of either random-donor or single-donor apheresis platelets, and in those requiring elective surgery.

Recombinant Factor VIIa

rFVIIa is licensed in Europe for use in GT patients with demonstrated refractoriness to platelet transfusions. It is thought to enhance thrombin generation by both tissue factor-dependent and -independent mechanisms. A commonly used dose is 90–120 µg/kg, administered by intravenous bolus injection. rFVIIa has a short half-life, and the dose may need to be repeated 2–4 hourly for several doses, or until the bleeding risk is minimized. Higher doses of up to 270 μg/kg given once have been used when the standard dose was not effective. rFVIIa is generally safe, but thrombotic complications have been recorded. It is not licensed for treatment of other platelet disorders, although there are some published data on its use in BSS. The decision to use rFVIIa off-licence must be balanced with the potential for antibody formation with repeated platelet transfusions [23, 24].

Management of Bleeding Episodes

Epistaxis/Gingival Bleeds/Tonsillar Bleed

For patients with acute bleeding who have a moderate to severe platelet disorder, it is important to have a low threshold for admission to hospital. Young children with epistaxis may lose much more blood than is clinically apparent. Treatment with local measures and systemic antifibrinolytics should be started immediately. When these measures fail to achieve hemostasis within 1–2 h, treatment includes platelet transfusions, rFVIIa or a combination. rFVIIa can be used in preference to platelet transfusion for non-life-threatening hemorrhage. Any life-threatening bleed should be treated with platelet transfusion. In severe cases, otolaryngology services (if available) should be involved in management of the bleeding site.

Menorrhagia

Young women with severe menorrhagia should be managed jointly with (pediatric) gynecology services (if available) to stop bleeding quickly. Therapy with oral antifibrinolytics is often useful and should be the initial therapeutic step. Failure to control bleeding is an indication for hormone therapy with either high-dose progesterone alone (e.g. norethisterone 5 mg every 4 h) or a combination of progesterone with estrogen. Commonly, bleeding severity will decrease within 24 h, so that a dose adjustment to 5 mg norethisterone twice a day continued for 3 weeks is justified. Menstrual bleeding of reduced severity will result on withdrawal of progesterone. Maintenance treatment with combined oral contraceptives can be initiated thereafter. Additional approaches to menorrhagia that may be useful include DDAVP or rFVIIa, or an intrauterine contraceptive device (Mirena®, levonorgestrel-releasing intrauterine system) for women who choose intrauterine contraception.

Dental Procedures

Dental procedures should be planned in advance and in consultation with a hematologist, whenever possible. Thresholds for platelet counts are similar to those recommended for patients with ITP. Mandibular blocks should be avoided. Local hemostatic measures and the use of oral or intravenous tranexamic acid are important therapeutic pillars. For patients with a less severe PFD (e.g. platelet secretion defect), DDAVP may be another agent of choice. rFVIIa may be used for prophylactic treatment in patients with GT and BSS. If bleeding is not controlled with several doses of rFVIIa or DDAVP, the patient should receive a platelet transfusion. Patients should be kept under close clinical supervision.

Minor Surgery

Minor surgical interventions such as wound closure, abscess drainage, removal of skin lesions, removal of ingrown toe nails, placement of ear tubes, correction of bone fractures, hernia repairs, skin biopsies, etc., can be treated with antifibrinolytics in most patients. Patients with a mild PFD may also benefit from DDAVP. Patients with GT or BSS or platelet refractoriness should additionally receive rFVIIa until the bleeding risk is minimized. If bleeding is not controlled (i.e. no response after two or three doses of rFVIIa or DDAVP), the dose of rFVIIa can be increased and platelets can be administered as necessary.

Major Surgery

Major surgery includes neurosurgery, thoracic, abdominal and pelvic surgery, vascular surgery, adenoidectomy, tonsillectomy, spinal/peridural anesthesia and solid organ biopsy. Most patients will profit from preoperatively initiated antifibrinolytics, continued for 7–14 days after surgery. Patients with a mild bleeding tendency may also be given one or possibly two doses of DDAVP, depending on previously known responses. Due to uncertainties concerning the efficacy of rFVIIa for treatment of severe PFDs, it is recommended that platelet transfusion be used for major surgery in patients with GT and BSS. A transfusion should be given immediately prior to the procedure and further doses given depending on clinical need. rFVIIa may be given for 48 h postoperatively as an adjunct.

Conclusion

Platelet disorders include thrombocytopenia, abnormalities of platelet function, or a combination of both. They present with the common symptom of mucocutaneous bleeding. Previous platelet counts and family studies may be helpful in distinguishing between congenital and acquired causes of thrombocytopenia. Congenital thrombocytopenias can be classified according to platelet size. Although ITP is the most common cause of thrombocytopenia in children, it is a diagnosis of exclusion. Most patients with ITP can be managed with observation alone and have an excellent outcome. Diagnosis of PFDs requires a systematic approach; algorithms aimed at guiding the process have been proposed. In GT, BSS and WAS, the bleeding tendency is usually severe and can be life-threatening. Far more frequent are patients with nonspecific PFD who manifest only with a mild bleeding diathesis that becomes problematic during episodes of hemostatic stress, such as surgery. Several hemostatic drugs are available that can reduce the need for blood products in the management of these disorders.

Acknowledgment

The authors would like to express their appreciation for the thoughtful comments provided by Drs. Margaret L. Rand (Toronto, Ont., Canada) and Sara J. Israels (Winnipeg, Man., Canada) who reviewed this chapter.

References

1 Jackson SP: The growing complexity of platelet aggregation. Blood 2007;109:5087–5095.
2 Biss TT, Blanchette VS, Clark DS, Wakefield CD, James PD, Rand ML: Use of a quantitative pediatric bleeding questionnaire to assess mucocutaneous bleeding symptoms in children with a platelet function disorder. J Thromb Haemost 2010;8:1416–1419.
3 Bowman M, Riddel J, Rand ML, Tosetto A, Silva M, James PD: Evaluation of the diagnostic utility for von Willebrand disease of a pediatric bleeding questionnaire. J Thromb Haemost 2009;7:1418–1421.
4 Konkle BA: Acquired disorders of platelet function. Hematology Am Soc Hematol Educ Program 2011;2011:391–396.
5 Cines DB, Bussel JB, McMillan RB, Zehnder JL: Congenital and acquired thrombocytopenia. Hematology Am Soc Hematol Educ Program 2004;2004:390–406.
6 Israels SJ, Kahr WH, Blanchette VS, Luban NL, Rivard GE, Rand ML: Platelet disorders in children: a diagnostic approach. Pediatr Blood Cancer 2011;56:975–983.
7 Harrison P, Mackie I, Mumford A, Briggs C, Liesner R, Winter M, Machin S, British Committee for Standards in Haematology: Guidelines for the laboratory investigation of heritable disorders of platelet function. Br J Haematol 2011;155:30–44.
8 Drachman JG: Inherited thrombocytopenia: when a low platelet count does not mean ITP. Blood 2004;103:390–398.
9 Cox K, Price V, Kahr WH: Inherited platelet disorders: a clinical approach to diagnosis and management. Expert Rev Hematol 2011;4:455–472.
10 Rodeghiero F, Stasi R, Gernsheimer T, Michel M, Provan D, Arnold DM, Bussel JB, Cines DB, Chong BH, Cooper N, Godeau B, Lechner K, Mazzucconi MG, McMillan R, Sanz MA, Imbach P, Blanchette V, Kühne T, Ruggeri M, George JN: Standardization of terminology, definitions and outcome criteria in immune thrombocytopenic purpura of adults and children: report from an international working group. Blood 2009;113:2386–2393.
11 Provan D, Stasi R, Newland AC, Blanchette VS, et al: International consensus report on the investigation and management of primary immune thrombocytopenia. Blood 2010;115:168–186.
12 Neunert C, Lim W, Crowther M, Cohen A, Solberg L Jr, Crowther MA: The American Society of Hematology 2011 evidence-based practice guideline for immune thrombocytopenia. Blood 2011;117:4190–4207.
13 British Committee for Standards in Haematology General Haematology Task Force: Guidelines for the investigation and management of idiopathic thrombocytopenic purpura in adults, children and in pregnancy. Br J Haematol 2003;120:574–596.

14 Carcao MD, Zipursky A, Butchart S, Leaker M, Blanchette VS: Short-course oral prednisone therapy in children presenting with acute immune thrombocytopenic purpura (ITP). Acta Paediatr Suppl 1998;424:71–74.
15 Bennett CM, Rogers ZR, Kinnamon DD, Bussel JB, et al: Prospective phase 1/2 study of rituximab in childhood and adolescent chronic immune thrombocytopenic purpura. Blood 2006;107: 2639–2642.
16 Aronis S, Platokouki H, Avgeri M, Pergantou H, Keramidas D: Retrospective evaluation of longterm efficacy and safety of splenectomy in chronic idiopathic thrombocytopenic purpura in children. Acta Paediatr 2004;93:638–642.
17 Jugenburg M, Haddock G, Freedman MH, Ford-Jones L, Ein SH: The morbidity and mortality of pediatric splenectomy: does prophylaxis make a difference? J Pediatr Surg 1999;34:1064–1067.
18 Stasi R, Stipa E, Masi M, Cecconi M, Scimo MT, Oliva F, Sciarra A, Perrotti AP, Adomo G, Amadori S, Papa G: Long-term observation of 208 adults with chronic idiopathic thrombocytopenic purpura. Am J Med 1995;98:436–442.
19 Bolton-Maggs PH, Chalmers EA, Collins PW, Harrison P, Kitchen S, Liesner RJ, Minford A, Mumford AD, Parapia LA, Perry DJ, Watson SP, Wilde JT, Williams MD, UKHCDO: A review of inherited platelet disorders with guidelines for their management on behalf of the UKHCDO. Br J Haematol 2006;35:603–633.
20 Alamelu J, Liesner R: Modern management of severe platelet function disorders. Br J Haematol 2010;149:813.
21 Nurden AT: Glanzmann thrombasthenia. Orphanet J Rare Dis 2006;1:10.
22 Lanza F: Bernard-Soulier syndrome (hemorrhagiparous thrombocytic dystrophy). Orphanet J Rare Dis 2006;1:46.
23 Almeida AM, Khair K, Hann I, Liesner R: The use of recombinant factor VIIa in children with inherited platelet function disorders. Br J Haematol 2003;121:477.
24 Poon MC, Demers C, Jobin F, Wu JW: Recombinant factor VIIa is effective for bleeding and surgery in patients with Glanzmann thrombasthenia. Blood;1999;94:3951–3953.

Abbreviations

ADP	Adenosine 5′-diphosphate
APLA	Antiphospholipid antibodies
APLS	Antiphospholipid syndrome
ARC	Arthrogryposis-renal dysfunction-cholestasis
ASA	Acetylsalicylic acid
aPTT	Activated partial thromboplastin time
ATP	Adenosine triphosphate
ATRUS	Amegakaryocytic thrombocytopenia with radioulnar synostosis
BSS	Bernard-Soulier syndrome
CAMT	Congenital amegakaryocytic thrombocytopenia
CBC	Complete blood count
COX	Cyclooxygenase
DDAVP	1-Deamino-8-D-arginine vasopressin (desmopressin)
ELISA	Enzyme-linked immunosorbent assay
FNAIT	Fetal and neonatal alloimmune thrombocytopenia
FPD/AML	Familial platelet disorder and predisposition to acute myelogenous leukemia
FVIII	Factor VIII
GP	Glycoprotein
GPS	Gray platelet syndrome
GT	Glanzmann thrombasthenia
HCV	Hepatitis C virus
HIV	Human immunodeficiency virus
HIT	Heparin-induced thrombocytopenia
HLA	Human leukocyte antigen
HUS	Hemolytic uremic syndrome
ICH	Intracranial hemorrhage
INR	International normalized ratio
ITP	Immune thrombocytopenia
IVIG	Intravenous immunoglobulin
LTA	Light transmission aggregometry
MDS	Myelodysplastic syndrome
MMR	Measles, mumps, rubella
MPV	Mean platelet volume
MYH9	Myosin heavy chain 9
NSAIDs	Nonsteroidal anti-inflammatory drugs
PBQ	Pediatric Bleeding Questionnaire
PFA-100®	Platelet function analyzer-100
PFD	Platelet function defect
PRP	Platelet-rich plasma
PT	Prothrombin time
rFVIIa	Recombinant activated factor VII
SLE	Systemic lupus erythematosus
TAR	Thrombocytopenia with absent radii
TEM	Transmission electron microscopy
THC2	Autosomal-dominant thrombocytopenia 2
TTP	Thrombotic thrombocytopenic purpura
TxA_2	Thromboxane A_2
VWD	von Willebrand disease
VWF	von Willebrand factor
WAS	Wiskott-Aldrich syndrome
WBC	White blood cell
XLT	X-linked thrombocytopenia

Chapter 6

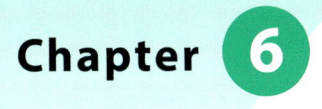

Managing Hemophilia in Children and Adolescents

Jeremy D. Robertson
Julie A. Curtin
Victor S. Blanchette

Introduction

Hemophilia is an X-linked recessive bleeding disorder caused by deficiency of FVIII (hemophilia A) or FIX (hemophilia B). Mutations in the *FVIII* or *FIX* genes, both located on the long arm of the X chromosome, are detectable in the majority of cases of hemophilia A or B, respectively. During normal hemostasis, FVIII and FIX form an enzymatic complex; thus, deficiency of either protein leads to a clinically similar phenotype, although there is some evidence to suggest that in the context of severe factor deficiency hemophilia B may be a subtly milder disorder than hemophilia A [1]. In contrast, deficiency of FXI (previously termed 'hemophilia C') is genetically and clinically distinct, and is discussed further in chapter 8. Similarly, 'acquired hemophilia' is a pathogenically unrelated autoimmune disorder, the management of which is discussed in chapter 9.

Hemophilia occurs in all racial groups with an estimated incidence of around 1/5,000 males for hemophilia A, and 1/30,000 for hemophilia B. As these are X-linked disorders, almost all severely affected individuals are male. The factor levels of heterozygous females are on average approximately half those of the normal population; however, females may be more severely affected through one of a variety of mechanisms (e.g. skewed X-inactivation, homozygosity, or chromosomal abnormalities such as Turner syndrome). Females with factor levels in the deficient range should be regarded as having hemophilia, as the approach to management is similar to that for males with corresponding levels of factor deficiency.

The clinical phenotype in hemophilia, although highly variable, is traditionally classified according to the baseline factor level (table 1). Affected individuals have a lifelong bleeding tendency that may manifest with spontaneous bleeding, particularly into joints and muscles of a severely affected individual, or as prolonged bleeding after surgery or trauma. Repeated bleeding into joints, the hallmark of severe hemophilia, results in chronic synovitis with destruction of bone and cartilage, ultimately leading to crippling

Table 1. Classification of hemophilia

	FVIII/FIX level	Clinical phenotype (untreated)
Severe	<0.01 IU/ml (<1%)	recurrent mucocutaneous, deep soft tissue and joint bleeding, often with minimal or no identifiable trauma (spontaneous); post-surgical bleeding can be life-threatening (e.g. after circumcision); progression to severe arthropathy due to recurrent hemarthrosis
Moderate	0.01–0.05 IU/ml (1–5%)	prolonged bleeding following trauma or surgery; spontaneous bleeding uncommon; joint bleeding uncommon
Mild	0.06–0.40 IU/ml (6–40%)	may be clinically silent in the absence of hemostatic challenge (surgery or trauma)

arthropathy. The routine use of regularly administered factor replacement therapy ('prophylaxis') has dramatically transformed the prognosis of hemophilia in countries with access to commercially produced factor concentrates.

General Management Principles

Hemostatic Management

Factor Replacement Therapy

Therapeutic products containing FVIII or FIX can be broadly divided into those which are plasma derived, and those manufactured using recombinant technology. Plasma-derived products can be subdivided according to 'purity' (i.e. the FVIII or FIX concentration relative to other plasma proteins), and the number of viral inactivation steps used during the manufacturing process. Recombinant products can also be subclassified according to production techniques (so-called first, second and third generation) and the genotype from which the product was derived (i.e. full length or B-domain deleted FVIII). For an up-to-date list of the various products currently available, the reader is referred to the World Federation of Haemophilia website (www.wfh.org, Registry of Clotting Factor Concentrates, ed 9, 2012). It should also be noted that a number of newer agents with potential benefits (such as longer half-life) are currently undergoing assessment in clinical trials. It is strongly recommended that recombinant products and virally inactivated plasma-derived products be prescribed in preference to FP or cryoprecipitate. One international unit (IU) is defined as the amount of FVIII/FIX in 1 ml of pooled normal plasma. The FVIII or FIX activity (IU/ml) of a factor concentrate is displayed on the vial label.

Adjuvant Therapy

There are a number of pharmacologic agents that can be useful for achieving or maintaining hemostasis, either alone or in combination with clotting factor therapy. The lysine analogue antifibrinolytic agents ε-aminocaproic acid and tranexamic acid inhibit the conversion of plasminogen to plasmin, thereby slowing fibrin dissolution at the site of clot formation. Antifibrinolytics are particularly useful for control of bleeding from mucosal surfaces (e.g. epistaxis, gum bleeding, menorrhagia), but are contraindicated in the setting of hematuria due to the potential for ureteric or intrarenal clot formation and obstruction. They can be administered orally, intravenously, or topically as a mouth rinse (table 2). Both agents are generally well tolerated, although dose-related gastrointestinal upset is common (particularly with ε-aminocaproic acid), and rapid intravenous infusion can cause dizziness and hypotension.

Desmopressin (1-deamino-8-D-arginine vasopressin, DDAVP) is a synthetic analogue of antidiuretic hormone (vasopressin) which elevates plasma VWF and FVIII levels, and increases platelet

Table 2. Comparison of lysine analogue antifibrinolytic agents

	Tranexamic acid	**Epsilon aminocaproic acid**
Trade names	Cyclokapron® (Pfizer, USA) Lysteda® (Ferring, Switzerland) Transamin® (Daiichi Sankyo, Japan) Espercil® (Grunenthal, Chile) Fermstrual™ (Manx Healthcare, UK) Traxyl™ (Nuvista, Bangladesh)	Amicar® (Xanodyne, USA)
Loading dose	Not usually required	50–100 mg/kg i.v. (over 1 h) or oral, 1–2 h before operation
i.v. dose	10 mg/kg q6–8 h	50 mg/kg q6–8 h
Oral dose	15–25 mg/kg q6–8 h	50 mg/kg q6–8 h
Topical	5% mouthwash[1] (50 mg/ml)	250 mg/ml solution

[1] 7.65 g of tranexamic acid powder combined with 150 ml of sterile water (final volume of 153 ml) creates a 5% solution (50 mg per ml).

adhesiveness via VWF-independent mechanisms which are not fully understood. DDAVP may avoid the need for clotting factor therapy in some patients with mild hemophilia A; however, individual responses vary and must be formally assessed with a test dose prior to administration for therapeutic purposes. Clinically meaningful responses are generally not seen in patients with a baseline FVIII level of <15% [2]. It must also be highlighted that DDAVP does not affect FIX level, and is therefore of no specific value in patients with hemophilia B. The dosing is discussed below (see 'Dosing in Patients without Inhibitors').

Topical hemostatic agents are various biological products that can be applied directly to a bleeding site to achieve or maintain hemostasis. In some centers, such agents are used routinely for dental procedures, circumcision, or orthopedic surgery, to reduce the requirement for factor replacement therapy. Fibrin sealants (also known as fibrin 'glues') are plasma-derived products incorporating a fibrinogen concentrate and a thrombin concentrate which are mixed at the time of application. Although such sealants can be prepared by blood banks from individual donations, commercial products prepared from pooled plasma are now widely available (e.g. Tisseel®, Evicel®), with viral inactivation incorporated into the manufacturing process. Topical thrombins (e.g. Evithrom®, Thrombi-Gel®) are typically provided as a lyophilized powder which is reconstituted with water prior to application (no exogenous fibrinogen). These agents are derived from human or bovine thrombin; however, a recombinant thrombin sealant has also recently become available (Recothrom™).

Prophylaxis

The observation that individuals with moderate hemophilia have few spontaneous bleeds, and that chronic arthropathy was less frequent and less severe in these patients, formed the hypothetical basis for prophylactic therapy in severe hemophilia. Prophylaxis refers to the regular infusion of factor replacement therapy primarily for the prevention of joint bleeding and its associated long-term sequelae. Primary prophylaxis is defined as regular continuous treatment commenced before age 3 years, prior to the onset of joint disease (determined by physical examination and/or imaging studies), and prior to the second clinically evident large joint bleed. In this context, 'continuous' implies receiving a minimum of a predetermined frequency of infusions for ≥45 weeks of the year under consideration. Regular continuous treatment commenced after ≥2 bleeds involving large joints, but before the onset of joint disease, is termed secondary prophylaxis, whilst that commenced to prevent progression of established joint disease is termed tertiary prophylaxis. Shorter-term regular treatment (e.g. weeks to months) to reduce the risk of recurrence following severe bleeding (such as iliopsoas or ICH) is termed intermittent (or periodic) prophylaxis [3].

There is now a sizeable body of evidence to suggest that prophylaxis is superior to 'on-demand' (episodic) treatment in patients with severe hemophilia for both reduction in bleeding rate and progression of joint disease, and that primary prophylaxis is superior to secondary prophylaxis in this regard [4, 5]. Thus, in countries without restricted access to clotting factor concentrates, primary prophylaxis has become the accepted standard of care for young boys with severe hemophilia. However, the optimal prophylaxis regimen remains the focus of ongoing investigation, and the benefits of more intensive replacement (e.g. 20–40 IU/kg every other day for hemophilia A) must be balanced against the cost of therapy, and the potential for greater reliance on surgically implanted venous access devices [5]. Pharmacokinetic studies have demonstrated that FVIII clearance varies considerably between individuals, raising the possibility that 'tailored' prophylaxis may improve resource utilization [6, 7].

Supportive Care

Comprehensive Care

Although treatment and prevention of bleeding through replacement of deficient clotting factor forms the basis of modern hemophilia care, management of the disorder is complex and requires the input of a multidisciplinary team with a high level of expertise. The core team is based at a designated HTC, and typically comprises a physician (usually a pediatrician and/or hematologist), a nurse coordinator, a physiotherapist, and a social worker or psychologist. Patients presenting at medical facilities distant from the HTC are usually managed by local medical staff in direct consultation with the HTC team. Comprehensive patient care also requires periodic input from other specialist teams, including (but not limited to) rheumatology, orthopedics, surgery, oral health, and genetics, as well as access to a specialized coagulation laboratory and a pediatric radiology service. Generally, patients with moderate or severe hemophilia should be assessed at the HTC at least twice a year, although more frequent review may be necessary for more complex patients such as those with inhibitors.

Routine Clinic Visits

The routine clinic visit provides an opportunity to review the patient and his/her family and their experience with hemophilia. It provides an opportunity for ongoing education of the family and identification of any intervention should it be required. The patient's bleeding frequency and treatment schedule should be reviewed. For patients on prophylaxis, breakthrough bleeds should be discussed, in particular with reference to the prophylaxis schedule. Venous access issues should be reviewed and discussed. Details of physical activity should be documented. Joint health should be formally assessed on a regular basis (e.g. every 6–12 months), and the recently validated Hemophilia Joint Health Score is useful in this context [8]. Oral health should be reviewed (see 'Dental Care' below). Older children and adolescents should be encouraged to wear an appropriately labeled medic-alert bracelet, and this can be reinforced during the clinic visit. Routine blood tests such as inhibitor screening are performed at regular intervals [9].

Dental Care

Prevention of dental problems is an essential component of care for persons with hemophilia. Good dental hygiene is important to avoid periodontal disease and associated procedures which may be associated with risk of bleeding. Persons with hemophilia should be regularly reviewed by a dentist at least annually. Should dental procedures be required, close liaison between the HTC and the dentist is required to determine what hemostatic cover (if any) is required. The dentist should avoid causing accidental damage to the oral mucosa in the course of treating dental problems. For minor procedures, antifibrinolytic therapy alone may suffice. Local hemostatic measures, including topical sealants and/or antifibrinolytics, and application of individually prepared mouth guards can reduce the requirement for clotting factor therapy. For more extensive dental procedures and certain nerve blocks used by dentists (e.g. inferior alveolar 'mandibular' block, lingual infiltration), raising the patient's factor level to 50% is advised to prevent potential serious complications from bleeding. For many patients with mild hemophilia A, this may be achieved with DDAVP. For patients with hemophilia B, moderate-severe hemophilia A, or those with a suboptimal DDAVP response, factor replacement therapy will be required (see 'Dosing in Patients without/with Inhibitors' below). Depending on the extent of the dental procedure(s), ongoing factor therapy may be required for several days to allow proper wound healing. Antifibrinolytics should be continued for 5–7 days to assist in maintenance of the clot.

Venous Access

Patients with moderate to severe hemophilia require frequent intravenous infusions of clotting factor for treatment or prevention of bleeding. Ideally, this is administered via peripheral veins, typically on the dorsum of the hand or the antecubital fossa using a small-gauge butterfly needle. However, in very young children this is often impractical due to the inability to reliably find a vein, or due to the child's lack of cooperation, and insertion of a CVC may be necessary. Furthermore, some older children and adults with needle-associated anxiety, scarred peripheral veins or upper limb arthropathy may also require a CVC, or occasionally, where local expertise permits, a surgically constructed arteriovenous fistula [10].

Options for CVC placement include a PICC, a centrally placed external catheter (tunneled or non-tunneled), or a fully implantable tunneled catheter ('port'). If the requirement for reliable venous access is temporary (e.g. short-term secondary prophylaxis after a significant bleed in a patient with moderate hemophilia), a PICC or non-tunneled catheter may be appropriate. For longer term venous access, a tunneled line is required, and a port is generally the preferred option (lower infection risk, minimal interference with daily activities). In young children, the placement of a CVC should always be viewed as a temporary measure, with a plan for transition to peripheral access as soon as practical. The port reservoir is usually placed in the subcutaneous tissue overlying the anterior chest wall, and is accessed under aseptic conditions using a specialized needle. Ports should only be accessed by individuals who have received appropriate training, and the site should be inspected regularly for signs of deterioration. There are a number of acute and chronic complications related to CVCs, in particular infection and thrombosis; for a detailed review of this topic, the reader is referred to previously published consensus guidelines [11].

Pain Management

Bleeding in children with hemophilia often causes pain, especially when the blood is accumulating in a confined space such as a joint cavity. While the primary treatment of the bleed with clotting factor concentrate is of utmost importance, and will result in reduction of the pain once the bleeding is stopped, there may be a need for analgesics to control the pain. Other measures such as ice packs, immobilization, and non-weight bearing also help in minimizing pain. If required, simple analgesia with paracetamol (acetaminophen) is often sufficient. When simple analgesia is not sufficient, the addition of oral opiates such as codeine, oxycodone, or tramadol may be considered. For acute severe pain, intravenous narcotics (e.g. morphine or fentanyl) may occasionally be necessary to achieve adequate pain control, and patient-controlled analgesia, in which a background opiate infusion is supplemented with regular small boluses as required, may be useful for older patients. NSAIDs are best avoided where possible, because their antiplatelet effect can exacerbate the bleeding risk. However, in patients with chronic hemophilic arthropathy (arthritis), short-term use of NSAIDs, in particular the selective COX-2 inhibitors (e.g. celecoxib, meloxicam, etoricoxib), may be indicated [12]. Distraction and play therapy are also very useful techniques in children to assist in managing their pain and distress, particularly in relation to venipunctures.

Inhibitors

Definitions

Patients with hemophilia are at risk of developing neutralizing alloantibodies ('inhibitors') against FVIII or FIX following exposure to clotting factor products administered for prevention or treatment of bleeding. Inhibitors present a significant management challenge for persons with hemophilia, as their presence reduces or abolishes the therapeutic response to factor replacement. The strength of inhibitory effect is measured in the laboratory using the Bethesda assay, in which one Bethesda unit (BU) corresponds to the amount of patient plasma required to neutralize 50% of the FVIII/FIX activity in normal plasma following a 2-hour incubation at body temperature. The currently accepted cutoff value for confirmation of an inhibitor is ≥0.6 BU using the Nijmegan modification of the Bethesda assay; however, it is well-recognized that some patients whose inhibitor level falls below 0.6 BU still exhibit suboptimal FVIII/FIX recovery, half-life, and/or clinical response, consistent with persistent inhibitory activity [Blanchette, pers. commun.].

A 'low-responder' inhibitor is defined as a level persistently <5 BU, while ≥5 BU at any time is considered a 'high responder', and corresponds to the inhibitor level at which treatment with even very high doses of clotting factor therapy becomes futile [Blanchette, pers. commun.]. In some patients, the high responder status only becomes apparent following reexposure to products containing FVIII/FIX, resulting in a sudden increase in inhibitor due to anamnesis.

Risk Factors

Most inhibitors develop during the first 20 exposures to factor concentrates, and rarely after 50 exposures; however, the risk is influenced by multiple genetic and environmental modifiers, and is therefore not uniform among patients with hemophilia. The cumulative incidence of inhibitor development in severe hemophilia A is around 20–30%, compared with 5–10% in mild-moderate subtypes, and only 3–5% for hemophilia B [13]. Probably the most important risk factor in hemophilia A is the type of *F8* gene mutation; those with large multi-domain gene deletions are at greatest risk (>50%), whilst those with missense mutations or small deletions/insertions have a relatively low risk [14]. Family history of inhibitors, ethnicity and certain genetic polymorphisms associated with immune function are other important genetic modifiers. Current evidence suggests that the most significant treatment-related risk factor is treatment intensity at initial exposure to clotting factor concentrate. The relative significance of other potential non-genetic risk factors, including severe infection or vaccination, type of factor concentrate (plasma derived versus recombinant), and mode of administration (bolus dosing versus continuous infusion), is yet to be determined.

Bypassing Agents

The presence of a high-level inhibitor in plasma renders factor replacement therapy ineffective. In this circumstance, products containing

Table 3. Currently available bypassing agents

Product type	aPCC	rFVIIa
Trade names	FEIBA NF	NovoSeven RT®
		Niastase RT®
Manufacturer	Baxter Bioscience Austria	Novo Nordisk Pharmaceuticals Denmark
FVIII content	1–6 IU/ml	none
Available strengths	500, 1,000, 2,500 U	1, 2, 5, 8 mg
Reconstituted volume	20–50 ml (25–50 U/ml)	1–8 ml (~1 mg/ml)
Infusion time	2 U/kg/min (25–50 min)	2–5 min
Typical treatment dose	50–100 U/kg q12 h (max. 200 U/kg/day)	90/kg q2 h (2–3 doses) or 270/kg (single dose)
Typical prophylaxis dose	70–100 U/kg 3–4 times/week	90/kg daily
Use with antifibrinolytics	no	yes
Use in hemophilia B with history of anaphylaxis	no	yes

preactivated clotting factors are necessary to achieve hemostasis, 'bypassing' the normal requirement for FVIII:FIX complex formation. There are two types of bypassing agents in common usage: plasma-derived aPCCs and rFVIIa. The potency of an aPCC is expressed in arbitrary bypassing 'Units' (U), determined by the manufacturer, while that of rFVIIa is typically expressed in micrograms (the corresponding IU content is also recorded on the vial). A comparison of the two agents currently available is provided in table 3. At appropriate doses, these agents show comparable effectiveness for the treatment of bleeding (see 'Dosing in Patients with Inhibitors' below).

Immune Tolerance Induction

The development of high-level inhibitors is a major complication for patients with hemophilia. ITI involves the regular administration of FVIII (or FIX) concentrates until the inhibitor is no longer detectable, typically at higher doses than those used for routine prophylaxis. ITI is the preferred management approach for patients with hemophilia A who develop this complication [15, 16]. The decision to attempt ITI for patients with hemophilia B must take into consideration the relatively high risk of severe reactions (including anaphylaxis and nephrotic syndrome) in this population, and the overall lower success rate as compared with hemophilia A. Patients undergoing ITI should be managed at their HTC.

Current consensus guidelines recommend delaying commencement of ITI until the inhibitor level falls below 10 BU, and exposure to FVIII-containing products (including FEIBA) should be avoided during this period [16]. Various schedules of ITI have been used, and the ideal schedule is yet to be determined; however, it has been shown that higher FVIII dose regimens (e.g. 200 IU/kg/day) are associated with less bleeding despite similar rates of ITI success using lower dose regimens (e.g. 50 IU/kg three times per week) [17]. Bleeding episodes while on ITI are typically managed with bypassing agents.

Prophylaxis

The issues surrounding prophylaxis in individuals with FVIII or FIX inhibitors are complex; however, there is emerging evidence that prophylaxis using bypassing agents may improve joint outcomes in this population [18, 19]. The dose and frequency must be tailored according to clinical response. For patients with severe recurrent bleeding, a regimen of rFVIIa (e.g. 90 μg/kg daily) or FEIBA (e.g. 75–100 U/kg 3–4 times per week) can be used in combination with standard ITI therapy [16, 19].

Management of Bleeding Episodes

Initial Assessment

Bleeding events still occur in patients with hemophilia despite prophylactic factor replacement. Appropriate management depends not only upon the hemophilia subtype and site of bleeding, but also the episode severity, identifiable precipitants (e.g. trauma), the patient's age and current place of residence, adequacy of venous access, presence or absence of inhibitors, previous history of bleeding at the same site, and the timing of onset in relation to prophylactic therapy. Minor bleeding episodes may respond to local hemostatic measures, with or without antifibrinolytics, and may not require clotting factor therapy. Similarly, DDAVP-responsive patients with mild hemophilia A can often be managed without factor replacement.

In many cases, the child will present to a medical facility distant to the HTC, or the child's parent will contact the HTC directly, and advice must be provided over the phone. If it is determined from this initial contact that factor replacement therapy is necessary, the appropriate dose should be administered without delay (the 'factor first' principle). When possible, this should occur in the home setting. Other important initial considerations include the applicability of basic first aid measures (e.g. ice, direct pressure, splinting etc.), appropriate analgesia, the requirement for transfer to a specialist pediatric facility, and the need for further follow-up or investigation (see 'Specific Sites of Bleeding' below).

Dosing in Patients without Inhibitors

Although it is practical to construct dosing regimens based on the site of bleeding, it must be highlighted that the assessment of bleed severity is subjective, and is influenced by the clinical context. In patients without inhibitors, the required dose of factor replacement therapy can be estimated from the suggested target factor level in plasma for any given bleeding episode (table 4). Whilst such a guideline can be very useful as a quick reference, therapy must always be tailored to individual circumstances and local resources, and requires a degree of clinical judgment. On average, 1 IU/kg of FVIII raises the plasma FVIII:C level by 2%. In contrast, 1 IU/kg of plasma-derived FIX concentrate raises the plasma FIX:C level by around 1% due to a lower in vivo recovery (resulting from reversible binding of FIX to vascular endothelium) and a larger volume of distribution (due to diffusion of FIX into extravascular tissues) as compared with FVIII. It is important to note that a 1 IU/kg infusion of BeneFIX® (recombinant FIX) produces a slightly lower FIX:C increment (approximately 0.8%) than plasma-derived FIX, possibly related to differences in post-translational modification [20].

Most minor bleeding episodes can be effectively managed with 1 or 2 doses of factor replacement, and monitoring of factor level is usually not necessary in this situation. More significant bleeding episodes (including joint bleeding) may require a more prolonged course of factor replacement therapy. If necessary, the intensity of treatment can be adjusted according to trough (pre-dose) factor levels. An inhibitor should be considered if the response to therapy is suboptimal, and a post-dose factor level ('recovery') should be measured. Often, a maintenance dose around half the initial loading dose is sufficient. The frequency of dosing depends on the clinical situation and the estimated half-life of the FVIII/IX product. Since the half-life is, on average, 2-fold higher for FIX versus FVIII products, the frequency of dosing with FIX is often 12–24 hourly, as compared to 8–12 hourly for FVIII, at least in the initial phases of treating severe bleeds, or in the context of prophylaxis for surgery. It should be highlighted that, in general, the half-life of infused FVIII/IX products is shorter in young children as compared to adolescents and adults, and is especially short in the immediate postsurgical period. Where stable factor levels are required for several days, a continuous infusion may be more practical and cost-effective.

Table 4. Suggested FVIII/FIX target levels by bleeding site

Bleeding site	Target factor level, IU/dl	Duration	Additional comments
Large joint, uncomplicated	40–60 20–40	1–2 days until recovery	early physiotherapy is important; splinting may be useful
Large joint, severe/complicated (e.g. hip/shoulder, tense effusion)	80–100 40–60	until improvement until recovery	ultrasound can be useful for confirmation of hip and shoulder bleeds; consider joint aspiration for pain refractory to factor replacement
Large joint, recurrent	40–60 20–40	until improvement during rehabilitation	consider adjustment to prophylaxis; consider joint imaging and synovectomy
Small joint (e.g. wrist, fingers)	20–30	1–2 days	protective splint may be useful
Muscle, uncomplicated	40–60	until recovery (e.g. 2–3 days)	early physiotherapy is important to avoid contracture, loss of function, or rebleeding
Muscle, severe/complicated (including iliopsoas)	80–100 30–60 20–40	1–2 days 3–7 days until rehabilitation complete	consider adjustment to prophylaxis; avoid activity that precipitated the bleed
Oral mucosa, severe	20–40	2–3 days	consider topical measures (e.g. fibrin sealant), antifibrinolytic therapy (oral and/or mouth rinse)
Soft tissue, uncomplicated	20–30	1–2 days	Factor therapy may not be required; compression bandage, ice and elevation may suffice
Compartment syndrome	80–100 40–60	until improvement until recovery	surgical consultation required: decompressive fasciotomy may be indicated
Epistaxis, severe	20–40	1–2 days	minor epistaxis may respond to local measures and/or antifibrinolytic therapy; consider surgical consultation
Throat/neck	80–100 40–60	until improvement until recovery	surgical consultation required; notify intensive care unit – risk of airway compression
Intracranial, suspected/at-risk	80–100	initial dose, pending neurologic assessment	decision to proceed with imaging (CT) depends on nature and timing of injury, clinical features to suggest bleeding (headache, vomiting, altered level of consciousness, seizure), and timing of prophylaxis prior to injury
Intracranial, confirmed	80–100 40–60	until improvement and/or completion of surgical intervention and invasive monitoring 1–3 weeks	basic life support measures; urgent neurosurgical consultation required; consider commencement of secondary prophylaxis or adjustment to existing prophylaxis regimen
Gastrointestinal, minor	20–30	1–2 days	factor therapy may not be required; consider antifibrinolytic therapy
Gastrointestinal, severe	80–100 40–60	until cessation of bleeding 1–2 weeks	gastroenterology consultation required; need to monitor hemoglobin

Table 4. Continued

Bleeding site	Target factor level, IU/dl	Duration	Additional comments
Hematuria, macroscopic	40–60	until cessation of bleeding (typically 3–5 days)	factor therapy may not be required; consider renal ultrasound and urine microscopy/culture; avoid antifibrinolytic therapy; maintain good urine output
Major trauma (e.g. car accident)	80–100	initial dose, pending clinical and radiological assessment	basic life support measures; consider relevant imaging studies (e.g. chest XR, cranial CT, abdominal CT or ultrasound); early surgical consultation

Note that these targets are only intended as a guide. Therapy must always be tailored to individual circumstances and local resources. On average 1 IU/kg of FVIII raises the plasma level by 2 IU/dl (2%); 1 IU/kg of FIX raises the plasma level by 1 IU/dl (1%) for plasma-derived concentrates and 0.8 IU/dl (0.8%) for BeneFIX® recombinant FIX.

DDAVP should always be considered as an alternative to clotting factor therapy in patients with mild hemophilia A who are known to respond to this agent [2]. The standard DDAVP dose is 0.3 μg/kg administered as a bolus subcutaneous injection without dilution (15 μg/ml vial), or as a slow intravenous infusion (over 30 min in 30–50 ml of isotonic saline, 4 or 15 μg/ml vial). The peak response occurs around 30–60 min after an intravenous dose, or 60–90 min after a subcutaneous dose [21]. An intranasal preparation is also available; however, there are limited data regarding the use of this product in children with hemophilia. Doses can be repeated safely every 24 h; the hemostatic response diminishes over time, and DDAVP is generally ineffective after 3–5 consecutive days of administration [21]. Adverse reactions associated with rapid intravenous infusion include tachycardia, flushing, headache, nausea and abdominal pain. DDAVP causes water retention and hyponatremia, so it is important to restrict fluid intake for 24 h after a dose, and sodium levels should be monitored where repeat dosing is being used. Due to the increased risk of hyponatremic seizures in young children, DDAVP is contraindicated in patients <2 years of age.

Dosing in Patients with Inhibitors

Minor bleeding in patients with inhibitors may still be effectively controlled with local hemostatic measures and antifibrinolytic therapy. DDAVP may also be considered in responsive patients with mild hemophilia A and a low-level inhibitor. When such measures fail, or are deemed inadequate for the type of bleeding, the options include high-dose factor replacement therapy or bypassing therapy (FEIBA or rFVIIa). The choice depends on inhibitor level, severity of bleeding, and previous therapeutic response. High-dose factor replacement is generally only feasible when the inhibitor level is <5 BU. Optimization of therapy using this approach requires some knowledge of an individual's FVIII (or FIX) recovery and half-life, such that dose and frequency can be adjusted accordingly. Home therapy is still a reasonable option for bleeds which are not life-threatening when a patient has previously been shown to respond to a given dose. Anamnesis in high responders will rapidly abolish the therapeutic response, and limits the utility of this approach in such patients. Plasmapheresis, with or without immunoadsorption, may be a short-term option in centers with the relevant expertise.

Bypassing therapy is required when high-dose factor replacement is considered insufficient, or is contraindicated due to a previous allergic reaction. The major determinant of which bypassing agent to use for initial treatment of a bleeding episode is the history of previous hemostatic response in that patient. Due to the risk of anamnesis, most centers avoid FEIBA in hemophilia A patients prior to commencing ITI, and in hemophilia B patients who are allergic to FIX. However, in most cases the choice of product is based on individual patient preferences. Importantly, neither agent is effective in all individuals, and patient responses to either agent can vary over time [22]. Furthermore, unlike standard replacement therapy, in which factor assays can be used to titrate the dose, there is no standardized laboratory test to quantify the activity of a bypassing agent in vivo. Therefore, apart from indirect measurements of overall hemostatic potential (such as thromboelastography or a thrombin generation assay), assessment of response to a bypassing agent must be based on clinical symptoms (especially pain) and signs of acute arthropathy (e.g. swelling, range of motion). Often, patients will have a supply of their preferred agent at home, allowing early treatment at the first sign of bleeding. If a patient is on regular prophylaxis with either agent, breakthrough bleeds can be managed initially with additional doses of the same agent. Failure to respond to one bypassing agent should prompt consideration of a switch to the alternative agent. In some instances, the bleeding may be refractory to either agent, and use of both agents in sequential fashion is appropriate in this context; however, close monitoring for thrombosis or consumptive coagulopathy (platelet count, fibrinogen, D-dimer, etc.) is required [23].

Previous studies have shown that effective hemostasis is achieved in >90% of mild-moderate bleeding episodes (i.e. not life-threatening or associated with severe pain) after 2–3 doses of 90 μg/kg rFVIIa, and that 270 μg/kg as a single dose is equally effective in this context [24]. To avoid product wastage, the dose is always rounded to the nearest whole vial size. Children have faster drug clearance; therefore, the high-dose regimen may be preferable at initiation of treatment, tapering to lower doses if ongoing treatment is required [24]. Comparative studies have shown that the clinical efficacy of a single dose of FEIBA at 75–100 U/kg is equivalent to that of 2 doses of rFVIIa 90–120 μg/kg for joint bleeding [25]. Due to the risk of thrombosis, FEIBA should not be given more frequently than every 12 h (maximum dose 200 U/kg/day). Furthermore, antifibrinolytic therapy can be used in combination with rFVIIa, but is currently not recommended in combination with FEIBA.

Specific Sites of Bleeding

Acute Hemarthrosis

All synovial joints are potentially at risk for bleeding in hemophilia; however, the most frequently affected are the 6 large hinge joints (ankles, knees, elbows), and, to a lesser extent, the 4 ball-and-socket joints (hips, shoulders). Bleeding causes synovial inflammation and hypertrophy, the precursor to hemophilic arthropathy; thus, early recognition and treatment are paramount. Older children may describe an unpleasant tingling sensation or stiffness prior to the onset of overt pain, swelling, or redness; however, in young children and infants reluctance to weight bear, pain on passive movement, or swelling that is warm to touch may be the only clues. The affected limb may be held in an antalgic (partially flexed) position, and there can be some associated muscle spasm. It may not always be possible to differentiate between a hemarthrosis and bleeding into the surrounding soft tissue; however, range of movement can be useful in this regard. Septic arthritis also occurs, albeit uncommonly, in patients with hemophilia, and should be considered when there is associated fever, constitutional symptoms, severe pain, or poor response to hemostatic therapy, with or without neutrophilia and elevated inflammatory markers.

Hemostatic treatment should be commenced at the first suspicion of bleeding (see table 4). Although factor replacement is the most effective way to relieve pain following hemarthrosis, analgesic medication should also be used when necessary (see 'Pain Management' above). Therapy should be continued until resolution of symptoms (typically 1–3 days). Persistence of symptoms beyond 3 days is unusual and should prompt careful reevaluation, including exclusion of a new inhibitor.

Routine diagnostic imaging during the assessment of an uncomplicated acute hemarthrosis is generally not needed; however, there are specific circumstances in which directed radiological investigation can be useful. Plain radiographs (X-rays) may be indicated to exclude an associated fracture if there is a history of significant trauma. Ultrasound examination may be useful for investigation of hip pain as joint bleeding may not be readily distinguished from other bleeds in this region (e.g. iliopsoas bleeding). Ultrasound examination can also be used at other sites to differentiate soft tissue bleeding from hemarthrosis, although in practice this is seldom necessary as management is guided by clinical findings. MRI can detect subtle changes such as ligamentous injury or early joint degeneration, and may be useful when the response to standard therapy appears suboptimal.

Joint aspiration (arthrocentesis) should be considered for large-volume (tense) hemarthrosis, lack of response after 24 h, pain which is not controlled by analgesia, or evidence of neurovascular compromise. If there are features to suggest septic arthritis, then joint aspiration (and culture of the synovial fluid) is essential. Joint aspiration should be performed under aseptic conditions by a clinician experienced in the technique. Factor levels should be maintained at 40–60 IU/dl for 2–3 days following the procedure. Ultrasound guidance is recommended for aspiration of the hip or shoulder joint.

Involvement of a physiotherapist to supervise rehabilitation following acute hemarthrosis is recommended by current consensus guidelines [26]. Initially, the affected joint should be rested entirely, then non-weight bearing for several days. Application of an ice pack, elevation of the affected joint, and a compression bandage can help to alleviate symptoms in some patients. Use of a splint (such as a 'soft' cast) can also be useful, and may be the only way to effectively immobilize and protect the joint in a young child. Isotonic exercises should be commenced once pain and swelling have subsided, generally after 1–2 days. Additional measures such as therapeutic ultrasound or transcutaneous electrical nerve stimulation may be used at the discretion of the physiotherapist. Resistance exercises and weight-bearing should be reintroduced gradually, with a rehabilitation program tailored to the individual.

Muscle Bleeding, Including Iliopsoas Bleeding

Delayed recognition or treatment of muscle bleeding can lead to long-term sequelae such as contracture, loss of function, and neurovascular compromise [27]. Muscle bleeds are usually trauma related (direct impact or strain injury); however, the precipitating event may not always be volunteered or recognized by the patient. A directed history is important as this will help to prevent recurrence. Pain on contraction of the affected muscle is the key finding; however, swelling, bruising and focal tenderness are also common. Neurovascular compromise distal to the bleeding site must be specifically excluded, particularly in the setting of anterior forearm or calf bleeds (see 'Compression of Vital Structures' below). Management of muscle bleeding requires appropriate clotting factor therapy (table 4), rest, elevation, graduated physiotherapy, and education to reduce the risk of recurrence. Compression, ice and splinting may be useful in some circumstances.

Recognition of iliopsoas bleeding is particularly important due to the frequency of serious complications associated with bleeding at this site. However, the iliopsoas muscle group is a deep structure, and bleeding may produce pain which is difficult to localize (hip, groin, thigh, lower abdomen or flank). Iliopsoas bleeding should be suspected when a patient presents with a partially flexed hip joint, and pain on passive extension. Altered sensation in the distribution of the femoral nerve may also be observed.

In contrast to acute hemarthrosis, radiologic imaging (particularly ultrasound) can be quite useful for the assessment of muscle bleeds (i.e. location, volume, progression), and is recommended for confirmation of iliopsoas bleeding. In addition to the treatment measures outlined above, iliopsoas bleeding requires 2–3 days of strict bed rest; thus, hospitalization should be considered.

Mucosal Bleeding

Prolonged oral mucosal bleeding is common in toddlers with moderate and severe hemophilia, and may be the first presenting symptom. The frenulum is a particularly susceptible site for bleeding. Oral bleeding is often manifested by a 'stop-start' pattern in patients with hemophilia which can continue for days if not appropriately managed. Initial oral bleeding should be managed with antifibrinolytic therapy and cold packs – ice blocks and cool teething rings can be helpful – and the patient should be encouraged to eat soft foods for 2–3 days to minimize the risk of recurrence. Antifibrinolytics can also be used as a mouthwash which is then swallowed (table 2). Unfortunately, very young children, in whom oral mucosal bleeding is common, are usually unable to hold the antifibrinolytic in their mouth for any significant period of time. If the bleeding continues or recurs over the next day, additional treatment to raise the factor level for 2–3 days is recommended. DDAVP is usually sufficient to manage oral mucosal bleeding in responsive patients with mild hemophilia A.

Epistaxis is common even in children without a bleeding disorder. Minor epistaxis can usually be managed with local pressure for sufficient time (at least 10 min). Factor therapy is rarely required except for severe bleeding. Topical agents such as petroleum jelly are useful to keep the nasal mucosa moist and prevent recurrence. Short-term use of topical steroids may be useful to reduce inflammation, and recurrent bleeding may respond to cauterization of mucosal blood vessels using silver nitrate.

Menorrhagia can occur in carrier females with low factor levels. This can usually be managed with antifibrinolytic therapy started at the onset of menstruation and continued until the end of the period. If this is insufficient to manage bleeding, the oral contraceptive pill is usually effective. In more severely affected patients, the active component of the oral contraceptive pill may be continued for several months at a time, with controlled withdrawal bleeds at a time suitable for the patient. If menorrhagia is not controlled by the above methods, it may be necessary to raise the factor level with DDAVP (hemophilia A) or factor concentrates (hemophilia B, or moderate-severe hemophilia A). In selected cases, use of an intrauterine contraceptive device such as a Mirena® can also be useful. Where available, the involvement of a pediatric gynecologist to provide expert advice and support is recommended. Iron deficiency is common in women with chronic menorrhagia, and regular monitoring of iron stores is appropriate in this patient group.

Compression of Vital Structures

Failure to recognize bleeding at sites adjacent to vital structures can result in rapid demise (i.e. the brain, airway, heart, or lungs), or severe and permanent loss of function (e.g. the spinal cord, eye, kidney, or peripheral neurovascular bundles). These are all medical emergencies, and mandate rapid administration of clotting factor (target factor level of 80–100 IU/dl) or bypassing therapy (where appropriate) in addition to life-support measures, confirmatory diagnostic imaging, and urgent consultation with the relevant surgical team. ICH is discussed below (see 'Intracranial Bleeding').

Upper airway obstruction may result from bleeding into the tongue, retropharyngeal space or soft tissues of the neck, and typically presents with stridor and progressive respiratory distress. Pain may be poorly localized, and in younger children this clinical picture may be confused with croup. A history of neck injury or oropharyngeal trauma (including vigorous coughing or iatrogenic injury) should be sought, and hemostatic therapy should be administered if there is any doubt prior to imaging studies.

Patients with hemophilia are at particular risk of compartment syndrome due to bleeding into the soft tissues of the wrist, anterior forearm or calf. Severe pain, tense swelling, paresthesia, and cool digits with slow capillary refill are key findings. Paresis and loss of arterial pulse are late findings, and the absence of these features does not exclude the diagnosis. The need for decompression fasciotomy may be averted if the condition is recognized early and treated with clotting factor therapy in addition to elevation of the affected limb.

Intracranial Bleeding

The reported incidence of ICH in hemophilia is highest during the neonatal period (3–4%, see 'Management of the Newborn' below), but remains a significant cause of mortality and long-term neurological morbidity in older children [28]. Suspected ICH is a medical emergency, and in all cases clotting factor therapy should be provided immediately, without waiting for results of imaging (table 4). Risk factors for ICH beyond the neonatal period include severe hemophilia, presence of inhibitors, absence of prophylaxis, previously confirmed ICH, a history of head trauma, and an altered level of consciousness [28]. Younger age is also a risk factor for ICH; however, this is not a useful discriminator when trying to make a decision regarding the need for diagnostic imaging. Other concerning symptoms at presentation include headache, vomiting, seizures and focal neurologic signs.

CT scanning, performed after factor replacement has been given, remains the imaging modality of choice for initial assessment; however, it must be highlighted that a negative scan does not exclude ICH, and patients (and their parents/caregivers) should be advised to return for medical assessment if there are new or persistent neurologic symptoms. There is a paucity of evidence regarding the role of imaging in asymptomatic patients presenting after minor head injury; however, it may be reasonable to defer CT in such patients, taking into account the timing of injury in relation to their last prophylaxis dose [28].

Patients with confirmed ICH require intensive factor replacement or bypassing therapy in addition to standard life-support measures. Neurosurgical consultation should be sought immediately, and transfer to the nearest HTC should be undertaken as soon as practical. Factor levels should be maintained at appropriate levels for 10–14 days, and continuous infusion allows efficient dose titration in this context. Following discharge from hospital, long-term secondary prophylaxis to prevent ICH recurrence is recommended in all patients, even those with inhibitors.

Gastrointestinal Bleeding

The causes of gastrointestinal bleeding (i.e. hematemesis, hematochezia or melena) in children with or without hemophilia are similar. However, swallowed blood (e.g. from epistaxis or a mouth bleed) warrants particular consideration in children with an underlying bleeding disorder, especially those with hemophilia. Furthermore, NSAIDs prescribed for pain associated with chronic synovitis may cause gastritis or ulceration which may predispose to bleeding. The approach to management and diagnostic workup depends on the site, volume and duration of bleeding; however, in all cases appropriate clotting factor therapy should be administered early (table 4). Careful attention to pulse, blood pressure and hemoglobin level is important as the degree of blood loss may initially be underestimated.

Macroscopic Hematuria

Hematuria in children with hemophilia is not an uncommon presentation. It is usually benign in nature. Initial assessment should include history and physical examination looking for possible precipitants (e.g. urinary tract infection), although in many cases no underlying cause will be identified. Investigations should include a urine culture and blood urea and creatinine. Renal ultrasound is not routinely indicated as a first-line test, but may be useful if there are any concerns about urinary obstruction. Painless hematuria in children with hemophilia should be initially managed with vigorous hydration, with the primary aim to maintain a good urine output. Admission and bed rest along with fluids are helpful. If there is pain, or persistent gross hematuria, treatment with factor concentrate should be considered (table 4). Antifibrinolytic therapy is contraindicated due to the potential for intrarenal or ureteric clots leading to urinary obstruction [3].

Management of Surgery and Other Invasive Procedures

Any surgery (or invasive procedure) in a patient with hemophilia must only be undertaken following consultation with the patient's HTC. There must be close liaison between the hematologist, the surgeon and the anesthetist. Formulation of an appropriate management plan for surgery requires prospective estimation of the anticipated bleeding risk; this is subjective and must take into account both surgical and patient-specific risk factors. Important surgical considerations include the experience of the operator, the anatomical site (in particular its accessibility and location with respect to vital structures), and whether significant bleeding occurs in non-hemophiliac patients undergoing the same procedure. The age of the child, relevant comorbidities, and the inhibitor status are important patient-specific factors. Surgery in patients with inhibitors should always be considered high risk.

The perioperative management plan should be clearly documented in the medical record, and should include the date and time of surgery, any required baseline laboratory tests, the timing of the preoperative loading dose, the dosing schedule during and after the procedure, the requirements for monitoring (e.g. factor levels), the requirement for adjuvant therapy, and the arrangements for follow-up on discharge. There should be adequate laboratory support for the monitoring of factor levels in the postoperative period. An inhibitor screen should be performed prior to any elective surgery.

Factor replacement therapy for surgery can be given by intermittent boluses or by continuous infusion; however, it should be highlighted that data to support specific dosing recommendations for various surgical procedures are scarce [29]. Examples of surgical protocols for port insertion (figure 1) and circumcision during the newborn period (figure 2) are provided for reference. Continuous infusion has the advantage of providing stable factor levels with overall less factor requirement and easier monitoring; however, it remains uncertain whether this mode of administration is associated with a higher incidence of inhibitor formation [30]. DDAVP may be adequate for responsive patients with mild hemophilia A undergoing low-risk procedures. Patients with high-level inhibitors (≥5 BU) require bypassing therapy for perioperative hemostasis, and currently this is administered as regular boluses (experience with continuous infusion in this setting is limited).

Chronic Complications of Hemophilia

Synovitis

Following a joint bleed, the synovial lining of the joint becomes inflamed, which results in an increased risk of recurrent bleeding. Acute synovitis should be managed with rest, splinting, and

> **Port insertion for** *(Patient Name)*
> **Diagnosis: severe hemophilia A**
> **Planned date of surgery:** *(Date)*
>
> Patient ID: Date of Birth: Weight:
>
> - The patient will be admitted the morning of the procedure.
> - Check that pharmacy has supplied the FVIII (_____ = brand name).
> - On admission, the child will need at least one peripheral cannula inserted.
> - Perform baseline aPTT, FVIII level and inhibitor screen.
> - Administer bolus dose of FVIII 50 IU/kg.
> - Blood should be taken 15 min after bolus from a different site for FVIII level (3.5 ml citrate tube – ensure the tube is filled with blood to the line and labelled).
> - Target FVIII level is between 90 and 110 IU/dL post-bolus.
> - Commence continuous FVIII infusion at a rate of 5 U/kg/h (Infusion should be written up as Factor VIII **250 units in 5 ml** (neat) and the rate written in the appropriate spots on the medication sheet). A 0.9% saline side line should also be written up to keep the vein open. Only make syringe up to **500 units in 10 ml each time**, so factor is not wasted if the rate changes.
> - If the post-bolus FVIII level is outside this range, an additional FVIII bolus or adjustment to infusion rate may be required: notify Dr _____ (via switchboard). The FVIII level is directly proportional to the infusion rate, so doubling the infusion rate should double the FVIII level.
> - The FVIII infusion should continue throughout the procedure and for 4–5 days post-op.
> - The peripheral cannula (I.V.) should be left in place for FVIII infusion post-op.
> - Commence oral tranexamic acid 25 mg/kg q8 h for 7–10 days.
> - Blood should be taken daily for the first 3–4 days postoperatively for FVIII levels.
> - The target levels are 80–120 IU/dL for the first 48 h, 60–80 U/mL for days 3–4.
> - After a few days of infusion, the half-life of FVIII tends to increase so that a lower infusion rate may achieve the same FVIII level.
> - The infusion can usually be discontinued after day 4, and once or twice daily boluses can be given over the next few days.
> - Usually, the patient can be discharged on day 5 if the port site is satisfactory.

Figure 1. Guide to surgical prophylaxis during port insertion. Adapted from current clinical practice at the Queensland Children's Haemophilia Centre, Brisbane, Qld., Australia. For hospitals not familiar with use of continuous intermittent (bolus) infusions of clotting factor concentrates should be used in the pre- and post-operative periods. For details please consult specific product inserts, or published *Guidelines for the Management of Hemophilia* [3].

prophylactic factor replacement. With repeated bleeding into the same joint, the synovium becomes chronically inflamed and hypertrophy develops, which is evident clinically by persistent swelling, and can be demonstrated with imaging such as MRI or ultrasound. Chronic synovitis should be proactively addressed to preserve joint function. Initially, this is best managed with intensification of prophylaxis (e.g. alternate days) and physiotherapy. Synovectomy (radioisotopic or surgical, depending on local resources and expertise) is indicated in persistent cases.

**Prophylaxis for neonatal circumcision
(Severe hemophilia A)**

Patient name:
Patient ID: Date of Birth: Weight:

- The patient will be admitted the morning of the procedure.
- Check that pharmacy has supplied the FVIII (_____ = brand name).
- Perform baseline aPTT, FVIII level and inhibitor screen.
- Administer bolus dose of FVIII 250 IU prior to the procedure.
- Commence oral tranexamic acid 1 h prior to the procedure (50 mg tid, 10 doses).
- Avoid topical sealants (to minimize exposure to plasma products).
- If necessary, administer a second bolus of FVIII 250 IU on day 2.

Figure 2. Guide to surgical prophylaxis during neonatal circumcision. Adapted from current clinical practice at The Israel National Hemophilia Center, Sheba Medical Center, Tel Hashomer, Israel.

Arthropathy

Chronic synovitis ultimately leads to localized destruction of cartilage and bone, resulting in loss of joint mobility and significant functional impairment. The problem is further compounded by wasting and contracture of surrounding muscle groups, producing a fixed flexion deformity, and osteoporosis of long bones due to lack of use. Plain radiographs (X-rays) will not detect arthropathy at an early stage; therefore, other imaging modalities are required for initial assessment. In centers with the relevant radiological expertise, ultrasound examination can be useful for early detection of soft tissue changes such as hemosiderin deposition or synovial hypertrophy. In contrast, MRI is more sensitive for osteochondral changes such as cartilage thinning, bony erosions or cysts. The major goals of therapy are to relieve pain, and to improve or preserve joint function. Specific COX-2 inhibitors and splinting can be useful for analgesia (see 'Pain management' above). A tailored physiotherapy program to maintain joint mobility and muscle strength prior to the onset of fixed deformity is important. When arthropathy is at an advanced stage, bracing, orthotics and mobility aids can facilitate independent functioning and resumption of normal daily activities. Options for surgical intervention include arthroscopic joint debridement, alignment osteotomy, arthrodesis or joint replacement. A detailed discussion of these procedures is beyond the scope of this text; however, for further information the reader is referred to a recent review of this topic [31].

Pseudotumors

Pseudotumors, a rare complication of hemophilia, result from repeated and unresolved soft tissue bleeding, usually into muscle. The hematoma becomes encapsulated and calcified, and the mass progressively enlarges and may destroy surrounding bone and tissue. The most commonly affected areas are the pelvis and the long bones. Initial therapy should involve intensive factor replacement; however, other treatments including aspiration, embolization, radiotherapy or surgery are often required. These lesions are highly vascular; thus, surgical intervention should only be undertaken at a tertiary HTC with appropriate multidisciplinary support.

Management of the Newborn with Suspected or Possible Hemophilia

Hemophilia may be suspected in a newborn due to the presence of unusual bleeding symptoms, a known family history, or both. A general overview of bleeding in the neonate is provided in chapter 4. Newborns with hemophilia are particularly prone to intra- and extracranial bleeding, and this risk is affected by mode of delivery, being highest for instrumental delivery (forceps or vacuum) and lowest for elective caesarean section or uncomplicated vaginal delivery. In addition to neurologic sequelae, loss of blood into the scalp or subgaleal space can be substantial. For this reason, instrumental delivery should be avoided in potentially affected infants (male fetus of a known or possible carrier).

At delivery, such infants should have cord blood collected for urgent factor assay, bearing in mind that results must be interpreted with reference to age-specific ranges (in normal newborns FVIII is elevated and FIX is reduced). Intramuscular vitamin K should be withheld pending these results (oral vitamin K can be given if there is likely to be significant delay) [32]. Subcutaneous vaccinations can be administered safely. Factor replacement therapy should be available for use in the event of bleeding; however, due to the lack of efficacy data and the unknown risk of inhibitor development, current guidelines do not support the routine use of prophylactic clotting factor therapy in neonates without additional risk factors (such as prematurity or traumatic delivery).

Iatrogenic hemorrhage is a genuine risk in newborns with hemophilia, and arterial puncture for blood sampling should be avoided. Prolonged pressure is usually adequate for achieving hemostasis following heel prick or venipuncture. Infants with nonspecific symptoms such as respiratory distress or poor perfusion should be investigated for occult bleeding (head, thorax, abdomen), and the threshold for diagnostic imaging should be low. Recently published guidelines also recommend that all infants with hemophilia should have a cranial ultrasound prior to discharge from hospital [32]. In addition, the newly diagnosed infant must be referred to the appropriate HTC so that timely follow-up can be arranged.

Conclusion

Modern hemophilia care has undergone considerable transformation in recent decades, largely due to the availability of safe, high-purity factor concentrates for treatment and prevention of bleeding. In countries with unrestricted access to factor concentrates, the prognosis for patients with hemophilia has improved dramatically. Furthermore, newer products now entering clinical trials offer the hope of less frequent treatment and more stable prophylaxis. Inhibitor development has become the most challenging complication facing hemophilia treaters in such countries, and ongoing research regarding inhibitor prevention and management is warranted. Whilst factor replacement remains the central pillar of hemophilia management, the involvement of an experienced physical therapist, along with other key members of the comprehensive care team, cannot be understated.

Acknowledgment

The authors would like to express their appreciation for the thoughtful comments provided by Drs. Manuel Carcao (Toronto, Ont., Canada), Chris Ludlam (Edinburgh, UK), Susan Baird (Edinburgh, UK), Paula Bolton-Maggs (Manchester, UK), Georges Rivard (Montreal, Que., Canada) and Gili Kenet (Tel Hashomer, Israel) who reviewed this chapter.

References

1 Santagostino E, Mancuso ME, Tripodi A, Chantarangkul V, Clerici M, Garagiola I, et al: Severe hemophilia with mild bleeding phenotype: molecular characterization and global coagulation profile. J Thromb Haemost 2010;8:737–743.
2 Seary ME, Feldman D, Carcao MD: DDAVP responsiveness in children with mild or moderate haemophilia A correlates with age, endogenous FVIII:C level and with haemophilic genotype. Haemophilia 2012;18:50–55.
3 Srivastava A, Brewer AK, Mauser-Bunschoten EP, Key NS, Kitchen S, Llinas A, et al: Guidelines for the management of hemophilia. Haemophilia 2013;19:e1–e47.
4 Iorio A, Marchesini E, Marcucci M, Stobart K, Chan AK: Clotting factor concentrates given to prevent bleeding and bleeding-related complications in people with hemophilia A or B. Cochrane Database Syst Rev 2011;9:CD003429.
5 Blanchette VS: Prophylaxis in the haemophilia population. Haemophilia 2010;16(suppl 5):181–188.
6 Collins PW, Bjorkman S, Fischer K, Blanchette V, Oh M, Schroth P, et al: Factor VIII requirement to maintain a target plasma level in the prophylactic treatment of severe hemophilia A: influences of variance in pharmacokinetics and treatment regimens. J Thromb Haemost 2010;8:269–275.
7 Valentino LA, Mamonov V, Hellmann A, Quon DV, Chybicka A, Schroth P, et al: A randomized comparison of two prophylaxis regimens and a paired comparison of on-demand and prophylaxis treatments in hemophilia A management. J Thromb Haemost 2012;10:359–367.
8 Feldman BM, Funk SM, Bergstrom BM, Zourikian N, Hilliard P, van der Net J, et al: Validation of a new pediatric joint scoring system from the International Hemophilia Prophylaxis Study Group: validity of the hemophilia joint health score. Arthritis Care Res 2011;63:223–230.
9 de Moerloose P, Fischer K, Lambert T, Windyga J, Batorova A, Lavigne-Lissalde G, et al: Recommendations for assessment, monitoring and follow-up of patients with haemophilia. Haemophilia 2012;18:319–325.
10 Valentino LA, Kawji M, Grygotis M: Venous access in the management of hemophilia. Blood Rev 2011;25:11–15.
11 Ewenstein BM, Valentino LA, Journeycake JM, Tarantino MD, Shapiro AD, Blanchette VS, et al: Consensus recommendations for use of central venous access devices in haemophilia. Haemophilia 2004;10:629–648.
12 Holstein K, Klamroth R, Richards M, Carvalho M, Perez-Garrido R, Gringeri A, et al: Pain management in patients with haemophilia: a European survey. Haemophilia 2012;18:743–752.
13 Berntorp E, Shapiro A, Astermark J, Blanchette VS, Collins PW, Dimichele D, et al: Inhibitor treatment in haemophilias A and B: summary statement for the 2006 international consensus conference. Haemophilia 2006;12(suppl 6):1–7.
14 Gouw SC, van den Berg HM, Oldenburg J, Astermark J, de Groot PG, Margaglione M, et al: F8 gene mutation type and inhibitor development in patients with severe hemophilia A: systematic review and meta-analysis. Blood 2012;119:2922–2934.
15 Hay CR, Brown S, Collins PW, Keeling DM, Liesner R: The diagnosis and management of factor VIII and IX inhibitors: a guideline from the United Kingdom Haemophilia Centre Doctors Organisation. Br J Haematol 2006;133:591–605.
16 DiMichele DM, Hoots WK, Pipe SW, Rivard GE, Santagostino E: International workshop on immune tolerance induction: consensus recommendations. Haemophilia 2007;13(suppl 1):1–22.
17 Hay CR, DiMichele DM: International Immune Tolerance S. The principal results of the International Immune Tolerance Study: a randomized dose comparison. Blood 2012;119:1335–1344.
18 Valentino LA: The benefits of prophylactic treatment with aPCC in patients with haemophilia and high-titre inhibitors: a retrospective case series. Haemophilia 2009;15:733–742.
19 Konkle BA, Ebbesen LS, Erhardtsen E, Bianco RP, Lissitchkov T, Rusen L, et al: Randomized, prospective clinical trial of recombinant factor VIIa for secondary prophylaxis in hemophilia patients with inhibitors. J Thromb Haemost 2007;5:1904–1913.
20 Morfini M, Laguna P, Leissinger C: Factor IX pharmacokinetics: differences between plasma-derived and recombinant products and the clinical and economic implications: a meeting report. Haemophilia 2008;14:873–875.
21 Mannucci PM: Hemostatic drugs. N Engl J Med 1998;339:245–253.
22 Berntorp E: Differential response to bypassing agents complicates treatment in patients with haemophilia and inhibitors. Haemophilia 2009;15:3–10.
23 Teitel J, Berntorp E, Collins P, D'Oiron R, Ewenstein B, Gomperts E, et al: A systematic approach to controlling problem bleeds in patients with severe congenital haemophilia A and high-titre inhibitors. Haemophilia 2007;13:256–263.
24 Sorensen B, Dargaud Y, Kenet G, Lusher J, Mumford A, Pipe S, et al: On-demand treatment of bleeds in haemophilia patients with inhibitors: strategies for securing and maintaining predictable efficacy with recombinant activated factor VII. Haemophilia 2012;18:255–262.
25 Astermark J, Donfield SM, DiMichele DM, Gringeri A, Gilbert SA, Waters J, et al: A randomized comparison of bypassing agents in hemophilia complicated by an inhibitor: the FEIBA NovoSeven Comparative (FENOC) Study. Blood 2007;109:546–551.
26 Hermans C, De Moerloose P, Fischer K, Holstein K, Klamroth R, Lambert T, et al: Management of acute haemarthrosis in haemophilia A without inhibitors: literature review, European survey and recommendations. Haemophilia 2011;17:383–392.
27 Sorensen B, Benson GM, Bladen M, Classey S, Keeling DM, McLaughlin P, et al: Management of muscle haematomas in patients with severe haemophilia in an evidence-poor world. Haemophilia 2012;18:598–606.
28 Traivaree C, Blanchette V, Armstrong D, Floros G, Stain AM, Carcao MD: Intracranial bleeding in hemophilia beyond the neonatal period – the role of CT imaging in suspected intracranial bleeding. Haemophilia 2007;13:552–559.
29 Hermans C, Altisent C, Batorova A, Chambost H, De Moerloose P, Karafoulidou A, et al: Replacement therapy for invasive procedures in patients with haemophilia: literature review, European survey and recommendations. Haemophilia 2009;15:639–658.
30 Batorova A, Holme P, Gringeri A, Richards M, Hermans C, Altisent C, et al: Continuous infusion in haemophilia: current practice in Europe. Haemophilia 2012;18:753–759.
31 Rodriguez-Merchan EC: Aspects of current management: orthopaedic surgery in haemophilia. Haemophilia 2012;18:8–16.
32 Chalmers E, Williams M, Brennand J, Liesner R, Collins P, Richards M, et al: Guideline on the management of haemophilia in the fetus and neonate. Br J Haematol 2011;154:208–215.

Abbreviations

aPCC	Activated prothrombin complex concentrate
aPTT	Activated partial thromboplastin time
CT	Computed tomography
COX	Cyclooxygenase
CVC	Central venous catheter
DDAVP	1-Deamino-8-D-arginine vasopressin (desmopressin)
DVT	Deep vein thrombosis
FP (FFP)	Frozen plasma (Fresh frozen plasma)
FVIII	Factor VIII
FIX	Factor IX
FXI	Factor XI
HTC	Hemophilia treatment center
ICH	Intracranial hemorrhage
ITI	Immune tolerance induction
MRI	Magnetic resonance imaging
NSAIDs	Nonsteroidal anti-inflammatory drugs
PICC	Peripheral inserted central catheter
rFVIIa	Recombinant activated factor VII
VWF	von Willebrand factor

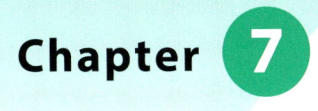

Chapter 7: von Willebrand Disease in Children

Vicky R. Breakey
Manuel Carcao

Introduction

VWD is the most common inherited bleeding disorder. It is estimated that up to 1% of all people are affected with VWD although only about 1/1,000 are symptomatic [1] and only 1/10,000 are likely to be followed in a bleeding disorders clinic. A deficiency or dysfunction of VWF results in defective primary hemostasis due to absent or abnormal platelet adhesion as well as decreased circulating FVIII. Despite its frequency, the majority of VWD is associated with a less severe bleeding phenotype than that of hemophilia. Type 1 VWD, the less severe quantitative defect, and the qualitative defects of type 2 VWD are associated mainly with mucocutaneous bleeding. Generally, only type 3 VWD, the rare but severe quantitative defect, is associated with significant bleeding and hemarthrosis.

In children, in the absence of a family history of the disease, the milder forms of VWD may not be diagnosed until there is a significant bleeding challenge. This may occur at the time of circumcision, dental work, surgery or menarche. Laboratory testing is imperative to make the diagnosis and to delineate the subtype of VWD. Treatment depends on the clinical severity, disease responsiveness and magnitude of bleeding/bleeding risk.

Pathophysiology of von Willebrand Disease

The first family of patients with VWD was reported from Finland by Dr. Erik von Willebrand in 1926. He noted an autosomal-dominant bleeding disorder in a family with multiple individuals that had significant bleeding with a prolonged bleeding time despite a normal platelet count. It later became apparent that although FVIII was also reduced, a distinct protein, VWF was diminished, dysfunctional or absent in those with the bleeding disorder.

In the mid-1980s, the VWF gene was identified on chromosome 12. The 178-kb gene is made up of 52 exons and codes for a protein of 2,050 amino acids. During its biosynthesis, the protein undergoes modifications that result in the production of VWF protein arranged into multimers

Figure 1. An area of endothelial cell loss with the sequence of events involved in the primary hemostatic event, platelet plug formation. The platelets initially adhere transiently to subendothelial VWF through the GpIb/IX receptor. This contact significantly slows the movement of the platelets that continue to roll across the subendothelium, maintaining an interaction with VWF and collagen through the GpIb/IX and platelet collagen receptor(s), respectively. Eventually, these contacts reach a threshold that signals the event of platelet activation. The platelets then adhere stably to the damaged vessel wall, and undergo an aggregation response through a platelet GP IIb/IIIa receptor-mediated event. Reproduced with permission from the World Federation of Hemophilia [2].

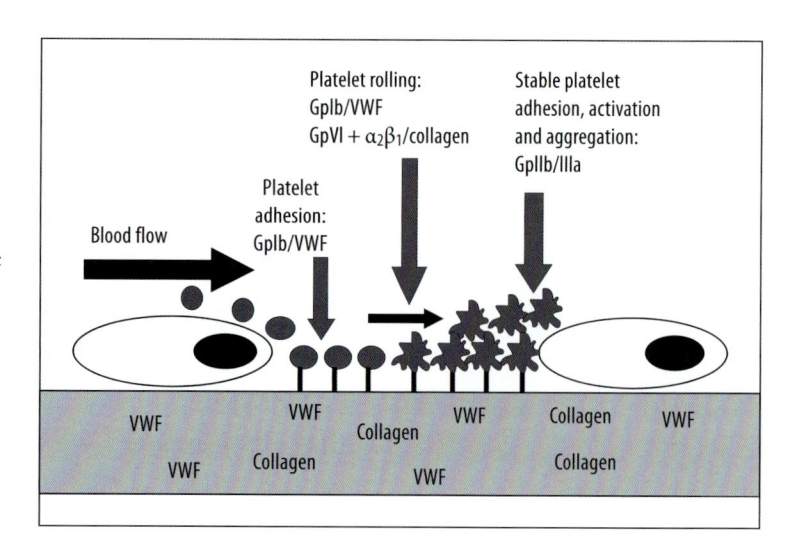

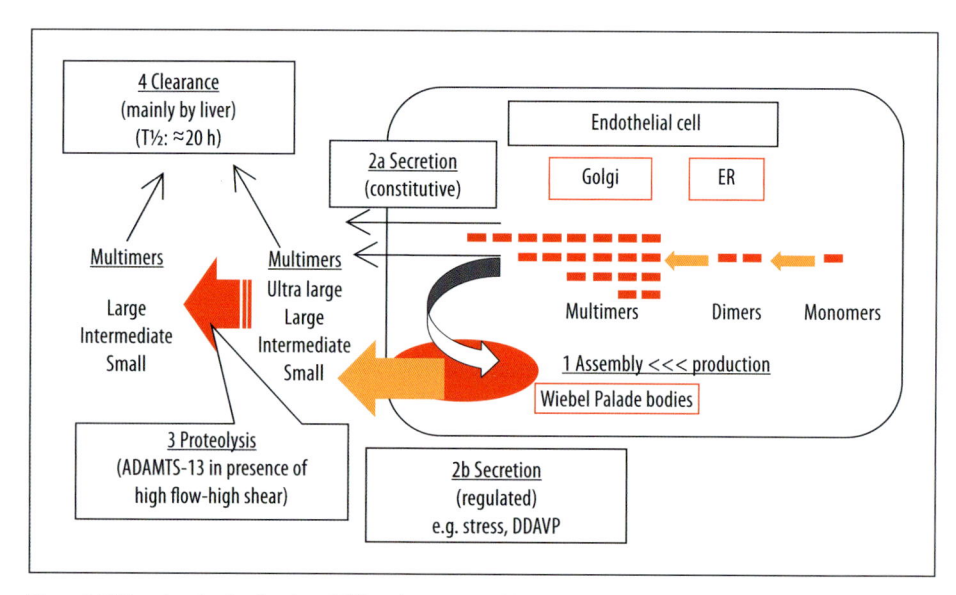

Figure 2. VWD can be related to disorders of VWF production, assembly, secretion or clearance.

that vary in size from dimers to polymers of up to 20 million Daltons in size. VWF is produced by both endothelial cells and by megakaryocytes. In these two cells, it is stored in distinct granules; Weibel-Palade bodies in the former and alpha granules in the latter.

Further research into the protein suggests three distinct functions: (1) to facilitate platelet adhesion to injured endothelium via GP Ib/IX and collagen, (2) to assist with the process of platelet aggregation through binding to the GP IIb/IIIa receptor, and (3) to carry FVIII and protect it from degradation by protein C (figure 1) [2]. VWD can be caused by disorders of VWF production, assembly, secretion or clearance (figure 2).

Table 1. Classification of VWD

Type	Basis of defect	Description
1	quantitative	partial deficiency of VWF
2A	qualitative	decreased VWF-dependent platelet adhesion and selective deficiency of high-molecular weight multimers
2B	qualitative	VWF increased affinity for platelet glycoprotein Ib
2M	qualitative	decreased VWF-dependent platelet adhesion without a selective deficiency of high-molecular-weight VWF multimers
2N	qualitative	markedly decreased binding affinity of VWF for Factor VIII
3	quantitative	severe deficiency of VWF

Clinical Presentation

In 2006, the ISTH VWD subcommittee published the generally accepted classification of VWD [3] (table 1).

Type 1 VWD

Type 1 VWD is the most common form of VWD accounting for approximately 75% of cases. Inheritance is autosomal-dominant, but incomplete penetrance and variable expressivity can obscure positive family histories. Patients with type 1 VWD may present with mucocutaneous bleeding, including excessive epistaxis, bruising and menorrhagia or may have prolonged bleeding after surgery. Clinically, there is a broad range of severity that generally correlates with the amount of functional VWF in the circulation.

Type 2 VWD

Type 2 VWD accounts for approximately 25% of cases. There are four subtypes of type 2 VWD: 2A, 2B, 2M and 2N, each having a different pathophysiological etiology and specific diagnostic findings (see 'Diagnosis'). Clinically, children with types 2A, 2B and 2M VWD present with increased mucocutaneous bleeding, similar to those with type 1 VWD. Children with type 2N present with a bleeding pattern more similar to that of mild to moderate hemophilia A. In adults, bleeding in type 2 VWD is often worse than in type I VWD. In general, severe bleeds such as ICH are rare in type 2 VWD, but are reported.

Type 3 VWD

Type 3 VWD is the most severe bleeding phenotype, due to severe deficiency of VWF (<5%). This autosomal-recessive condition is very rare, occurring in only one to three per million. Its highest incidence is in regions where consanguinity is common. In addition to severe mucocutaneous bleeding, there can be repeated bleeding into muscles and joints. As in hemophilia, the complications of hemarthrosis include severe arthritis and sometimes result in chronic disability. ICH and other severe bleeds, although still rare, are more commonly reported in type 3 VWD.

Diagnosis

The diagnosis of VWD is based on the patient's bleeding history, a family history of bleeding and laboratory investigations that are consistent with a quantitative or qualitative abnormality of VWF.

Personal and Familial Bleeding History

Both a personal and family history of bleeding is important (chapter 3). Ideally, the history is taken objectively, with a focus on both unprovoked bleeding and the response to bleeding challenges (surgeries, tooth extractions, etc.). For women, a detailed menstrual history is important. The use of a validated bleeding score is helpful to maintain consistency amongst care givers. In pediatrics, the PBQ can be used to identify children with increased bleeding (chapter 3) [4].

Family history of bleeding is also important, although as mentioned, may not always be present

Table 2. VWD laboratory investigations

	Type 1	Type 2				Type 3
		2A	2B	2M	2N	
VWF:Ag	↓	↓	↓	↓	↓/N	↓↓↓
VWF:RCo	↓	↓↓	↓↓	↓↓	↓/N	↓↓↓
FVIII:C, IU/mL	↓/N	↓/N	↓/N	↓/N	0.05–0.4	0.05–0.1
VWF:RCo/VWF:Ag ratio	N	<0.6	<0.6	<0.6	N	N/A
Multimers	N	abN	abN	N	N	absent
RIPA	N	↓	↑	↓	N	absent

↓ = Slightly reduced; ↓↓ = moderately reduced; ↓↓↓ = extremely reduced; N = normal; abN = abnormal; N/A = not applicable.

in type 1 VWD. Dominant types of VWD may be present in each generation, with multiple people affected. Both type 2N and type 3 VWD are autosomal-recessive conditions, so a family history of bleeding may be absent but consanguinity is often noted.

Laboratory Investigations

Some nonspecific laboratory investigations can suggest VWD.

Complete Blood Count

Anemia may be present in patients arising from excessive blood loss and there may also be evidence of iron deficiency (microcytosis and hypochromasia) if the blood loss is chronic. Thrombocytopenia can be seen in type 2B VWD.

Activated Partial Thromboplastin Time

In most persons with VWD the aPTT is normal and as such the aPTT is not a good screening test for VWD. Exceptions to this are severe forms of VWD that result in very low levels of FVIII:C. This includes type 3 VWD, type 2N VWD and severe forms of types 1 and 2 VWD.

Bleeding Time

This is no longer readily available in most centers and is not considered a good screen for VWD due to its low sensitivity and specificity (chapter 3).

Platelet Function Analyzer (PFA-100®)

This has been validated as an in vitro method for assessing primary hemostasis in children [5]. Although it has been shown to be more sensitive than the bleeding time as a screen for VWD [6], its use remains controversial and many centers prefer to do specific testing for VWD rather than rely on the PFA-100® as a screening test (chapter 3).

It is important to recognize that these nonspecific investigations may be completely normal in VWD and, therefore, specific tests of VWF and FVIII are required. Specific initial tests to investigate the diagnosis of VWD include: the VWF antigen assay (VWF:Ag), the ristocetin cofactor assay (VWF:RCo) and factor VIII (coagulant) level (FVIII:C). A guide to interpretation of these test results can be seen in table 2. The results of VWD testing can be influenced by both preanalytic and patient-related factors that should be considered during interpretation. Care must be taken to ensure that the blood draw is not traumatic and that the samples are not shaken or agitated as this may initiate clotting and result in both VWF and FVIII being consumed. Samples must be processed within 2 h to prevent degradation of VWF. If this is not feasible, plasma should be separated promptly at room temperature, and the plasma should be centrifuged thoroughly to remove platelets and then frozen. Frozen plasma can be transported to a reference laboratory at or below –40°C.

VWF levels are affected by a number of physiological parameters. ABO blood type affects VWF levels; individuals who are type O blood type will have VWF levels that are 20–25% lower than non-O blood type individuals [7]. Whether blood type should be taken into consideration in diagnosing VWD remains debatable although we suggest, for practical reasons, the criteria to diagnose VWD be the same regardless of blood type (see section below regarding the diagnosis of type 1 VWD). Other parameters that might affect VWF levels include states of high estrogen levels (e.g. pregnancy or when taking oral contraceptive pills), hypothyroidism (decreases levels of VWF), stress (including struggling or crying in children at the time of phlebotomy) or acute illness which usually increases VWF levels.

Type 1 VWD

The diagnosis of type 1 VWD is often challenging due to the lack of a definitive cut-off that separates normal from abnormal VWF:Ag and VWF:RCo levels, the impact of blood group type on these levels and the variability in test results in the same individual over time [8]. In a prospective study of 58 children ages 2.5–17 years, the 95% lower confidence limit for VWF:Ag was 0.37 IU/ml (group O) and 0.5 IU/ml (non-group O). Comparable values for VWF:RCo were 0.42 IU/ml (group O) and 0.51 IU/ml (non-group 0) [6]. Based on such studies, many clinicians have suggested using ABO-specific reference ranges to diagnose type 1 VWD. Yet this might be impractical and ignore the fact that bleeding manifestations in a person are likely to be proportional to their level of VWF irrespective of their blood group. VWF:Ag cutoff levels that have been proposed to differentiate normal from type 1 VWD have included 0.3, 0.4 and 0.5 IU/ml [9]. We suggest that a cutoff level of 0.4 IU/ml is most practical and avoids under- or overdiagnosing VWD as would likely occur if cutoff levels of 0.3 or 0.5 IU/ml were used. Also, the ratio of VWF:RCo/VWF:Ag in type 1 VWD is >0.6 which differentiates this from type 2 VWD [9]. Borderline testing should be repeated at least once for confirmation before making a diagnosis. We suggest that a laboratory diagnosis of type 1 VWD requires at least two VWF:Ag levels of <0.4 IU/ml or two VWF:RCo levels of <0.4 IU/ml plus one VWF:Ag level of <0.4 IU/ml [6]. Test results may vary in the same individual over time, leading to uncertainty in diagnosis and frustration in patients/families [8].

Type 1C VWD

Although not included in the 2006 classification, type IC VWD is now well described and deserves mention due to its particular clinical/treatment implications [10]. This disorder, which comprises approximately 15% of cases of type 1 VWD, is due to increased VWF clearance. Typical laboratory findings include low VWF:Ag and proportionately low VWF:RCo activity with a low or normal FVIII:C level. A high VWF propeptide/VWF:Ag ratio is very helpful in diagnosis, but is not widely available [11]. There may be persistence of larger than normal size VWF multimers. Practically, a DDAVP challenge test is most helpful, as patients with type 1C VWD show an exaggerated response to DDAVP at 1 h postadministration, but have a marked reduction at the 4-hour mark due to accelerated clearance. Genetic analysis and the identification of missense mutations known to cause type 1C VWD in exons 26, 27 and 37 can confirm this condition.

Type 2 VWD

When the VWF:RCo/VWF:Ag ratio is <0.6, type 2 VWD should be considered and additional testing performed. VWF multimers should be assessed by gel electrophoresis (figure 3). Decreased VWF multimers suggest type 2A or type 2B VWD. In type 2A VWD, the high molecular weight multimers are missing due to an inability to make these forms or because of premature degradation by ADAMTS13. In contrast, type 2B VWD patients do not show the high molecular weight forms as they spontaneously bind to platelets and

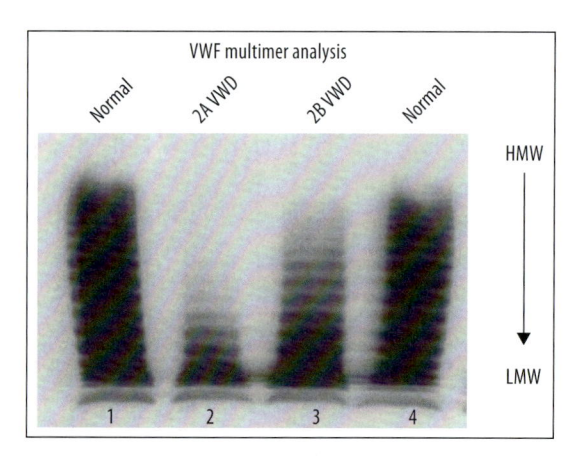

Figure 3. Example of VWF multimer analysis. Plasma VWF multimer patterns in normal plasma (lanes 1 and 4), in type 2A plasma (lane 2) and type 2B plasma (lane 3) [2]. HMW = High molecular weight; LMW = low molecular weight.

are cleared from the circulation. To differentiate 2B from 2A VWD, a RIPA test may be performed. Under normal conditions, the addition of ristocetin to PRP induces platelet-clumping. This activity is generally reduced in most VWD patients (including patients with types 2A and 2M VWD). In type 2B VWD, there is hyper-responsiveness to ristocetin (increased RIPA test) due to enhanced binding of VWF to platelet GP Ib/IX receptors (gain of function mutation).

The diagnosis of type 2N VWD can be challenging and cases may be misdiagnosed as having mild/moderate hemophilia A (in males) or as hemophilia carriers (in females). The VWF:Ag and VWF:RCo may be slightly low, borderline or normal. The diagnosis of type 2N VWD should be suspected when the FVIII:C level is disproportionately low relative to the VWF:Ag level or when there is consanguinity suggesting an autosomal recessive inheritance. An ELISA-based FVIII binding assay can be done to determine if VWF binds FVIII abnormally to confirm the diagnosis; however, the binding assay is not generally available except in research laboratories so confirmation by genetic testing is preferred (see below). Type 2N VWD should be considered in cases labeled as having mild hemophilia A in whom a hemophilia mutation cannot be identified, or in those that do not respond well to a recombinant or plasma-derived FVIII concentrate that does not contain VWF.

Type 3 VWD

Type 3 VWD is diagnosed when the VWF:Ag and VWF:RCo levels are <0.05 IU/ml. The FVIII:C is usually between 0.01 and 0.10 IU/ml, VWF multimers are absent and there can be a history of consanguinity. Genetic testing may be pursued for prenatal counseling in families with an affected child and who are planning to have additional children.

Genetic Testing for VWD

Genetic mutation analysis is not part of the routine diagnostic testing for VWD, as it is limited by the size and complexity of the gene [12]. Approximately 35% of patients with type 1 VWD have no identifiable mutation in the promoter, coding region or splice sites of the VWF gene, suggesting that there may be other genes that affect VWF production and clearance. Despite the challenges, there are a number of situations in which genetic testing can confirm the diagnosis when standard approaches are not able to provide a definitive diagnosis. This includes type 2N disease (caused by mutations in exons 18–24) as well as type 2B or 2M VWD where mutations occur in exon 28 and for prenatal diagnosis for type 3 VWD as mentioned above.

Management

Prevention of bleeding is important for patients with VWD. Patients should be advised to avoid ASA and other antiplatelet medications (e.g. NSAIDs). Protective gear, such as helmets for bike riding, should be recommended. In addition, optimal dental care is important, as the increased mucocutaneous bleeding can result in patients avoiding routine brushing leading to dental caries and the need for dental extractions over time [13]. Despite these precautions, medical therapies are often needed to control bleeding in patients with VWD.

In general, patients with VWD do not need routine treatment. Treatment is necessary to prevent operative bleeding, manage bleeding during childbirth or miscarriage and in the event of excessive mucosal bleeding such as menorrhagia or epistaxis. Many practical reviews of VWD treatment have been published [14, 15]. Medical therapies for prevention/control of bleeding in VWD can be divided into two types: non-specific adjunctive therapies that provide hemostatic support (antifibrinolytics, estrogens, fibrin sealants) and treatments that directly increase levels of VWF and FVIII (DDAVP, VWF/FVIII concentrates, cryoprecipitate).

Nonspecific Adjunctive Therapies
Antifibrinolytics

Two antifibrinolytics are used for patients with VWD, tranexamic acid and EACA. Their mechanism of action is inhibition of plasminogen. They are contraindicated in patients who are felt to have an elevated risk of thrombosis, patients with clinical disseminated intravascular coagulation and in patients with gross hematuria. Metabolism is renal, so doses should be adjusted in renal impairment. Antifibrinolytic treatment should continue for up to 1 week after a procedure depending on the procedure and the inherent risk of bleeding. Dosing of antifibrinolytics is detailed below.

Tranexamic Acid. 10 mg/kg i.v. (maximum 50 mg/dose) prior to procedure and 3–4 times daily postoperatively until able to tolerate orally. By mouth, 25 mg/kg/dose (maximum 1.5 g/dose) can be given 3–4 times daily. Tranexamic acid is available in 500-mg tablets. For young children the intravenous solution can be given by mouth.

EACA. 100 mg/kg i.v./p.o. every 4–6 h (maximum 30 g/day). EACA is available in suspension (250 mg/ml) and 500 and 1,000 mg tablets.

Estrogens

In women with menorrhagia, estrogens can be given to regulate ovulation cycles and increase VWF and FVIII levels. Standard oral contraceptive pills that contain estrogen can be used (see section on menorrhagia).

Fibrin Sealants

This topical remedy contains both fibrinogen and thrombin and can be applied directly to sites of bleeding during surgery. These agents are commercially available and guidelines for administration are detailed in the product insert and should be followed.

Treatments that Directly Increase Levels of VWF and FVIII
Desmopressin

DDAVP is a synthetic form of vasopressin that acts to stimulate the release of VWF from endothelial cells. DDAVP is often sufficient treatment for mild cases of VWD. DDAVP can be used to treat active bleeding and to prevent bleeding associated with dental procedures, minor surgeries and menorrhagia. Because DDAVP can exacerbate thrombocytopenia in type 2B VWD, it is generally contraindicated in this condition. It is not beneficial for type 3 VWD.

It is important to know a patient's responsiveness to DDAVP, as approximately 20% of patients with type 1 VWD are considered nonresponders. A DDAVP challenge test should be done following diagnosis. In this test, a dose of 0.3 μg/kg of DDAVP (maximum 20 μg) is given intravenously or subcutaneously and the response is assessed. Response to DDAVP is classified according to peak FVIII:C and VWF:RCo levels at 1 h. In addition, a 4-hour sample is important to detect those patients with exaggerated clearance of VWF (e.g. type 1C VWD). A complete response following a dose of DDAVP is defined as VWF:RCo and FVIII:C levels ≥0.5 IU/ml while a partial response is defined as VWF:RCo and FVIII:C levels of >0.3 IU/ml

[16]. Some clinicians have suggested that to be classified as a 'responder' the patient needs to at least double their VWF:RCo from baseline. DDAVP can be used to manage most bleeds and most surgical procedures in complete responders whereas it would be limited to minor bleeds and surgeries in partial responders.

As the response to DDAVP has been shown to improve with age, children assessed to be DDAVP nonresponders at a young age (<10 years of age) should undergo a repeat DDAVP challenge test at an older age.

DDAVP can be administered subcutaneously, intranasally or intravenously. Standard DDAVP dosing is 0.3 µg/kg i.v./s.c. (maximum dose 20 µg). Intranasal dosing usually consists of administering 300 µg (one 150-µg puff into each nostril) for older children and adults and 150 µg (1 puff) for younger children.

The side effects of DDAVP are generally mild and transient and include tachycardia, flushing and headache. An important but rare side effect of DDAVP is seizures which can occur because of the antidiuretic properties of DDAVP that can lead to fluid overload and consequent hyponatremia. For this reason, DDAVP should generally be limited to once daily administration and should be used with extreme caution in very young children (<3 years) or in elderly patients. In both groups fluid intake should be restricted for 12 h following administration and isotonic fluid solutions are recommended. With repeated exposure to DDAVP, stores of VWF become reduced. Consequently, after multiple consecutive days of DDAVP use, the hemostatic effect of DDAVP is diminished in many patients (a phenomenon known as 'tachyphylaxis'). A study by Mannucci et al. [17] showed a 30% fall in the response to DDAVP after the second day of DDAVP administration. Further use of DDAVP after the second day should be individualized and based on the laboratory measurement of VWF:RCo, taking into consideration the clinical indication for which ongoing hemostatic cover is needed. If clinically significant tachyphylaxis occurs, one option is to use an alternating combination of a VWF concentrate and DDAVP.

VWF/FVIII Concentrates

When the DDAVP response is insufficient or contraindicated, VWF concentrates can be used. There are several plasma-derived VWF-containing concentrates. These are differentiated by the ratio of VWF to FVIII. Haemate-P (Humate-P®) has a VWF:FVIII ratio of 2.5:1 whereas other VWF-containing concentrates (e.g. Wilate® and Alphanate®) have ratios of about 1:1. All of these products undergo one or more viral inactivation steps to minimize risk of blood-borne infections. Dosing for VWF concentrate is as follows: Dose (IU VWF:RCo) = desired % increase in VWF:RCo (IU/dl) × body weight (kg)/1.5. Replacement should be given every 8–12 h, as needed.

VWF concentrates are generally well tolerated with minimal complications or side effects. Although the product is virally inactivated, a small theoretical risk of transmitting infection persists. For this reason, susceptible patients who are hepatitis A and/or B antibody negative should be immunized prophylactically. There have been a small number of thromboembolic events reported in patients who are treated with VWF concentrates, mainly in patients with other risk factors. In addition, there is a small risk of intravascular hemolysis in patients treated with high doses and/or for long periods of time due to the presence of isoagglutinins (anti-A and anti-B) in the product. Inhibitors to VWF are rare, but have been reported in patients with type 3 VWD.

Cryoprecipiate

Cryoprecipitate is a nonvirally inactivated (though viral screened) blood product that contains VWF, FVIII, fibrinogen and FXIII. In patients with VWD, it should only be used if DDAVP is insufficient and VWF concentrates are not available. Cryoprecipitate is dosed at 1 unit per 5–10 kg body weight and should be infused over 10–30

Table 3. Suggested durations of VWF replacement for different types of surgical procedures

Major surgery 7–14 days*	Minor surgery 1–5 days*	Other procedures, if uncomplicated, single VWF treatment
Cardiothoracic	Biopsy: breast, cervical	Cardiac catheterization
Cesarean section	Complicated dental extractions	Cataract surgery
Craniotomy	Gingival surgery	Endoscopy (without biopsy)
Hysterectomy	Central line placement	Liver biopsy
Open cholecystectomy	Laparoscopic procedures	Lacerations
Prostatectomy		Simple dental extractions

* Individual cases may need longer or shorter duration depending on the severity of VWD and the type of procedure. From Nichols et al. [18].

min. In most developed countries, cryoprecipitate is no longer used routinely in the management of VWD due to the higher risk of transmission of infection.

Perioperative Management

Treatment of VWD prior to invasive procedures to prevent excessive perioperative blood loss is important. The management guidelines from the American National Heart, Lung and Blood Institute (NHLBI) suggest that all major procedures should be treated in institutions with access to 24-hour laboratory services and an expert clinical team whenever feasible [18]. Specific treatment plans should be based on laboratory testing of the response of VWF:RCo and FVIII activity levels to DDAVP or to VWF concentrate.

Depending on the extent of the invasive procedure and the patient's known response to DDAVP, either DDAVP or factor concentrates may be used. DDAVP should be given 1 h prior to dental/surgical intervention and can be given daily for several days afterwards. Factor concentrates are utilized when DDAVP response is inadequate or insufficient for the expected bleeding risk. General recommendations for dosing of VWF concentrates for surgery aim to raise FVIII and VWF to adequate levels to allow for perioperative hemostasis [18].

More specific recommendations for perioperative management are illustrated in tables 3 and 4. In general, for prophylaxis of major surgery, initial target VWF:RCo and FVIII activity levels should be at least 1.0 IU/ml. Subsequent dosing should maintain levels above a trough of 0.50 IU/ml for at least 7–10 days. VWF:RCo levels should not exceed 2.0 IU/ml, and FVIII:C levels should not exceed 2.5 IU/ml to decrease the risk of thrombosis. Common procedures in children not listed in the table 3 include tonsillectomy and circumcision. We suggest that these should be managed with 4–7 days of VWF replacement for tonsillectomy and a single VWF treatment for circumcision (a second dose postsurgery may be considered). In these scenarios the use of antifibrinolytics is strongly recommended.

Management of Menorrhagia in VWD

Management of menorrhagia can be considered in both the acute and chronic settings. This subject has recently been reviewed and a consensus guideline has been published by an international expert panel [19].

Acute menorrhagia in girls with VWD can be severe and may lead to severe, symptomatic anemia and the need for blood transfusion and hospitalization. Management of such cases ideally requires consultation from both gynecology and hematology services. Usually high-dose intravenous or oral estrogens are prescribed to control bleeding in conjunction with hemostatic therapies (0.3 μg/kg of DDAVP in girls responsive to DDAVP or VWF concentrates 50 VWF:RCo IU/kg in those who are insufficiently responsive to DDAVP) and intravenous tranexamic acid (10 mg/kg every 8 h).

Table 4. Initial dosing recommendations for VWF concentrate replacement for prevention or management of bleeding

Major surgery/bleeding	
Loading dose*	40–60 IU/kg
Maintenance dose	20–40 IU/kg every 8–24 h
Monitoring	frequent VWF:RCo and FVIII trough and peak levels
Therapeutic goal	trough VWF:RCo and FVIII >0.50 IU/ml for 7–14 days
Safety parameter	do not exceed VWF:RCo 2.0 IU/ml or FVIII 2.5–3.0 IU/ml
May alternate with DDAVP for latter part of treatment	
Minor surgery/bleeding	
Loading dose*	30–60 IU/kg
Maintenance dose	20–40 IU/kg every 12–48 h
Monitoring	VWF:RCo and FVIII trough and peak, at least once
Therapeutic goal	trough VWF:RCo and FVIII >0.5 IU/ml for 3–5 days
Safety parameter	do not exceed VWF:RCo 2.0 IU/ml or FVIII 2.5–3.0 IU/ml
May alternate with DDAVP for latter part of treatment	

* Dosing is in VWF:RCo International Units (IU) per kilogram body weight. From Nichols et al. [18].

Should these measures fail then gynecological surgical measures may be needed. Once bleeding is controlled, the patient is generally transitioned to combined oral contraceptive pills. Oral tranexamic acid (25 mg/kg/dose every 8 h) may be continued. Careful monitoring of the hemoglobin level is required. Ondansetron may be used to control nausea, if needed. In general, dilatation and curettage (D&C), endometrial ablation and hysterectomy are avoided in pediatric and adolescent patients.

For girls with chronic menorrhagia a number of options exist: (1) oral contraceptive pills, (2) antifibrinolytics such as tranexamic acid, and (3) DDAVP for those girls who respond to DDAVP. DDAVP responders may be treated with intranasal DDAVP alone or in combination with an antifibrinolytic agent or oral contraceptive pills. Combined oral contraceptive pills will also help to regulate menstrual cycles and decrease menstrual flow. The choice of pill should be tailored to the individual patient, considering side effects, such as weight gain. In the setting of anovulatory bleeding, higher doses of estrogen may be required. Finally, in situations where side effects from oral contraceptives are not tolerated or compliance is an issue, a levonorgestrel-releasing intrauterine device, such as Mirena® can be considered. These devices must be inserted by an experienced practitioner and adolescent girls may need sedation to facilitate insertion.

Prophylaxis in VWD

The issue of long-term prophylaxis for VWD is controversial. Studies suggest VWD prophylaxis to be safe and suggest benefit however definitive trials are lacking at this time.

Conclusion

VWD is a common bleeding disorder with a wide spectrum of clinical severity. Clinical suspicion is often based on patient history and/or family history of mucocutaneous bleeding. Laboratory investigations are needed to confirm the diagnosis and the specific subtype. Many therapies are available and treatment strategies must take into account the pathophysiology of the individual's VWD and its responsiveness to therapy as well as the expected severity of the bleed/bleeding challenge. The role for prophylaxis in VWD is still under study.

Acknowledgment

The authors would like to express their appreciation for the thoughtful comments provided by Drs. Paula James (Kingston, Ont., Canada), David Lillicrap (Kingston, Ont., Canada) and Rochelle Winikoff (Montreal, Que., Canada) who reviewed this chapter.

References

1 Bolton-Maggs PH, Lillicrap D, Goudemand J, Berntorp E: von Willebrand disease update: diagnostic and treatment dilemmas. Haemophilia 2008;14(suppl 3):56–61.
2 Lillicrap D: The basic science, diagnosis and clinical management of von Willebrand disease. Treatment of hemophilia (monograph). 2008;35. World Federation of Hemophilia, Montreal, Canada. Available online at: http://www1.wfh.org/publication/files/pdf-1180.pdf.
3 Sadler JE, Budde U, Eikenboom JC, Favaloro EJ, Hill FG, Holmberg L, et al: Update on the pathophysiology and classification of von Willebrand disease: a report of the subcommittee on von Willebrand factor. J Thromb Haemost 2006;4:2103–2114.
4 Bowman M, Riddel J, Rand ML, Tosetto A, Silva M, James PD: Evaluation of the diagnostic utility for von Willebrand disease of a pediatric bleeding questionnaire. J Thromb Haemost 2009;7:1418–1421.
5 Carcao MD, Blanchette VS, Dean JA, He L, Kern MA, Stain AM, et al: The platelet function analyzer (PFA-100®): a novel in-vitro system for evaluation of primary haemostasis in children. Br J Haematol 1998;101:70–73.
6 Dean JA, Blanchette VS, Carcao MD, Stain AM, Sparling CR, Siekmann J, et al: Von Willebrand disease in a paediatric-based population – comparison of type 1 diagnostic criteria and use of the PFA-100® and a von Willebrand factor/collagen-binding assay. Thromb Haemost 2000;84:401–409.
7 Jenkins PV, O'Donnell JS: ABO blood group determines plasma von willebrand factor levels: a biologic function after all? Transfusion 2006;46:1836–1844.
8 Abildgaard CF, Suzuki Z, Harrison J, Jefcoat K, Zimmerman TS: Serial studies in von Willebrand's disease: variability versus 'variants'. Blood 1980;56:712–716.
9 Dutt T, Burns S, Mackett N, Benfield C, Lwin R, Keenan R: Application of UKHCDO 2004 guidelines in type 1 von Willebrand disease – a single centre paediatric experience of the implications of altered or removed diagnosis. Haemophilia 2011;17:522–526.
10 Haberichter SL, Balistreri M, Christopherson P, Morateck P, Gavazova S, Bellissimo DB, et al: Assay of the von Willebrand factor (VWF) propeptide to identify patients with type 1 von Willebrand disease with decreased VWF survival. Blood 2006;108:3344–3351.
11 Robertson JD, Yenson PR, Rand ML, Blanchette VS, Carcao MD, Notley C, et al: Expanded phenotype-genotype correlations in a pediatric population with type 1 von Willebrand disease. J Thromb Haemost 2011;9:1752–1760.
12 James P, Lillicrap D: The role of molecular genetics in diagnosing von Willebrand disease. Semin Thromb Hemost 2008;34:502–508.
13 Carcao MD, Seary ME, Casas M, Winter L, Stain AM, Judd P: Dental disease in type 3 von Willebrand disease: a neglected problem. Haemophilia 2010;16:943–948.
14 Mannucci PM: Treatment of von Willebrand's disease. N Engl J Med 2004;351:683–694.
15 Rodeghiero F, Castaman G, Tosetto A: How I treat von Willebrand disease. Blood 2009;114:1158–1165.
16 Castaman G, Lethagen S, Federici AB, Tosetto A, Goodeve A, Budde U, et al: Response to desmopressin is influenced by the genotype and phenotype in type 1 von Willebrand disease (VWD): results from the European study MCMDM-1VWD. Blood 2008;111:3531–3539.
17 Mannucci PM, Bettega D, Cattaneo M: Patterns of development of tachyphylaxis in patients with haemophilia and von willebrand disease after repeated doses of desmopressin (DDAVP). Br J Haematol 1992;82:87–93.
18 Nichols WL, Hultin MB, James AH, Manco-Johnson MJ, Montgomery RR, Ortel TL, et al: von Willebrand disease (VWD): Evidence-based diagnosis and management guidelines, the national heart, lung, and blood institute (NHLBI) expert panel report (USA). Haemophilia 2008;14:171–232.
19 James AH, Kouides PA, Abdul-Kadir R, Dietrich JE, Edlund M, Federici AB, et al: Evaluation and management of acute menorrhagia in women with and without underlying bleeding disorders: consensus from an international expert panel. Eur J Obstet Gynecol Reprod Biol 2011;158:124–134.

Abbreviations

aPTT	Activated partial thromboplastin time
ASA	Acetylsalicyclic acid
DDAVP	1-Deamino-8-D-arginine vasopressin (desmopressin)
EACA	Epsilon-aminocaproic acid (Amicar)
ELISA	Enzyme-linked immunosorbent assay
FVIII	Factor VIII
FXIII	Factor XIII
FVIII:C	Factor VIII coagulant
GP	Glycoprotein
ICH	Intracranial hemorrhage
ISTH	International Society on Thrombosis and Haemostasis
IU	International unit
NSAIDs	Nonsteroidal anti-inflammatory drugs
PBQ	Pediatric Bleeding Questionnaire
PFA-100®	Platelet function analyzer-100
PRP	Platelet-rich plasma
RIPA	Ristocetin-induced platelet aggregation
VWD	von Willebrand disease
VWF	von Willebrand factor
VWF:Ag	VWF antigen
VWF:RCo	VWF activity (ristocetin cofactor assay)

Chapter 8: Rare Congenital Factor Deficiencies in Childhood

Frederico Xavier
Victor S. Blanchette

Introduction

Rare inherited coagulation disorders beyond FVIII and FIX deficiencies and VWD present clinical challenges in both diagnosis and management. These conditions have variable correlations between the circulating coagulation factor level and the clinical bleeding phenotype; in addition, due to the rarity of these disorders, clinical management guidelines are sparse or lacking depending on the condition. In this chapter, we review the clinical features, laboratory findings and treatment options for very rare congenital bleeding disorders including deficiencies in FV, FVII, FX, FXI, FXIII, fibrinogen, prothrombin and combined deficiencies of the vitamin K-dependent coagulation factors (table 1) [1–3]. The physiologic expected level for each coagulation factor must be considered when diagnosing these disorders, and results must be compared with age-matched normal ranges (appendix). An algorithm for diagnosis of coagulation disorders in children with bleeding symptoms is available in chapter 3. Recommendations for therapy will be made throughout this chapter according to published data and the authors' clinical experience for each deficiency. A general prescriptive hierarchy should be followed based upon the safety of replacement products with regard to blood-borne pathogens: recombinant products are the first choice for treatment, followed by pathogen-inactivated, plasma-derived concentrates. As a last choice due to a potential risk of transmission of a blood-borne pathogen, blood products such as FP or cryoprecipitate may be used and should be pathogen inactivated whenever possible.

Factor XI Deficiency

The major biological function of FXI is the activation of FIX (see chapter 2). Another function of FXI is sustaining thrombin generation initiated by the tissue factor/FVIIa complex. FXI is produced in the liver and circulates in the plasma

Table 1. Genetics, epidemiology and management options for rare congenital factor deficiencies

Factor	Estimated prevalence	Hemostatic level	Half-life of transfused factor	Factor replacement therapy
Prothrombin	extremely rare	20–30 IU/dl	3-4 days	PCCs; FP
FV	1:1,000,000	15–20 IU/dl	36 h	FP
FV + FVIII combined	1:1,000,000	as for individual factors	as for individual factors	FP + FVIII concentrate (chapter 6)
FVII	1:500,000	15–20 IU/dl	4–6 h	rFVIIa; plasma-derived, pathogen-inactivated FVII concentrates; PCCs; FP
FX	1:500,000	15–20 IU/dl	40–60 h	PCCs; FP
FXI	depends on ethnicity[1]	15–30 IU/dl	40–70 h	FP; plasma-derived, pathogen-inactivated FXI concentrates
FXIII	1:2,000,000	not known	11–14 days	rFXIII; plasma-derived, pathogen-inactivated FXIII concentrates; cryoprecipitate; FP

Fibrinogen
  Afibrinogenemia
  Hypofibrinogenemia
  Dysfibrinogenemia
	
	rare
	extremely rare
	rare
		50 g/dl	2–4 days	Plasma-derived, pathogen-inactivated fibrinogen concentrates; cryoprecipitate; FP

[1] Common in Ashkenazi Jews.

forming a complex with HMWK. FXI deficiency is a coagulopathy found predominantly, but not exclusively, in individuals of Ashkenazi Jewish descent with incidences as high as 8–9% in this population. There are two common mutations found in Ashkenazi Jewish populations (type II and type III); the type II mutation is prevalent in Iraqi Jews, who represent the ancient Jewish gene pool [4].

FXI deficiency is inherited as an autosomal trait with more than 200 different mutations described in the FXI gene, located on chromosome 4q35 (www.factorXI.org) [4]. Homozygotes or heterozygotes are identified by severe or partial deficiency of FXI coagulant levels, respectively; homozygotes generally have levels of <15% or <15 IU/dl, while heterozygotes have levels >15 but <70 IU/dl [5]. Bleeding symptoms are very heterogeneous. For the 125 subjects with FXI deficiency studied by the EN-RBD, FXI levels (IU/dl; 95% CI) for asymptomatic subjects and those with grade I, II, and III bleeding (table 2) were 26

Table 2. Assigned categories of clinical bleeding severity

Clinical bleeding severity	Definition
Asymptomatic	No documented bleeding episodes
Grade I bleeding	Bleeding that occurred after trauma or drug ingestion (antiplatelet or anticoagulant therapy)
Grade II bleeding	Spontaneous minor bleeding: bruising, ecchymosis, minor wounds, oral cavity bleeding, epistaxis and menorrhagia
Grade III bleeding	Spontaneous major bleeding: intramuscular hematomas requiring hospitalization, hemarthrosis, CNS, GI and umbilical cord bleeding

(14–39), 26 (13–38), 25 (11–39), and 25 (9–41), respectively [6]. Coagulation FXI activity level does not predict clinical bleeding severity [6]. In most families, levels <20 IU/dl are reported without excessive bleeding, while in others excessive bleeding may occur [4].

Clinical Presentation

FXI deficiency is generally associated with a mild bleeding tendency that most commonly manifests as delayed bleeding after injury, trauma, surgery, dental extractions and childbirth. Chronic epistaxis and menorrhagia may occur, whereas excessive bleeding from minor injury is unusual. Easy bruising is common. Spontaneous bleeding, except for menorrhagia, is rare even in patients with severe FXI deficiency (defined as FXI <10 IU/dl generally seen in individuals with two abnormal FXI genes) [2]. Bleeding is usually injury related particularly when it afflicts tissues containing activators of fibrinolysis, such as oral cavity, nose, oral-pharyngeal and urinary tract [4]. Bleeding is less common at other sites of trauma for example during orthopedic surgery, appendectomy, circumcision, or cutaneous lacerations. Some patients with very low FXI levels may not bleed following trauma, while others, exhibit variable bleeding over time even when provoked by similar hemostatic challenges. Bleeding, once it occurs, will persist until treated; bleeding may occur at the time of injury or several hours later.

Diagnosis

Patients with congenital FXI deficiency manifest an isolated prolongation of the aPTT. All patients with severe FXI deficiency exhibit an aPTT value >2 standard deviations above the normal mean [4]. Heterozygotes may have a slightly prolonged aPTT or values within the normal range. Confirmation of the disorder requires demonstration of reduced levels of coagulant FXI in a clotting assay on two or more occasions and absence of an alternative cause for the laboratory abnormality (e.g. liver disease, lupus anticoagulant, etc.). FXI antigen levels are necessary only in rare cases of a qualitative deficiency. Family studies are recommended to provide additional evidence of an inherited condition. Because severe FXI deficiency can remain asymptomatic until unmasked by an injury, it is essential for all those of Ashkenazi Jewish descent who require surgery to have an aPTT [4], and if prolonged, an FXI activity should be performed to rule out a deficiency state.

Management

Spontaneous bleeding, except menorrhagia, is rare in patients with severe FXI deficiency, and if it occurs, it usually abates without therapy. Oral antifibrinolytics are useful to ameliorate menorrhagia [4]. FXI replacement therapy is only necessary in individuals with clinically significant bleeding or as hemostatic coverage for major surgery. As FXI levels do not necessary correlate with the risk for bleeding, important aspects to be considered when assessing the need for treatment include personal and family history of bleeding, the severity of bleeding, individual event or planned procedure. Prior to planned surgery, several factors should be considered including deciding whether the procedure is clearly indicated, the type and site of surgery, the previous bleeding history, exclusion of other bleeding abnormalities (e.g. VWD) and cessation of antiplatelet agents and/or other NSAIDs, if utilized [7].

For high-risk surgical procedures associated with high levels of local fibrinolysis (e.g. neurosurgery, ophthalmic surgery, tonsillectomy/adenoidectomy and surgery of the genitourinary tract, prostatectomy and removal of molar/wisdom teeth) in patients with severe FXI deficiency, or for individuals with a prior history of significant clinical bleeding, pre- and postoperative replacement therapy should be given. Assessment of cardiac function in these patients is important as it may guide the selection of replacement product utilized; for example, FP has a larger volume compared to FXI concentrate. The risk of thrombosis when using FXI concentrate may also be related to poor cardiac function. Fibrin glue can be used as an adjunctive hemostatic agent. For urological procedures, flushing the bladder with tranexamic or aminocaproic acid-containing solutions can also be used. Factor replacement is not indicated for dental extraction and skin biopsies, but antifibrinolytic agents should be utilized [4]. Clinical management of difference scenarios in FXI deficiency is published [7].

The standard therapy for replacement of FXI is FP (20 ml/kg to start), and as discussed previously, this should be pathogen inactivated whenever possible; large volumes may be required in severely deficient patients. Additionally, plasma-derived FXI concentrates have been available since the 1980s; replacement therapy commonly aims to increase the circulating FXI level to approximately 45 IU/dl for 7 days (major surgery) or 30 IU/dl for 5 days (minor surgery; table 3). The plasma half-life of FXI is approximately 45 h; if prolonged coverage is required, bolus infusions should be given on alternate days in conjunction with monitoring peak and trough levels to adjust dosing amount and frequency. FXI replacement in patients at high risk for thromboembolic complications, such as the elderly, those with presence of cardiovascular diseases and other prothrombotic conditions, should be utilized with caution, as the literature demonstrates a 10% risk of arterial and venous thrombosis after replacement therapy in these patients [8].

Replacement therapy for patients with a history of an FXI inhibitor consists of the use of rFVIIa and/or antifibrinolytic agents during procedures and in the postoperative period according to the associated bleeding risk [4].

Factor VII Deficiency

Among the rare congenital bleeding disorders, FVII deficiency is the most frequent; the true incidence is difficult to determine due to either individuals with few to no clinical symptoms and mild deficiencies. The incidence of clinically significant FVII deficiency is estimated to be one per 500,000 births with no racial or ethnic group predilection. FVII deficiency exhibits a clinically variable bleeding pattern ranging from severe life-threatening or organ-specific hemorrhage, such as cerebral, GI, and hemarthrosis, to other minor bleeding symptoms [3, 9].

Clinical Presentation

The International Registry on Congenital FVII Deficiency reports a common discordance between the clinical bleeding phenotype and circulating FVII activity levels, more significant bleeding manifestations among females, and frequent surgery-related bleeding, which may often serve as the diagnostic trigger in previously asymptomatic individuals [3, 10]. Some authors suggest staging based on the patient's bleeding history as outlined in table 2 [6].

Diagnosis

FVII deficiency is characterized by an isolated prolongation of the PT; liver disease and vitamin K deficiency must be excluded. Rarely, cases of acquired FVII antibody/inhibitor are described. FVII inhibitors are detected via a 1:1 mixing study with normal plasma which demonstrates lack of correction. A FVII activity assay is commonly available and has been standardized to reduce the variability of inter-laboratory determinations particularly of low to very low plasma FVII levels. Molecular diagnosis is available, with a broad spectrum of mutations having been characterized in the FVII gene, located on chromosome 13. The International FVII Study Group website can be found at www.targetseven.org. Virtually all patients with moderate and severe disease have been found to be either homozygotes or double heterozygotes for a FVII mutation. Interestingly, phenotypic-genotype correlations are at times difficult to make as even patients homozygous for the same mutation do not always present with the same bleeding severity [10].

Management

As observed by the EN-RBD, patients with FVII deficiency with levels above 25 IU/dl remain asymptomatic [6]. Replacement therapy for patients with FVII deficiency should be individualized and is dependent on the bleeding history, severity of the deficiency, site of bleeding, type of

Table 3. Dosing and therapeutic target levels for the rare coagulation factor deficiency

Concentrate, trade name[1]	Dosing[2]

FXI
Hemoleven® (LFB, France), FXI Concentrate (BPL, UK)
	Dose (IU): desired % (IU/dl) FXI increase × kg BW/2
	Therapeutic target:
	    Major surgery: ~45 IU/dl for 7 days
	    Minor surgery: ~30 IU/dl for 5 days

FVII concentrate Provertin-Um TIM 3® (Baxter), Hemofactor® HT (Grifols)	Hemarthrosis: 10 IU/kg BW Surgery: 30–40 IU/kg BW every 4–6 h for up to 10 days Alternatively 30–40 IU/kg BW twice per day
rFVIIa, Novoseven® (Novo Nordisk)	Surgery or bleeding: 15–30 µg/kg BW every 4–6 h until hemostasis is achieved (dosing for hemophilia patients with inhibitors is detailed in chapter 6)

Fibrinogen
RiaSTAP® (CSL Behring), Haemocomplettan® P (CSL Behring)
	When baseline fibrinogen level is known:
	Dose (mg/kg BW): [Target level (mg/dl) – measured level (mg/dl)]/1.7 (g/dl per mg/kg BW); for example: target level 100 mg/dl, measured level 20 mg/dl, BW 20 kg; dose: (100 – 20 mg/dl)/1.7 = 47.1 mg/kg BW; 47.1 × 20 kg BW = 942 mg
	When baseline fibrinogen level is not known:
	    Initial dose: 70 mg/kg BW
	    Maintenance dose: 50 mg/kg BW
	Therapeutic target:
	    Major bleeding: Target plasma fibrinogen level of 150 mg/dl for 7 days
	    Minor bleeding: Target plasma fibrinogen level of 100 mg/dl for 5 days

FXIII
Fibrogammin® (CSL Behring), Corifact® (CSL Behring)
	Fibrogamin-P:
	Prophylaxis: 10 IU/kg BW, approximately once a month. Should be guided by the most recent trough FXIII activity level to maintain a trough FXIII activity level of approximately 5–20 IU/dl. The interval should be shortened if spontaneous hemorrhage develops.
	Surgery: up to 35 IU/kg BW to obtain normal FXIII levels. Required efficacy should be maintained by repeated injection until the wound has healed completely.
	Therapy: 10–20 IU/kg BW. Daily for severe hemorrhage and extensive hematoma until bleeding has stopped.
	Corifact:
	    Prophylaxis: Initial dose: 40 IU/kg BW. Subsequent dosing should be guided by the most recent trough FXIII activity, to maintain a trough FXIII activity level of approximately 5–20 IU/dl.
	    No controlled trials demonstrating a direct benefit of treatment of bleeding episodes with Cortifact.

rFXIII (Catridecacog®, Novo Nordisk)	Prophylaxis: 35 IU/kg BW (currently approved in Europe for patients over 6 years of age)
PCCs	For treatment and/or prevention of bleeding in patients with congenital FII, FVII, FX and familial vitamin K deficiency. The recommended dose of PCCs depends on the amount of each factor in the specific product. It should be emphasized that not only is there a marked difference in factor content between the different commercial preparations, but factor content can also vary between product lots produced by the same manufacturer. (Note: Some PCCs do not contain an acceptable concentration of FVII for clinical use in patients with FVII deficiency.)

[1] The trade name list is <u>not</u> complete. Readers should refer to the local reference for products available in their country.
[2] In general, dosing regimen should be individualized based on body weight (BW), laboratory values and the patient's clinical condition.

intervention required (i.e. major or minor surgery) and presence of comorbidities [11]. When treatment is required, safety of replacement products specifically in terms of viral transmission risk should be considered.

rFVIIa is the treatment of choice, but certain features, such as the short in vivo half-life and the increased clearance in young children, influence the treatment plan. The recommended dose is 15–30 µg/kg every 4–6 h; it is important to note that these doses are significantly lower than those used in hemophilia patients with inhibitors. A recent report from the International FVII Study Group demonstrated the safety and efficacy of rFVIIa for surgical prophylaxis, provided that minimally effective doses are used [11]. Only patients with a FVII activity <20 IU/ml were included in this analysis. The minimally effective dose, calculated with respect to the time period for the highest risk for bleeding (the operative day), was estimated to be 13 μg/kg followed by at least two more administrations per day, especially for patients who underwent major surgical procedures. For those undergoing endoscopic procedures with biopsies, catheter insertions or single dental extractions, FVII replacement for a 24-hour period was found to be safe and effective (average total dose of rFVIIa of 20 μg/kg, possibly divided into more than one administration) [12].

If rFVIIa is not available, other alternatives exist and include plasma-derived, pathogen-inactivated FVII concentrates, PCCs containing FVII and FP (table 3). Thrombotic episodes (particularly DVT) have been reported in 3–4% of patients with FVII deficiency, particularly in those requiring surgery and replacement treatment, but 'spontaneous' thrombosis may occur as well [13]. Plasma-derived, pathogen-inactivated FVII concentrate is effective and may be favored over rFVIIa because of a longer half-life and use of a non-activated zymogen; however, a low risk of the transmission of blood-borne agents may still exist, dependent upon the specific viral inactivation processes utilized. Both plasma-derived FVII concentrate and PCCs contain other vitamin K-dependent factors in higher concentration than FVII, potentially increasing the risk for thrombosis [10]. FP, 10–15 ml/kg, continues to be used in developing countries, the most significant associated difficulties being blood volume overload, inability to achieve and maintain hemostatic levels, and a relatively high risk for transmission of blood-borne infections.

Prophylaxis has not been infrequently utilized in FVII-deficient patients; it is mainly used in toddlers prone to severe and frequent bleeding or those with a significant bleeding history such as those with recurrent hemarthroses or other chronic recalcitrant bleeding symptoms unresponsive to usual therapy such as clinically significant epistaxis [9]. Another indication for prophylactic use of replacement of FVII is in females with menorrhagia when antifibrinolytic and hormonal therapies fail to control bleeding (rFVIIa 15–30 μg/kg every 4–6 h). Standard management of women with FVII deficiency during pregnancy is not well established with a range of treatment options reported including use of FP, rFVIIa for labor and delivery, and tranexamic acid for the peripartum period [14].

Monitoring of replacement treatment in FVII deficiency is achieved via the FVII activity assay. Routine bedside monitoring may be accomplished with the PT in some cases as its normalization approximately correlates with hemostatic levels. FVII levels of approximately 50% are associated with the 'normal' PT range [10].

With appropriate management, FVII deficiency is associated with a good prognosis and a life expectancy similar to that of normal individuals. For 203 subjects with FVII deficiency studied by the EN-RBD, FVII levels (IU/dl; 95% CI) for asymptomatic subjects and those with grade I, II, and III bleeding (table 2) were 25 (15–35), 19 (8–30), 13 (2–25), and 8 (0–21), respectively [6].

Fibrinogen Disorders

Fibrinogen is a dimeric, soluble molecule, composed of three pairs of polypeptide chains; it is the precursor of insoluble fibrin that is required for the formation of the hemostatic plug in conjunction with platelets (chapter 2). In vivo, thrombin catalyzes the conversion of fibrinogen to fibrin. Other fibrinogen functions include platelet aggregation, native thrombin sink, and fibrinolysis. Its multitude of functions explains the variety of symptoms from bleeding to thrombotic phenotypes seen with some fibrinogen disorders [15].

The normal plasma fibrinogen concentration is approximately 150–400 mg/dl. Fibrinogen is produced in the liver, and its production may be increased up to 20-fold designating it as an acute-phase reactant. It has a half-life of approximately 4 days. Fibrinogen disorders can be divided accordingly to fibrinogen quantity (afibrinogenemia and hypofibrinogenemia), activity (dysfibrinogenemia) or both (hypodysfibrinogenemia). Quantitative fibrinogen deficiencies are the result of mutations affecting fibrinogen synthesis or processing, while qualitative defects are caused by mutations leading to abnormal polymerization, cross-linking or assembly of the fibrinolytic system. The pattern of inheritance varies according to the defect involved. A list of mutations can be found at: www.geht.org/databaseang/fibrinogen. The fibrinogen locus comprises three genes coding for fibrinogen-γ, -α and -β, clustered in a region of approximately 50 kb on the long arm of chromosome 4q23-q32. For the 26 subjects with a fibrinogen deficiency reported by the EN-RBD, fibrinogen levels (mg/dl; 95% CI) for asymptomatic subjects and those with grade I, II, and III (table 2) bleeding were 113 (23–204), 73 (0–164), 33 (0–126), and zero (0–91), respectively [6]. A strong association was observed between clinical bleeding severity and fibrinogen level [6].

Afibrinogenemia

Afibrinogenemia is a rare congenital bleeding disorder transmitted as an autosomal recessive trait with variable penetrance. Its incidence is estimated to be 1 in 1,000,000 births with a higher incidence in consanguineous marriages. Most cases are double-heterozygous, resulting in a hypofibrinogenemic state with clinical symptoms manifesting with levels below 100 mg/dl [6]. Afibrinogenemia is diagnosed when the circulating fibrinogen level is undetectable.

Patients may be diagnosed early in life because of prolonged bleeding from the umbilical stump. However, the diagnosis may be delayed, occurring only following a significant hemostatic challenge such as surgery or trauma. According to multiple international registries (Iran, Italy and North American Registries) the most common bleeding presentations are umbilical stump bleeding (~85% of cases) followed by skin and musculoskeletal bleeds. Other systems may also be affected, and patients may experience hemorrhage in the GI and genitourinary tracts as well as antepartum, postpartum hemorrhage and first-trimester abortion. These registries also document ICH as a major cause of death. TEs may occur both prior to and after fibrinogen replacement therapy in such patients and, therefore, close observation and monitoring are strongly recommended.

Hypofibrinogenemia

Inheritance is autosomal, and patients are usually heterozygous for fibrinogen mutations with fibrinogen levels ~50 mg/dl. Patients frequently have a mild bleeding phenotype or are asymptomatic. Typically, diagnosis is delayed, occurring only following a significant hemostatic challenge such as surgery or injury. Among bleeding symptoms, menorrhagia and intramuscular hemorrhage are most common, followed by GI bleeding.

Dysfibrinogenemia

Patients with dysfibrinogenemia can present clinically as either a hemorrhagic or thrombotic disorder. The inheritance pattern is autosomal dominant. The ISTH Registry reports postpartum thrombosis, spontaneous abortions and stillbirths in its database associated with dysfibrinogenemia [15]. An abnormal fibrinogen may result in thrombosis due to its incapacity to bind to thrombin, resulting in accumulation of thrombin, leading to the development of an abnormal fibrin sheath resistant to plasmin, or due to its abnormal binding to platelets.

Diagnosis

Global screening tests, such as PT, aPTT, and TT in patients with hypo-/afibrinogenemia all require the production of a fibrin clot as an end point, and therefore will be prolonged in patients with hypofibrinogenemia or afibrinogenemia. The diagnosis of afibrinogenemia is established by demonstrating trace or absent plasma immunoreactive fibrinogen.

Initial screening tests for dysfibrinogenemia should include the fibrinogen concentration, as determined by both immunologic (antigenic) and clotting methods ('clottable' fibrinogen), TT and reptilase time. In dysfibrinogenemias, levels of functional fibrinogen (i.e. clottable fibrinogen) are usually low or normal, but the total fibrinogen concentration is usually normal or elevated when measured immunologically (e.g. ELISA; a ratio of 1:2 between the assays is confirmatory for dysfibrinogenemia). A specific prothrombotic condition of dysfibrinogenemia, fibrinogen Oslo I, is characterized by normal/shorter TT due to its increased capacity to bind to stimulated platelets. Molecular and genetic tests remain largely limited to research institutions [16].

Management

There are three options for treating disorders of fibrinogen: fibrinogen concentrates, cryoprecipitate and FP. Hemostatic levels are achieved once fibrinogen activity levels reach 100–150 mg/dl [17]. Plasma-derived fibrinogen concentrates exhibit a decreased risk of transfusion-transmitted infections relative to FP and require a decreased infusion volume to achieve a hemostatic level. For fibrinogen concentrates, the initial pediatric dose is 70 mg/kg and 50 mg/kg for maintenance, wound healing, or prophylaxis (table 3). Adult dosage is 8–10 g as loading and 3–4 g (approximately 50 mg/kg) every 2–4 days as maintenance [18]. Doses are targeted to achieve a fibrinogen activity level at 100 mg/dl (pediatric patients with life-threatening hemorrhage may require 200 mg/kg initially), and continuous infusions have also been described [19].

If fibrinogen concentrate is unavailable, cryoprecipitate can be used. One unit of cryoprecipitate from a single donor contains 200–300 mg of fibrinogen. The pediatric dose is 1 unit of cryoprecipitate per 5–10 kg body weight to raise the fibrinogen concentration by 50–100 mg/dl. FP can also be used at a dose of 10–15 ml/kg and should be pathogen inactivated if available.

The plasma half-life of fibrinogen is ~3–4 days, thereby allowing every other day replacement therapy. For prophylactic replacement in cases of recurrent bleeding in important sites, weekly infusions should be considered. For pregnancy, fibrinogen levels should be maintained at or above 50 mg/dl during the first and second trimesters, at or above 100 mg/dl in the late third trimester and at or above 150 mg/dl during labor and delivery [19]. The risk of TEs associated with afibrinogenemia and fibrinogen replacement therapy should be kept in mind when caring for patients with fibrinogen defects.

Factor XIII Deficiency

FXIII plays a pivotal role in coagulation through covalent linkage of fibrin to α_2-plasmin inhibitor creating a fibrin web resistant to fibrinolysis via plasmin. FXIII circulates in plasma as a tetrameric molecule (FXIII-A2B2) composed of two potentially active A subunits (FXIII-A) and two B subunits (FXIII-B) [20]. FXIII deficiency results in unstable clot formation with dissolution 24–48 h after initial formation due to weak fibrin crosslinking.

FXIII deficiency is transmitted as an autosomal recessive trait, and severe patients have either homozygous or compound heterozygous mutations. FXIII-A deficiency has an incidence of 1:2,000,000 births, and severe FXIII-B deficiency has only been documented in 4 cases to date [21]. FXIII-A deficiency is divided into type I (quantitative defect) as a result of a production defect, and type II (qualitative defect) which results from a normal or near normal concentration of functionally defective subunit A.

Initial symptoms may occur early in life including ICH and/or umbilical stump hemorrhage or abnormal healing. Delayed and repeated bleeding from superficial wounds is common. FXIII also plays a role in angiogenesis, thereby providing the pathophysiologic explanation for observed poor wound healing and recurrent spontaneous miscarriages. Individuals who carry one abnormal gene (heterozygous) are as yet uncharacterized due to the lack of large population-based studies. According to the ISTH, FXIII deficiency may represent the most commonly underdiagnosed rare congenital bleeding disorder [22].

Clinical Presentation

FXIII deficiency may be suspected in neonates with ICH and/or prolonged bleeding or poor healing from the umbilical stump. Due to the autosomal recessive nature of the condition, it is not uncommon for the child to be the product of a consanguineous marriage. Other presentations may include delayed bleeding after surgery or trauma (a typical history would be a patient that has to return several times to a dental clinic for bleeding after a dental extraction), recurrent spontaneous miscarriages and ICH. ICH can reach incidences as high as 25–30% in some registries, and is the main cause of death and disability among patients with this condition. For the 33 subjects with FXIII deficiency studied by the EN-RBD, FXIII levels (IU/dl; 95% CI) for asymptomatic subjects and those with grade I, II, and III bleeding (table 2) were 31 (11–51), 17 (0–37), 3 (0–24), and zero (0–11), respectively. A strong association was found between clinical bleeding severity and FXIII coagulation factor level [6].

Diagnosis

Standard screening tests of coagulation including the PT, aPTT, TT and fibrinogen level are all normal even in cases of severe FXIII deficiency. Historically, the urea clot solubility test was used to screen for FXIII deficiency but as it is only sensitive to severe deficiencies (<5 IU/dl), the test is no longer recommended [21].

The ISTH recommends that the following algorithm should be used for diagnosis of FXIII deficiency [21]:

– An initial screen using a quantitative functional FXIII activity assay (measurement of ammonia release during transglutaminase and/or measurement of labeled amine incorporated to a protein substrate).
– After a positive screening test, proceed with the measurement of plasma FXIII-A_2B_2 antigen.
  • If FXIII-A_2B_2 antigen is decreased: measure FXIII-A antigen (including platelet FXIII-A) and FXIII-B antigen. Also perform binding studies with FXIII-A and FXIII-B to exclude non-neutralizing autoantibodies.
  • If FXIII-A_2B_2 antigen is normal: suspect FXIII-A deficiency type II or exclude a neutralizing antibody against FXIII-A using mixing studies.
– Additional studies: evaluation of fibrin cross-linkings by SDS PAGE analysis; molecular genetic tests.

Management

The clinical severity of FXIII deficiency requires treatment with regular prophylaxis from the time of diagnosis for all patients with severe disease (<1 IU/dl) and for all symptomatic patients regardless of severity [2]. Regular prophylaxis is feasible as effective hemostatic levels of FXIII may be as low as 2–5 IU/dl, and the plasma half-life is 11–14 days. Accordingly, replacement material can be infused at intervals as long as every 20–30 days.

Three types of FXIII-containing products are available: FP, cryoprecipitate, and pasteurized plasma concentrates (Fibrogammin®-P, CSL Behring UK, Ltd., also known as Corifact®, CSL Behring LLC, Kankakee, Ill., USA). The pasteurized concentrate, when available, is preferred to FP and cryoprecipitate. The recommended dosages for Corifact®/Fibrogammin®-P are detailed in table 3. The FXIII concentrate half-life is 11–14 days. If pasteurized plasma concentrate is unavailable, the recommended dose for FXIII replacement (every 20-30 days) is 15–20 ml/kg for FP, or 1 unit of cryoprecipitate per 10 kg. For acute bleeding episode, a single dose of FP of 2–3 ml/kg can be sufficient to raise the FXIII level to >5 IU/dl, often adequate to achieve initial hemostasis.

Severe FXIII-deficient women require prophylactic replacement therapy during pregnancy to prevent spontaneous abortion and miscarriage. Optimal dosing of FXIII in this clinical situation has not yet been standardized. The goal is to maintain FXIII levels above 10 IU/dl. One study suggested infusions of Fibrogammin®-P 250 IU weekly before 23 weeks gestation, and subsequently 500 IU weekly [23]. The same study recommended achieving FXIII levels above 30 IU/dl during labor, achieved with a 'bolus' of 1,000 IU just prior to initiation of labor.

Recently, a new rFXIII product developed by Novo Nordisk, known as Catridecacog® has been approved for prophylactic FXIII replacement therapy in Europe and Canada. Catridecacog® is identical in structure and function to the human FXIII-A subunit. Catridecacog® is indicated for use in patients over 6 years of age or >20 kg with FXIII-A subunit deficiency, and is administered as a monthly i.v. infusion of 35 IU/kg [24]. Transient, non-neutralizing, low-titer anti rFXIII antibodies developed in 4/41 patients, none of whom experienced allergic reaction, bleeding episodes requiring treatment, or changes in FXIII pharmacokinetics. Once rFXIII is widely available, it may become standard therapy for FXIII replacement due to its manufacture through recombinant technology. This product is not indicated in the rare patients with FXIII-subunit deficiency.

Other Rare Inherited Coagulation Disorders

Factor V Deficiency

FV deficiency is inherited in an autosomal recessive manner with a prevalence of ~1 in 1 million births [25]. The bleeding phenotype of FV deficiency is variable; heterozygotes are often asymptomatic, whereas homozygotes and compound heterozygotes exhibit bleeding symptoms ranging from mild to severe. For the 50 subjects with FV deficiency studied by the EN-RBD, FV levels (IU/dl; 95% CI) for asymptomatic subjects and those with grade I, II, and III bleeding (table 2) were 12 (0–34), 6 (0–28), zero (0–23), and zero (0–19), respectively [6]. A poor association was found between FV activity level and clinical bleeding severity [6]. This lack of correlation may result from the availability of small amounts of FV in platelets in some patients with congenital FV deficiency; in addition, reduced plasma levels of total and free tissue factor pathway inhibitor antigen decreases the FV requirement for minimal thrombin generation in FV-deficient plasmas to <1 IU/dl [6]. The majority of severe cases are characterized by an extremely low FV activity and antigen levels (<1 IU/dl).

Clinical Features

FV-deficient patients are likely to present with clinical bleeding at an early age from sites including skin and mucosal surfaces. Cases with very low FV levels are at risk for hemophilic-like bleeding into joints, muscles and the CNS. Due to the small number of patients reported, an improved clinical characterization of the deficiency is needed.

Diagnosis

Screening laboratory tests reveal a prolongation of the PT and aPTT, with a normal TT. Measurement of FV activity or antigen is required for confirmation after excluding other causes of factor deficiencies including liver disease or acquired antibodies to coagulation factors such as with lupus anticoagulants or specific factor inhibitors with mixing studies required.

Management

For mild episodes of bleeding, antifibrinolytic agents (tranexamic acid or aminocaproic acid) may be sufficient. For severe bleeding episodes or preventive treatment prior to high-risk medical interventions, FP should be administered to achieve FV levels to or above 20 IU/dl activity (FP transfusion of 15–20 ml/kg). Standard protocols recommend loading doses of 20 ml/kg of FP prior to surgery and maintenance with 15–20 ml/kg every 24 h until recovery [25]. The half-life of FV ranges from 12 to 36 h.

Combined FV and FVIII Deficiency

Combined FV and FVIII deficiency is an extremely rare condition (1:2,000,000 births) and unique among rare bleeding disorders as the condition results from an abnormality in the FV and FVIII intracellular transport pathway due to defects in proteins, specifically LMAN1 and MCFD2, which are encoded by two different genes found on chromosome 18q21 and chromosome 2p21, respectively [26]. This rare condition is more common (1:1,000,000) in Mediterranean countries and individuals of Middle Eastern Jewish descent.

Clinical Features

A mild to moderate bleeding phenotype usually corresponds with activity levels below 25 IU/dl and manifests as easy bruising, gingival bleeding and epistaxis, or bleeding after surgery, dental extraction or trauma; menorrhagia and postpartum hemorrhage are also described. Severe cases usually manifest with activity levels below 15 IU/dl [6]. For the 18 subjects with combined deficiencies of FV and FVIII studied by the EN-RBD, factor levels (IU/dl; 95% CI) for asymptomatic subjects and those with grade I, II, and III bleeding (table 2) were 43 (25–62), 34 (16–52), 24 (5–44), and 15 (0–37), respectively [6]. The most commonly reported clinical symptom other than excessive bleeding after invasive procedures is mucosal bleeding. Hemarthroses, typical in hemophilia A, occur in less than one third of these patients.

Diagnosis

Screening coagulation tests reveal a prolongation of both the PT and aPTT. Specific factor analyses reveal decreased FV and FVIII levels of approximately 5–20 IU/dl.

Management

Treatment is dependent on the level of each factor, the type of bleeding episode or required procedure [26]. Treatment of bleeding episodes requires a source of both FV and FVIII; replacement of FV is achieved through use of FP (see above) with replacement of FVIII through the use of FP, desmopressin (DDAVP) or FVIII concentrates (recombinant or plasma-derived FVIII products; see chapter 6 for details). Due to the shorter half-life of FVIII relative to FV (table 1), FP should be not be administered to maintain the FVIII level, as it may lead to volume overload. Therefore, for major bleeding events and surgical procedures, replacement of FVIII should be guided by protocols utilized for hemophilia A treatment, whereas FV replacement should be administered as FP every 12 h, targeting a minimal activity level of 25 IU/dl [26].

Prothrombin Deficiency

Prothrombin (FII) deficiency is among the rarest of all bleeding disorders, occurring in approximately 1 in 1–2 million births. Prothrombin is a vitamin K-dependent glycoprotein whose activated form is thrombin, a pivotal enzyme responsible for cleaving fibrinogen to fibrin, and subsequently contributing to the formation of a stable fibrin clot. Patients with activity levels ~20–40 IU/dl are without clinical bleeding symptoms. Prothrombin has a half-life of approximately 3 days. The inheritance of prothrombin deficiency is autosomal recessive; the gene resides on chromosome 11p11.2 with more than 40 mutations having been described. Hypoprothrombinemia and dysprothrombinemia have been reported [27].

Clinical Features

Symptoms usually correlate with the level of the functional protein. Patients who are homozygous or compound heterozygous may present with moderate to severe bleeding symptoms as early as the neonatal period. The most common manifestations include easy bruising, gingival bleeding, menorrhagia, epistaxis or bleeding after surgery, dental extraction, or postpartum hemorrhage. Hemarthroses, umbilical cord bleeding, and ICH are also described in severe cases.

Diagnosis

Low prothrombin activity typically prolongs both the aPTT and PT. Functional and antigenic assays are required for diagnosis (hypo- and dysprothrombinemia).

Management

No purified prothrombin concentrates are available, making PCCs and FP the mainstay of treatment. Severe bleeding episodes can be treated with FP at 15–20 ml/kg, which should result in an increase in prothrombin levels by 25 IU/dl. For prophylaxis in high-risk surgical interventions, a loading dose of 15–20 ml/kg of FP followed by 3–6 ml/kg every 12–24 h may be adequate for hemostasis. PCCs are the preferred option when volume overload is a concern (table 3). The minimal hemostatic level is somewhat higher for prothrombin (20–30 IU/dl) than for most other rare inherited congenital disorders (15–20 IU/dl) [27]. For mild bleeding episodes, antifibrinolytic agents (tranexamic acid or aminocaproic acid) may be used.

Factor X Deficiency

FX is a vitamin K-dependent glycoprotein synthesized in the liver. FX is the initial common pathway enzyme. FX deficiency is inherited as an autosomal recessive condition estimated to occur in 1:1,000,000 births with up to 1:500 people being carriers. The majority of reported genetic alternations are missense mutations, duplications and partial deletions, with most patients usually compound heterozygous; homozygous defects are more prevalent in offspring of consanguineous marriage [28]. Internationally, efforts are being made to identify those genotypes associated with ICH to standardize prophylactic therapy for specific mutations.

Clinical Features

FX deficiency results in a variable bleeding tendency; patients with severe deficiency (<1 IU/dl) tend to experience the most severe symptoms of the rare coagulation disorders, similar to those observed with FVIII and FIX deficiency. Severe clinical symptoms including ICH, GI bleeding and hemarthrosis, are uncommon in patients with FX levels >2 IU/dl. Patients with 1–5 IU/dl activity are considered moderate with regard to their bleeding symptoms, 6–10 IU/dl are mild, and levels above 20 IU/dl are infrequently associated with clinical bleeding. Patients with severe FX deficiency may present in the neonatal period with bleeding with circumcision, umbilical stump separation most commonly at 7–14 days, ICH or GI bleeding. Moderately affected patients may be recognized only after hemostatic challenge, such as surgery, trauma or menses. Mild FX deficiency may be diagnosed during routine screening or due to a known family history. For the 34 subjects with FX deficiency studied by the EN-RBD, FX levels (IU/dl; 95% CI) for asymptomatic subjects and those with grade I, II, and III bleeding (table 2) were 56 (29–83), 40 (14–67), 25 (0–52), and 10 (0–39), respectively [6].

Diagnosis

Screening tests reveal prolongation of both the PT and aPTT that correct with 1:1 mixing with normal plasma. For final diagnosis, liver disease and vitamin K deficiency must be excluded. Diagnostic tests for FX deficiency include immunological or functional assays. Two sub-classifications exist: type

I and type II. Type I deficiency is characterized by proportionally low functional activity and antigen levels. Type II deficiency consist of a dysfunctional FX protein characterized by a near-normal level of the antigenic level with a disproportionally reduced functional activity [29].

Management

FX deficiency can be treated in a way similar to prothrombin deficiency, although the plasma half-life of FX of 40–60 h is shorter than that of prothrombin. A FX activity of 10–40 IU/dl is considered hemostatic. There is no licensed purified FX concentrate product available; one product is currently in clinical development. Treatment is based on blood-derived products containing FX such as the above-mentioned investigational product, PCCs and FP. Daily infusions of PCCs or FP (15–20 ml/kg) are necessary when prolonged hemostatic coverage is required to maintain an FX level >20 IU/dl. Patients should be closely monitored to avoid FII, FVII, and FIX levels to accumulate above 150 IU/dl.

Familial Deficiency of Vitamin K-Dependent Clotting Factors

Hereditary combined deficiency of FII, FVII, FIX and FX is a very rare autosomal recessive bleeding disorder (1:2,000,000). The disorder also involves the vitamin K-dependent naturally occurring anticoagulants, proteins C, S and Z, in addition to the vitamin K-dependent bone proteins. This combined deficiency results from a defective carboxylation step in the vitamin K-dependent factors due to mutated genes responsible for encoding either of two enzymes involved in this process: GGCX and VKOR complex. This condition is reported in less than 30 families worldwide. The diagnosis should be considered only after other more common causes of combined vitamin K deficiency such as liver disease, vitamin K antagonist (i.e. warfarin) overdose, and malabsorption (inflammatory bowel disease or celiac disease) have been ruled out (see chapter 9).

Clinical Features

Vitamin K-dependent clotting factor deficiency was first described in 1966 in a 3-month-old girl with multiple episodes of spontaneous bleeding and easy bruising. Patients may exhibit a severe bleeding phenotype that includes early ICH identical to that observed in hemorrhagic disease of the newborn period prior to routine vitamin K prophylaxis. Some cases also are associated with dysmorphic features (warfarin embryopathy like), developmental delay, skeletal defects, osteoporosis and a high incidence of miscarriages. The severity of symptoms may be affected by diet, gut microflora and genetic penetrance of the mutation. Anecdotal cases of thrombosis likely due to associated deficiencies of proteins C and S, are reported.

Diagnosis

After excluding other causes of vitamin K deficiency, genotyping of VKOR complex and GGCX is strongly recommended. A vitamin K assay, if available, may be useful; however, final diagnosis requires genetic confirmation. Screening laboratory tests reveal a prolonged PT and aPTT.

Management

Administration of large doses of vitamin K is the current standard of care; however, bleeding symptoms may still be observed. Administration of an oral dose of 10 mg twice or three times per week usually avoids frequent mucocutaneous bleeding [30]. Alternatively, if not tolerated orally, the same dose of vitamin K may be regularly administered intravenously at intervals which are based on PT-INR values. Despite the generally acknowledged efficacy of vitamin K, a fixed therapeutic schedule does not exist. Sequential transfusions of PCCs would be the treatment of choice during bleeding events (table 3). Standardized treatment for vitamin K-dependent clotting factor deficiency is not available, and current therapeutic schedules are derived from the reversal of vitamin K agonists, with a suggested dose of 500 IU given intravenously (median 8.8 IU/kg) for an INR below 5. The risk of thrombosis must be considered [30]. If PCCs are not available, FP (15–20 ml/kg) prior to medical interventions or to treat acute severe hemorrhagic episodes is recommended.

As rFVIIa and vitamin K have differing onset of actions (4 and 24 h, respectively), their combined use via simultaneous infusion may result in a sustained normalization of clotting times in cases of major bleeding, life-threatening bleeding episodes and more complex surgical procedures [30].

Plasminogen Activator Inhibitor Type 1 Deficiency

This condition was first identified in 1989; its true incidence is unknown due to the lack of sensitive/discriminatory PAI-1 activity assays [31]. PAI-1 deficiency usually manifests as a mild to moderate bleeding phenotype with rare spontaneous bleeding episodes. PAI-1 is involved in downregulation of the fibrinolytic pathway. The half-life of PAI-1 is short, ~10 min; it is encoded by a gene localized on chromosome 7q21.3-22.

Clinical Features

PAI-1 deficiency is most commonly manifested by delayed bleeding after hemostatic challenge including trauma, dental extraction, or an invasive medical intervention. Menorrhagia and abnormal bleeding in pregnancy may also occur.

Diagnosis

Diagnosis is challenging and requires a combination of the clinical history, laboratory evaluation, and at times a trial of antifibrinolytic therapy. Patients with PAI-1 activity assays <1 IU/dl in association with low antigen levels are most easily diagnosed, but those with dysfunctional proteins with normal antigens may be difficult. Diagnosis of PAI-1 deficiency should be pursued after other bleeding disorders including platelet function defects have been excluded [31].

Management

Therapy is mainly based on antifibrinolytic agents (aminocaproic or tranexamic acid) for prevention or control of bleeding. Menstruating females with menorrhagia may require initiation of antifibrinolytic agents a few days prior to the menstrual cycle [31].

Conclusion

Diagnosis and treatment of rare bleeding disorders represent significant challenges to the pediatric hematologist. Often, inadequate information exists for these disorders due to their rarity. The diagnosis of a rare bleeding disorder should be considered in all children with unusual bleeding symptoms, and urgent diagnosis is required to institute appropriate care. Pediatricians caring for populations where consanguinity is common should have heightened awareness of these disorders. Neonatal ICH is one of the most severe bleeding events associated with a significant risk of morbidity and mortality and requires emergent evaluation, diagnosis and treatment in these populations; the most common disorders in this clinical situation to consider include but are not limited to FXIII, FVII, FX deficiencies and afibrinogenemia. Management for each specific deficiency is outlined above and includes involvement of a pediatric hematologist knowledgeable in this field. It is important to consider a complete coagulation evaluation in offspring of consanguineous unions. Particular issues are observed in females with rare bleeding disorders due to menstruation, pregnancy, and childbirth, and require careful management in conjunction with an obstetrician/gynecologist.

Acknowledgment

The authors would like to express their appreciation for the thoughtful comments provided by Drs. Paula Bolton-Maggs (Manchester, UK) and Amy Shapiro (Indianapolis, Ind., USA) who reviewed this chapter.

References

1 Blanchette VD, Dean J, Lillicrap D: Rare Congenital Hemorrhagic Disorders; in Lillyman J, Hann I, Blanchette V: Coagulation Disorders. London, Churchill Livingstone, 1999.
2 Bolton-Maggs P: The rare inherited coagulation disorders (review). Pediatr Blood Cancer 2013;60(suppl 1):S37–S40.
3 Peyvandi F, Bolton-Maggs PH, Batorova A, De Moerloose P: Rare bleeding disorders. Haemophilia 2012;18(suppl 4):148–153.
4 Seligsohn U: Factor XI deficiency in humans. J Thromb Haemost 2009;7(suppl 1):84–87.
5 Emsley J, McEwan PA, Gailani D: Structure and function of factor XI. Blood 2010;115:2569–2577.
6 Peyvandi F, Palla R, Menegatti M, Siboni SM, et al: Coagulation factor activity and clinical bleeding severity in rare bleeding disorders: results from the European Network of Rare Bleeding Disorders. J Thromb Haemost 2012;10:615–621.
7 Bolton-Maggs PH: Factor XI deficiency – resolving the enigma? Hematology Am Soc Hematol Educ Program 2009:97–105.
8 Gomez K, Bolton-Maggs P: Factor XI deficiency. Haemophilia 2008;14:1183–1189.
9 Lapecorella M, Mariani G: Factor VII deficiency: defining the clinical picture and optimizing therapeutic options. Haemophilia 2008;14:1170–1175.
10 Mariani G, Bernardi F: Factor VII deficiency. Semin Thromb Hemost 2009;35:400–406.
11 Mariani G, Dolce A, Batorova A, Auerswald G, et al: Recombinant, activated factor VII for surgery in factor VII deficiency: a prospective evaluation – the surgical STER. Br J Haematol 2011;152:340–346.
12 Mariani G, Dolce A, Napolitano M, Ingerslev J, et al: Invasive procedures and minor surgery in factor VII deficiency. Haemophilia 2012;18:e63–e65.
13 Mariani G, Herrmann FH, Schulman S, Batorova A, et al: Thrombosis in inherited factor VII deficiency. J Thromb Haemost 2003; 1:2153–2158.
14 Kulkarni AA, Lee CA, Kadir RA: Pregnancy in women with congenital factor VII deficiency. Haemophilia 2006;12:413–416.
15 Acharya SS, Dimichele DM: Rare inherited disorders of fibrinogen. Haemophilia 2008;14:1151–1158.
16 de Moerloose P, Neerman-Arbez M: Congenital fibrinogen disorders. Semin Thromb Hemost 2009;35:356–366.
17 Sorensen B, Larsen OH, Rea CJ, Tang M, Foley JH, Fenger-Eriksen C: Fibrinogen as a hemostatic agent. Semin Thromb Hemost 2012;38:268–273.
18 Bornikova L, Peyvandi F, Allen G, Bernstein J, Manco-Johnson MJ: Fibrinogen replacement therapy for congenital fibrinogen deficiency. J Thromb Haemost 2011;9:1687–1704.
19 Mensah PK, Oppenheimer C, Watson C, Pavord S: Congenital afibrinogenaemia in pregnancy. Haemophilia 2011;17:167–168.
20 Hsieh L, Nugent D: Factor XIII deficiency. Haemophilia 2008;14: 1190–1200.
21 Kohler HP, Ichinose A, Seitz R, Ariens RA, Muszbek L, Factor XIII and Fibrinogen SSC Subcommittee of the ISTH: Diagnosis and classification of factor XIII deficiencies. J Thromb Haemost 2011;9:1404–1406.
22 Muszbek L, Bagoly Z, Cairo A, Peyvandi F: Novel aspects of factor XIII deficiency. Curr Opin Hematol 2011;18:366–372.
23 Asahina T, Kobayashi T, Takeuchi K, Kanayama N: Congenital blood coagulation factor XIII deficiency and successful deliveries: a review of the literature. Obstet Gynecol Surv 2007;62:255–260.
24 Inbal A, Oldenburg J, Carcao M, Rosholm A, Tehranchi R, Nugent D: Recombinant factor XIII: a safe and novel treatment for congenital factor XIII deficiency. Blood 2012;119:5111–5117.
25 Huang JN, Koerper MA: Factor V deficiency: a concise review. Haemophilia 2008;14:1164–1169.
26 Spreafico M, Peyvandi F: Combined factor V and factor VIII deficiency. Semin Thromb Hemost 2009;35:390–399.
27 Meeks SL, Abshire TC: Abnormalities of prothrombin: a review of the pathophysiology, diagnosis, and treatment. Haemophilia 2008; 14:1159–1163.
28 Brown DL, Kouides PA: Diagnosis and treatment of inherited factor X deficiency. Haemophilia 2008;14:1176–1182.
29 Nance D, Josephson NC, Paulyson-Nunez K, James AH: Factor X deficiency and pregnancy: preconception counselling and therapeutic options. Haemophilia 2012;18:e277–e285.
30 Napolitano M, Mariani G, Lapecorella M: Hereditary combined deficiency of the vitamin K-dependent clotting factors. Orphanet J Rare Dis 2010;5:21.
31 Mehta R, Shapiro AD: Plasminogen activator inhibitor type 1 deficiency. Haemophilia 2008;14:1255–1260.

Abbreviations

aPTT	Activated partial thromboplastin time
BW	Body weight
CNS	Central nervous system
DDAVP	1-Deamino-8-D-arginine vasopressin (desmopressin)
DVT	Deep vein thrombosis
ELISA	Enzyme-linked immunosorbent assay
EN-RBD	European Network of Rare Bleeding Disorders
FP (FFP)	Frozen plasma (Fresh frozen plasma)
FII	Factor II (prothrombin)
FV	Factor V
FVII	Factor VII
FVIII	Factor VIII
FIX	Factor IX
FX	Factor X
FXI	Factor XI
FXII	Factor XII
FXIII	Factor XIII
GGCX	γ-Glutamyl carboxylase
GI	Gastrointestinal
HMWK	High-molecular-weight kininogen
ICH	Intracranial hemorrhage
INR	International normalized ratio
ISTH	International Society on Thrombosis and Haemostasis
NSAIDs	Nonsteroidal anti-inflammatory drugs
PAI-1	Plasminogen activator inhibitor type 1
PCC	Prothrombin complex concentrate
PT	Prothrombin time
rFVIIa	Recombinant activated factor VII
rFXIII	Recombinant factor XIII
TE	Thromboembolism/thromboembolic event
TT	Thrombin time
VKOR	Vitamin K epoxide reductase
VWD	von Willebrand disease

Chapter 9

Acquired Bleeding Disorders in Children

Riten Kumar
MacGregor Steele

Introduction

Acquired bleeding disorders in children are rare and therefore often difficult to diagnose and manage. A correct diagnosis requires a detailed medical history, family history, physical examination and laboratory investigations. Given the paucity of randomized controlled trials or prospective cohort studies, it is difficult to make evidence-based treatment guidelines. Recommendations made in this chapter have been extrapolated from the adult literature.

Disseminated Intravascular Coagulation

DIC is a form of consumptive coagulopathy that is characterized by the dysregulated systemic activation of coagulation and impairment of fibrinolysis. DIC results in the widespread deposition of fibrin, occlusion of small- to medium-sized blood vessels and may eventually result in multiorgan failure. Concurrent consumption of platelets and clotting factors from the ongoing coagulation may result in hemorrhage, thereby complicating the clinical picture and laboratory evaluation (algorithm 1). DIC rarely occurs in isolation and is usually secondary to an underlying pathology. The most common cause of DIC in children is sepsis. In addition, a wide spectrum of disorders such as malignancy, trauma and vascular anomalies have also been implicated (table 1). These conditions result in activation of the coagulation system by release of inflammatory cytokines and exposure of blood to tissue factor released from damaged or tumor cells.

Clinical Presentation

Clinical presentation of DIC is often complicated by the underlying pathology. DIC may be non-overt (compensated), manifesting as laboratory abnormalities alone, or overt (decompensated), where laboratory abnormalities are associated with symptoms of bleeding and/or microvascular thrombosis. Bleeding, in the form of oozing from venipuncture sites, postoperative bleeding, petechiae and ecchymosis has been reported in about 50% of pediatric patients with DIC; whereas, symptomatic thrombosis is

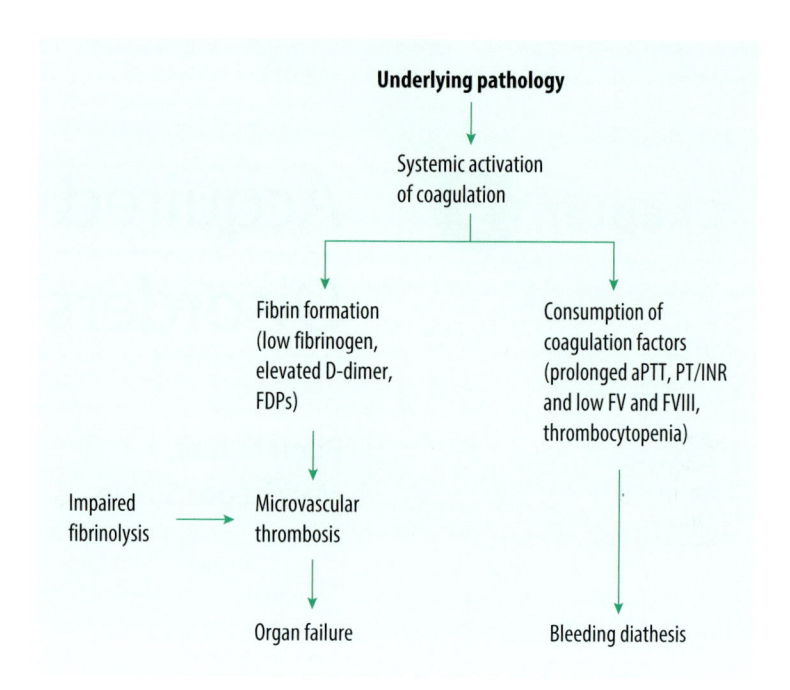

Algorithm 1. Mechanism of disseminated intravascular coagulation.

seen in about 5% of pediatric DIC patients [1]. Untreated, overt DIC may eventually progress to multiorgan failure.

Purpura fulminans, a particularly severe form of DIC, is characterized by skin infarction and necrosis. It is commonly associated with meningococcal and herpes zoster infection (where it may be associated with acquired protein S and protein C deficiency). Neonatal purpura fulminans usually occurs in patients with inherited protein C and rarely protein S deficiency (homozygotes and compound heterozygotes) (see chapter 10 for details).

Diagnosis

No single laboratory test can establish or rule out the diagnosis of DIC. Common laboratory manifestations of DIC include:

Complete Blood Count and Peripheral Smear
Thrombocytopenia from thrombin-induced platelet aggregation is seen in nearly 50% of patients with DIC. The peripheral smear may show evidence of microangiopathic hemolysis in the form of fragmented red blood cells (schistocytes) (figure 1).

Coagulation Testing
Prolonged PT/INR and aPTT from increased consumption and impaired synthesis of coagulation factors is reported in 50–60% of patients. FV and FVIII levels are both reduced in DIC (this may help differentiate DIC from coagulopathy of liver disease where FVIII levels are often elevated). There is elevation of FDPs including D-dimer, with reduced fibrinogen levels (fibrinogen is an acute phase reactant, and occasionally fibrinogen levels may be normal). Thrombin time may be prolonged secondary to low fibrinogen levels and/or interference of the high molecular weight FDPs on the thrombin used for the test. Reduction in plasma native anticoagulants (protein C, protein S and antithrombin) has also been described.

Table 1. Clinical conditions associated with disseminated intravascular coagulation

Sepsis
  Gram-negative organisms *(Neisseria meningitis, Haemophilus influenza)*
  Gram-positive organisms (group B *Streptococcus, Staphylococcus*)
  Viral (dengue fever)
  Rickettsiae (Rocky Mountain spotted fever, typhus)
  Protozoan (malaria)
Trauma
  Massive tissue injury/surgery
  Head injury
  Fat embolism
Malignancy
  Acute promyelocytic, monoblastic or myelocytic leukemia
  Solid tumors
Obstetric complications
  Placental abruption
  Amniotic fluid embolism
  Pre-eclampsia (HELLP syndrome, hemolysis, elevated liver enzymes, low platelets)
Reaction to toxins
  Snake venom, drugs, amphetamines
Vascular anomaly
  Giant hemangioma (Kassabach-Merritt syndrome)
Miscellaneous
  Acute hemolytic transfusion reaction
  Transplant rejection
  Severe allergic reaction
Specific neonatal DIC
  Sepsis
  Birth asphyxia
  Necrotizing enterocolitis
  Respiratory distress syndrome
  Metabolic conditions (e.g. galactosemia)
  Hereditary protein C/protein S deficiency

International Society on Thrombosis and Haemostasis Algorithm

Recently, the scientific subcommittee of the ISTH has recommended a 5-step algorithm to diagnose overt DIC, based on laboratory tests that are routinely available in most hospitals (table 2) [2]. The presence of a condition known to predispose to DIC is a prerequisite for the algorithm. Several adult studies have demonstrated that the ISTH DIC score reliably predicts mortality. While not prospectively validated in children, a recent retrospective pediatric study has shown that a one point increase in the ISTH DIC score was associated with a 1.35-fold increase in mortality after adjusting for baseline demographics, initial severity of illness and hemodynamic status [3]. Of note, the score should be interpreted with caution in children younger than 6 months of age, since several coagulation parameters do not reach adult values until 6 months of age. Diagnostic scores for DIC in neonates and low birth weight infants have previously been described [4]. Given the dynamic nature of DIC, repeated scores with clear trends are preferred over a single value.

Management

Given the paucity of pediatric literature and prospective randomized studies, it is difficult to make evidence-based treatment recommendations. The cornerstone for treatment of DIC remains the treatment of the underlying condition (e.g. antibiotic therapy for sepsis and chemotherapy for underlying malignancy). The following general guidelines have been extrapolated from published adult guidelines and should be individualized based on the patient's presentation and clinical status [5].

Blood Component Therapy

Transfusion of platelets and plasma products (FP/cryoprecipitate) should be based on symptoms of bleeding and not abnormal laboratory values. However, asymptomatic patients who are thought to be at high risk of bleeding (postoperative patients or patients scheduled to undergo an invasive procedure) may be candidates for replacement therapy as well. Reasonable goals for such patients are to maintain the platelet count >30–50 × 10^9/l, fibrinogen >1 g/l and aPTT less than double the normal range. Cryoprecipitate or fibrinogen concentrate may be considered in patients with severe hypofibrinogenemia (<1 g/l), that does not improve despite FP infusion (refer to the appendix for dosing guidelines).

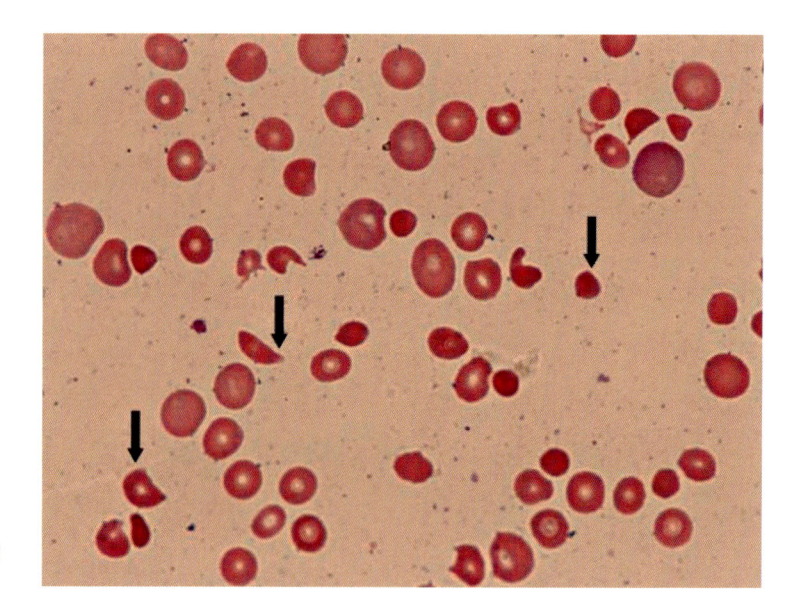

Figure 1. Microangiopathic hemolytic anemia. Peripheral blood smear from a patient with microangiopathic hemolytic anemia showing helmet cells, schistocytes and microspherocytes. Courtesy of William Brien, MD, FRCP, Division of Pathology and Laboratory Medicine, Hospital for Sick Children.

Table 2. ISTH Diagnostic Scoring system for overt (uncompensated) DIC

1. Risk assessment: Does the patient have an underlying disorder?
   If yes: proceed; if no: do not use this algorithm
2. Order global coagulation tests: platelet count, PT, fibrinogen, fibrin degradation products (D-dimer)
3. Score global coagulation results:
   – Platelet count (>100 = 0; <100 = 1; <50 = 2)
   – Elevated fibrin-related marker (no increase = 0; moderate increase = 2; strong increase = 3)
   – Prolonged PT (<3 s = 0; >3 but <6 s = 1; >6 s = 2)
   – Fibrinogen level (>1 g/l = 0; <1 g/l = 1)
4. Calculate score
5. Interpretation of score
   – If total score ≥5: compatible with overt DIC; repeat score daily
   – If total score <5: suggestive (not affirmative) for non-overt DIC; repeat in 1–2 days

Reproduced with permission from Taylor et al. [2].

Anticoagulation

Patients with DIC presenting with limb or life-threatening arterial, symptomatic venous TEs or purpura fulminans may be candidates for anticoagulation. Given its short half-life and reversibility, an infusion of UFH (see chapter 16 for doses) may be preferred over LMWH. Thromboembolism with concurrent bleeding may warrant a trial of prophylactic doses of UFH (10 U/kg/h). Anti-Xa levels (or an aPTT that has been correlated to the therapeutic anti-Xa) should be closely followed in these patients given the increased risk of hemorrhage (see chapter 16 for details).

Recombinant Factor VIIa

Some data suggests a potential role of rFVIIa (NovoSeven®) in adult DIC patients with uncontrolled bleeding, but pediatric data is anecdotal and conflicting [6]. However, in situations of significant bleeding despite replacement of blood components, rFVIIa may be tried. The recommended dose for hemophilia patients with inhibitor is 90 µg/kg/dose q2 h. Whether the same dose or a lower dose is needed for patients with DIC is not clear as no evidence-based data exist. If rFVIIa is considered, most experts consider using a lower dose of rFVIIa in DIC (20 µg/kg/dose). Treatment with rFVIIa may result in an increased risk of thrombosis, including stroke and it should be used with caution. To ensure maximum efficacy, platelet count, acidosis and hypothermia should be corrected prior to infusion of rFVIIa.

Protein C Concentrate
Neonatal purpura fulminans in patients with hereditary protein C deficiency requires the replacement of protein C either from FP or human plasma-derived, viral inactivated protein C concentrate (Ceprotin®) (50–100 U/kg q6–12 h), in addition to anticoagulation (see chapter 10 and appendix for details).

Recombinant Human Activated Protein C
The use of activated protein C is not recommended in pediatric patients with DIC [7].

Antifibrinolytics
The use of antifibrinolytics is contraindicated in patients with DIC.

Other Agents
The use of antithrombin has not been systematically studied in pediatric DIC. Newer anticoagulants directed against the tissue factor-FVIIa complex (nematode anticoagulant protein C2) remain investigational.

Thrombotic Microangiopathic Disorders

Thrombotic microangiopathic disorders are characterized by thrombosis in medium and small sized blood vessels with resulting thrombocytopenia, microangiopathic hemolytic anemia and end organ damage. HUS and TTP are the classic variants of this condition. While both conditions present with microangiopathic hemolytic anemia and thrombocytopenia, their epidemiology, pathophysiology and management are distinct.

Hemolytic Uremic Syndrome

HUS is defined by the simultaneous occurrence of thrombocytopenia, microangiopathic hemolytic anemia and renal dysfunction. A prospective surveillance study estimated the incidence of HUS to be 0.7 per 100,000 children younger than 16 years of age with nearly 70% of the cases occurring in children younger than 5 years [8]. Ninety percent of HUS is caused by shiga toxin (verotoxin) producing serotypes of *Escherichia coli* (STEC-HUS), the prototype being *E. coli* 0157:H7; although other serotypes and bacteria (including invasive pneumococcal infection) have also been implicated. The verotoxin causes direct injury to the vascular endothelium resulting in formation of platelet-fibrin thrombi with subsequent thrombotic injury to the microvasculature, classically the kidney. HUS remains the most common cause of acute and chronic renal failure requiring dialysis in the pediatric population.

Approximately 10% of pediatric HUS is classified as aHUS or diarrhea-negative HUS as it does not occur after infection with verotoxin-producing bacteria. These are a heterogeneous group of disorders that typically occur secondary to inherited or acquired defects in complement regulation. Mutations have been identified in genes encoding complement regulators (CFH, CFI, CFHR, MCP), as well as complement activators CFB and C3. In addition, mutations in the thrombomodulin gene have also been implicated [9]. Recently, a novel subtype of aHUS characterized by both the deficiency of CFHRs (CFHR1 and CFHR2) and CFH autoantibody positivity has been described (DEAP-HUS). aHUS may also occur as a complication of HSCT, solid organ transplantation, autoimmune disorders or secondary to certain medications (mitomycin C, cyclosporine). Defective intracellular cobalamin reduction/cofactor function may result in aHUS. Details of the pathophysiology of aHUS have been reviewed elsewhere [9, 10].

Clinical Presentation
The rate of STEC-HUS following *E. coli* 0157:H7 infection ranges from 8% to 18%. After ingestion of *E. coli* there is usually an incubation period

of 3–8 days after which symptoms typically start with watery diarrhea progressing to bloody diarrhea in about 48 h. Only 30% of the patients have concurrent fever. Pallor and oliguria or anuria eventually develops. Renal complications requiring dialysis are seen in 50–60% of the patients and acute hypertension is seen in about 30% of the patients. Seizures, lethargy, irritability and other neurological complications may be noted in 25–50% of the patients.

Bleeding, despite significant thrombocytopenia, is rare, and generally restricted to mucocutaneous symptoms such as petechiae and ecchymosis. Long-term renal sequelae of STEC-HUS include hypertension, low glomerular filtration rate and proteinuria. Severity of acute illness, neurological symptoms and need for initial dialysis are thought to be associated with poor prognosis.

The renal, neurological and hematological manifestations of aHUS are similar to STEC-HUS. In contrast, aHUS is characterized by familial inheritance, frequent relapses, progression to end-stage renal disease in 50% of the cases, high rate of recurrence post-renal transplant (30–100%) and poor long-term prognosis.

Diagnosis

CBC and Peripheral Smear

Anemia and thrombocytopenia are present. Peripheral blood smear shows schistocytes, helmet cells and polychromasia (figure 1), consistent with microangiopathic hemolytic anemia. Serum LDH is elevated and serum haptoglobin is low. Direct antiglobin test (Coomb's test) is negative.

Coagulation Testing

PT (INR), aPTT and fibrinogen are typically normal (this may help differentiate STEC-HUS from DIC).

Microbiological Testing

Stool culture for *E. coli* and direct evaluation of shiga toxin through PCR should be carried out. Given that STEC-HUS is not always preceded by diarrhea, stool evaluation should be done even in the absence of diarrhea. Urine culture is recommended as STEC-HUS has been reported after urinary tract infections.

Renal Function Testing

Renal abnormalities include proteinuria, hematuria and acute renal failure. Renal function needs to be closely monitored. Renal biopsy is not required for diagnosis. However, when performed, biopsy findings typically show thickening of arterioles and capillaries, endothelial swelling and detachment and subendothelial protein deposition.

Atypical HUS

The European pediatric study group on HUS has recommended suspecting aHUS when the following features are present: presentation before 6 months of age, insidious onset, previous episode of HUS, previous unexplained anemia, family history of HUS or HUS post-transplantation [11]. In a patient with suspected aHUS, measurement of plasma concentrations of C3, C4, CFH, CFH antibodies, CFI and CFB levels and surface expression of MCP on mononuclear leukocytes is recommended. In addition genetic mutation analysis for susceptibility genes CFH, CFI, CFHR1–5, CFB, MCP and C3 may be undertaken [9]. Details of laboratories offering these tests can be found at http://espn.cardiff.ac.uk.

Management

General Guidelines

Fluid replacement and early volume expansion in the pre-HUS diarrhea phase may be beneficial and has been associated with lower rates of oligoanuria, need for dialysis and shorter duration of hospitalization. Management of acute renal failure remains the cornerstone for therapy of STEC-HUS. Electrolyte management, antihypertensive therapy and dialysis should be guided by a pediatric nephrologist. Peritoneal and hemodialysis are equally effective.

Blood Component Therapy

Packed red blood cells and platelet transfusions should be reserved for symptomatic patients only. Platelet transfusions carry a theoretical risk of exacerbating the microvascular thrombosis in STEC-HUS. FP may not be beneficial in patients with STEC-HUS, though it has role in the management of aHUS.

Antibiotics

Currently, antibiotics are not recommended with the exception being aHUS associated with invasive pneumococcal disease. The role of antibiotics may be re-evaluated in the future as several studies show an increased risk of HUS with the use of antibiotics in the diarrhea phase but other studies including a recent meta-analysis have not shown this association.

Anticoagulation

In the absence of symptomatic venous TE, anticoagulation is not recommended in STEC-HUS [12].

Miscellaneous

Strict isolation of hospitalized patients to reduce person-to-person transmission is recommended as soon as the diagnosis is made. Antimotility agents are not recommended. Steroids and shiga toxin binding agent (Synsorb-PK) have not been found to be beneficial. Novel therapies, including vaccination, monoclonal shiga toxin antibody and shiga toxin receptor analogs remain investigational.

Atypical HUS

Guidelines for the management of patients with aHUS have been elaborated by European pediatric study group on HUS [11]. In summary, aggressive and early plasmapheresis remains the cornerstone of management of aHUS. Plasma exchange with 1.5 times the plasma volume should be performed daily for 5 days, followed by 5 sessions per week for 2 weeks, and then 3 sessions per week for 2 weeks.

Hematological remission is defined as platelet counts >150 × 10^9/l for 2 weeks with no evidence of hemolysis as determined by the presence of fragmented red cells, elevated LDH and low haptoglobin. Renal transplantation has been performed in patients with aHUS, though recurrence rates post-transplant are high, particularly in patients with CFH, and CFI mutations. Combined renal-liver transplant (given that CFH and CHI are synthesized in the liver) remains investigational. Case reports and phase II clinical trials show efficacy with use of the eculizumab, a humanized monoclonal antibody against complement C5. Two international multicenter prospective phase II open-label clinical trials in adolescent and adult aHUS patients are currently underway.

Thrombotic Thrombocytopenic Purpura

TTP has been historically characterized by the pentad of microangiopathic hemolytic anemia, thrombocytopenia, fever, neurological deficit and renal impairment. The availability of appropriate therapy and urgency to treat may warrant a less stringent definition; and the presence of thrombocytopenia and microangiopathic hemolytic anemia in the absence of an alternate etiology may be sufficient to make a presumptive diagnosis of TTP and initiate therapy [13]. TTP is rare, with an incidence of 1 in 4–11 million; with less than 5% of cases occurring in children.

ADAMTS13 and Thrombotic Thrombocytopenic Purpura

ADAMTS13 (a disintegrin and metalloprotease with thrombospondin type 1 motif, member 13) is a metalloprotease enzyme responsible for cleaving ULVWF into smaller inactive monomers. The gene for ADAMTS13 has been localized to 9q34. TTP is thought to result from either the congenital (Upshaw-Schülman syndrome) or acquired (idiopathic TTP) deficiency of ADAMTS13. In the absence of the protease, platelets bind to the ULVWF

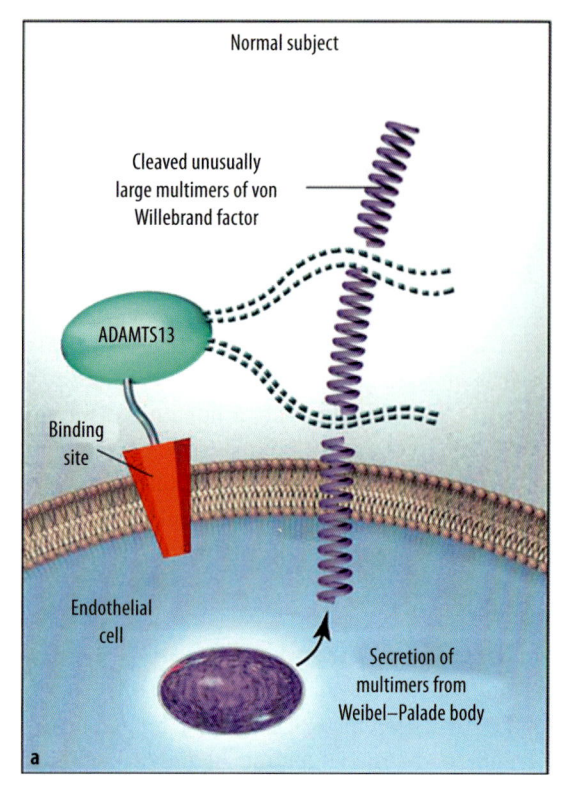

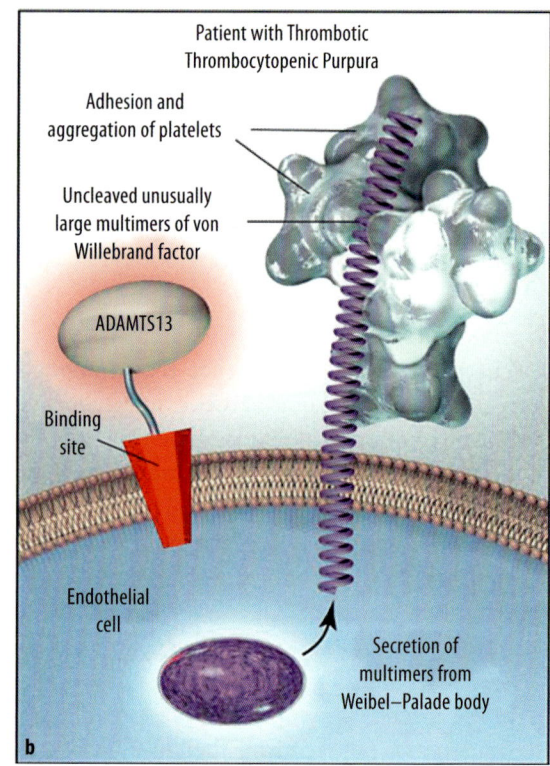

Figure 2. Postulated mechanism of thrombotic thrombocytopenic purpura. **a** In normal subjects ULVWF secreted by the Weibel-Palade bodies of the endothelial cells are cleaved by ADMTS13. **b** In subjects with TTP, ADAMTS13 may be congenitally deficient (Upshaw-Schülman syndrome) or secondary to acquired inhibitors (idiopathic TTP). In such subjects, there is formation of platelet-ULVWF microthrombi in terminal arterioles and capillaries resulting in symptoms of TTP. Modified from Moake [14], with permission.

resulting in the formation of platelet-VWF microthrombi (as opposed to platelet-fibrin microthrombi in HUS) in the terminal arterioles and capillaries resulting in thrombocytopenia, anemia and end-organ infarction (figure 2) [14].

Upshaw-Schülman syndrome is an autosomal-recessive condition, often presenting in the neonates who are homozygous or compound heterozygous for mutations in the ADAMTS13 gene, with less than 10% (0.1 U/ml) ADAMTS13 activity. Parents of such infants are usually asymptomatic, though they have low ADAMTS13 activity (about 0.5 U/ml). Adolescents and adults usually develop TTP secondary to acquired inhibitors (IgG subclass) to ADAMTS13. These antibodies may develop idiopathically or secondary to autoimmune conditions, specifically SLE. TTP has also been described after HSCT and certain medications (i.e. clopidogrel, ticlopidine).

Clinical Presentation

Clinical presentation of TTP can be nonspecific and variable depending on the age of the patient and site of microvascular thrombi. Upshaw-Schülman syndrome classically presents in the early neonatal period with anemia, thrombocytopenia and severe hyperbilirubinemia, often warranting exchange transfusion. Thrombocytopenia may be severe and bleeding symptoms including IVH has been described. Diagnosis is often delayed and is made after the infants present with recurrent episodes of anemia and thrombocytopenia.

Developmental delay has also been noted in these infants, and is thought to be secondary to leukoencephalopathy and kernicterus. A 'late-onset phenotype' of Upshaw-Schülman syndrome characterized by mild thrombocytopenia during childhood and exacerbations associated with pregnancy and infections has also been described [15].

Bleeding is the most common manifestation of idiopathic pediatric TTP and can occur as petechiae, gingival bleeding, purpura and epistaxis. CNS manifestations including altered mental status, ICH, seizures and hemiparesis may occur. General symptoms including fever, abdominal symptoms, nausea and vomiting have also been described.

Diagnosis
CBC and Peripheral Smear
At presentation, most children have evidence of Coomb's negative microangiopathic hemolytic anemia. Peripheral smear shows schistocytes, helmet cells, anisocytosis and poikiloctosis (figure 1). Anemia can be severe and hemoglobin concentrations below 5 mg/dl have been described. Thrombocytopenia is also severe, with presenting platelet counts often less than 20×10^9/l. Serum LDH is elevated and haptoglobin is low. Patients presenting with idiopathic TTP should be evaluated for SLE (antinuclear antibody and anti-ds DNA).

Coagulation Testing
PT (INR), aPTT and fibrinogen are usually normal (this may help differentiate TTP from DIC).

Renal Function Testing
Renal abnormalities including hematuria, proteinuria and elevated creatinine have been described.

ADAMTS13 Testing
ADAMTS13 level and inhibitors to ADAMTS13 can be measured in specialized laboratories. However, the utility of measuring ADAMTS13 remains unclear. While low ADAMTS13 may help differentiate TTP from HUS, several conditions including sepsis, neoplasms, aHUS and liver cirrhosis can result in low ADAMTS13 levels as well. Also, there are conflicting reports regarding ADAMTS13 activity in newborns. In summary, when available, ADAMTS13 activity and inhibitors should be measured, but this should not delay initiation of therapy when there is high clinical suspicion.

Genetic Testing
ADAMTS13 gene sequencing may be pursued for patients with suspected Upshaw-Schülman syndrome.

Management of Upshaw-Schülman Syndrome
Blood Component Therapy
FP replacement remains the treatment modality of choice for infants with Upshaw-Schülman syndrome. Replacement of 10–15 ml/kg of FP is usually sufficient to bring patients into remission. Most infants will require FP infusion every 2–3 weeks to remain in remission. Currently, chronic regular FP transfusions are the only available treatment for Upshaw-Schülman syndrome.

Management of Idiopathic (Acquired) TTP
Plasmapheresis
Plasmapheresis remains the cornerstone for management of idiopathic TTP and has reduced the mortality from 90% to less than 10%. It is thought to act by replenishing ADAMTS13, as well as removing ULVWF multimers and ADAMTS13 antibodies. It should be initiated as soon as the diagnosis of TTP is seriously considered. Bouw et al. [16] recommends daily plasmapheresis (exchange volume: 40–60 ml/kg) until resolution of clinical symptoms and correction of thrombocytopenia.

Blood Component Therapy
Plasmapheresis is superior to FP infusion for idiopathic TTP. However, FP infusions may be a reasonable alternative until plasmapheresis is initiated. There have been case reports of clinical

deterioration and death in patients with TTP after platelet transfusion. As such, platelet transfusion should be restricted for symptomatic bleeding patients.

Immunosuppressive Agents

Steroids (prednisone 2 mg/kg/day) are often used as in conjunction with plasmapheresis for patients with idiopathic TTP, though efficacy has not been systematically evaluated in randomized studies. Rituximab, a monoclonal anti CD-20 antibody has been studied in patients with idiopathic TTP and shown to be effective. It is reasonable to consider treatment with rituximab (375 mg/m^2 × 4 weekly doses) in patients with relapsing/refractory TTP.

Cyclosporine, vincristine and cyclophosphamide have all been used in patients with relapsing/ refractory TTP. Paradoxically, cyclosporine has also been associated with post-transplant TTP.

Antiplatelet Agents
Antiplatelet agents are not recommended.

Splenectomy
Splenectomy acts by depleting B cell reservoirs and may benefit patients with idiopathic relapsing/refractory TTP. There have been no pediatric studies of splenectomy in TTP.

Coagulopathy of Chronic Liver Disease

CLD has historically been considered to be the prototype of acquired bleeding disorders. Recent studies, however, underline a shifting paradigm in this dogma [17, 18]. The liver is responsible for synthesis of both pro- and anticoagulant factors, thrombopoetin and proteins of fibrinolysis. Patients with CLD may have thrombocytopenia secondary to splenic sequestration and decreased thrombopoetin production. They also have elevated levels of FVIII and VWF. Recent reviews have therefore alluded to a 'rebalanced state' of the coagulation system secondary to this simultaneous impact on both pro- and anticoagulant pathways (table 3). This rebalanced state, however, is more labile and can result in bleeding associated with invasive procedures, associated vitamin K deficiency, renal dysfunction and variceal bleeding resulting from local vasculopathy.

Conventional tests of hemostasis such as the PT and aPTT, although significantly prolonged, do not accurately predict the bleeding risk in patients with CLD. Global tests of hemostasis such as thromboelastography and thrombin generation times have been reported to be grossly normal. Recent studies have also indicated that the prolonged PT does not protect CLD patients from venous TEs. In fact, the incidence of venous TEs in patients with CLD is reported to be higher than the general population with PVT, DVT and PE being the common manifestations [19].

Clinical Presentation

The coagulopathy of chronic liver disease is recognized in cirrhosis, whose common causes in young infants include biliary atresia, inborn errors of metabolism, familial cholestatic diseases, intestinal failure-associated liver disease and idiopathic neonatal hepatitis. In older children and adolescents, causes of cirrhosis include

Table 3. Rebalanced hemostasis in chronic liver disease

Factors promoting bleeding	Factors promoting thrombosis
↓ Synthesis of FII, V, VII, IX, X, XI, XIII	↓ Synthesis of protein C, protein S and antithrombin
Hypofibrinogenemia	↑ FVIII
Dysfibrinogenemia	↑ VWF
↓ Synthesis of TAFI and α$_2$-antiplasmin	↓ Synthesis of ADAMTS13
↓ Clearance of t-PA	↓ Synthesis of plasminogen
↓ Thrombopoetin production	
Platelet sequestration in spleen	
Acquired platelet dysfunction	

Modified with permission from Roberts et al. [17].

autoimmune hepatitis, primary sclerosing cholangitis, and less commonly, chronic hepatitis B and C, nonalcoholic fatty liver disease and cystic fibrosis liver disease.

Bruising, purpura, ecchymosis, epistaxis, and bleeding from gums may be seen in children with cirrhosis. Interestingly, it is often abnormal coagulation parameters tested prior to an invasive procedure that prompts a hematology consult. Bleeding from esophageal varices is primarily the result of a mechanical breach in the variceal wall resulting from increased intraluminal pressure and mural thinning related to increasing venous diameter. The extent to which coagulopathy contributes to variceal hemorrhage is unclear.

Diagnosis

CBC and Peripheral Smear

Mild to moderate thrombocytopenia may be present. Peripheral smear in patients with advanced liver disease may show target cells.

Coagulation Testing

PT (INR) is typically prolonged secondary to impaired synthesis of coagulation factors and/or vitamin K deficiency resulting from cholestasis. PT is used in both the Childs-Pugh score for prognosis of CLD and the pediatric end-stage liver disease score for ranking of pediatric patients awaiting transplant [19]. aPTT and D-dimer may be normal to slightly prolonged and the fibrinogen levels may be low. Factors V and VII are particularly sensitive indicators of liver protein synthesis and may be used as a guide to the severity of liver disease. It is important to note that the PT (INR), aPTT, platelet count and fibrinogen levels do not accurately predict bleeding in patients with CLD.

Management

There is little data on the management of coagulopathy in children with CLD who present with variceal bleeding or during liver transplantation and liver biopsy. Management of variceal bleeding relies on vasoactive drugs to reduce variceal pressure, and endoscopic occlusion of the varices with band ligation or sclerotherapy. The following recommendations for treatment of coagulopathy are based on studies of adult patients and on clinical experience [19].

Blood Component Therapy

FP should be used in patients with overt bleeding or for patients with an INR >1.5 prior to an invasive procedure, though normalization of PT (INR) without causing significant volume overload is difficult. A reasonable initial infusion of 15 ml/kg can be given (range 10–20 ml/kg) with follow up PT (INR). When used prior to an invasive procedure, it is important to replace FP as close to the procedure as possible (given that the correction is usually short-lived).

Maintaining a platelet count greater than 50×10^9/l during overt bleeding or prior to an invasive procedure is recommended. Of note, response to platelet transfusion may be markedly less than expected secondary to splenic sequestration of transfused platelets. Cryoprecipitate should be considered in patients with severe hypofibrinogenemia (<1 g/l) and bleeding patients (dose of cryoprecipitate is outlined in the appendix).

Vitamin K

Despite a paucity of evidence, it is reasonable to replace vitamin K deficiency in CLD. Current UK guidelines recommend 0.3 mg/kg (maximum 10 mg) of vitamin K three times a week (p.o., i.v. or s.c.) for all patients admitted into intensive care [20].

Recombinant Factor VIIa (rFVIIa)

In adult patients with CLD and variceal bleeding, two randomized controlled trials have demonstrated no efficacy of rFVIIa in control of bleeding, prevention of rebleeding and overall mortality. A recent meta-analysis evaluating the role of prophylactic rFVIIa prior to liver biopsy and transplant in adults did not demonstrate an efficacy with regards to red blood cell units transfused and mortality [21]. Though the risk of thrombosis was not greater with rFVIIa use, there was a trend towards more serious adverse effects occurring in patients receiving rFVIIa.

Despite lack of evidence for rFVIIa in bleeding pediatric patients with CLD, it might be considered if there is failure to control bleeding with standard therapy or there are concerns of volume overload. The recommended dose of rFVIIa is unclear but most experts would consider using a low dose of rFVIIa in CLD (20 μg/kg/dose). Treatment with rFVIIa may result in an increased risk of thrombosis.

Antifibrinolytic Agents

Antifibrinolytic agents such as tranexamic acid have been shown to reduce the need for blood transfusion in patients undergoing liver transplant without increasing the risk of TEs. No randomized controlled trials have evaluated the role of antifibrinolytic agents in variceal bleeding. Tranexamic acid (10 mg/kg/dose i.v. q6–8 h; 25 mg/kg p.o. q8 h maximum dose 1,500 tid) or ε-aminocaproic acid (50 mg/kg/dose, p.o. q4–6 h; maximum daily dose 30 g) can be considered for mucous membrane bleeding, and has been reported for the management of bleeding from gastric antral vascular ectasia associated with cirrhosis.

Prothrombin Complex Concentrate

PCC is a plasma-derived, viral-inactivated product containing FII, FVII, FIX, FX, protein C, protein S and traces of antithrombin, heparin and vitronectin. There are no randomized controlled trials evaluating the use of PCC in patients with CLD. The Italian Society of Transfusion Medicine and Immunohematology has recommended PCC as a second-choice alternative to FP in adult patients with severe liver disease and serious bleeding or in preparation of surgery [22]. They recommend an initial dose of 20–25 IU/kg with a follow-up INR in 30–60 min to guide further dosing. Given the high risk of thrombosis and limited pediatric experience, PCCs should be used with extreme caution and only if bleeding cannot be controlled with any of the above-mentioned modalities.

Bleeding in Chronic Renal Failure

Bleeding is a common and serious complication in patients with CRF, though its incidence has decreased with the advent of improved dialysis techniques and routine use of erythropoietin for management of anemia. The pathophysiology of bleeding is thought to be multifactorial. Platelet dysfunction, abnormal platelet-vessel wall interaction, the presence of uremic toxins, and anemia have been implicated as contributory factors (table 4). In addition, thrombocytopenia may also be present in patients with CRF, though the platelet counts are rarely less than 100×10^9/l. Bleeding in patients with CRF usually manifests as mucocutaneous bleeding including easy bruising, petechiae, epistaxis and bleeding from venipuncture sites. More serious bleeds, specifically, gastrointestinal hemorrhage has been described in up to one third of patients with CRF.

Diagnosis

Treatment is usually reserved for symptomatic patients. However, laboratory evaluation may be helpful in predicting the risk of bleeding with invasive procedures.

CBC and Peripheral Smear

Mild to moderate thrombocytopenia is common in patients with CRF. Peripheral smear may show a reduced mean platelet volume, a finding that is thought to be inversely related to bleeding time.

Coagulation Testing

aPTT, PT (INR) and TT are usually within normal limits. Bleeding time was historically thought to be the best laboratory test for predicting bleeding in patients with uremia. However,

Table 4. Mechanisms affecting hemostasis in uremia

Platelet dysfunction: reduction in: dense granule content, intracellular ADP and serotonin, and release of platelet α-granule protein and β-thromboglobulin; enhanced intracellular c-AMP; defective cyclooxygenase activity; abnormalities in mobilization of platelet calcium, arachidonic acid metabolism and ex vivo platelet aggregation.

Defects in platelet-vessel wall interaction: abnormal platelet adhesion, altered VWF, and increased formation of vascular prostacyclin (PGI2).

Abnormal production of nitric oxide

Uremic toxins

Anemia: altered blood rheology, defective platelet diffusivity, decreased release of ADP by erythrocytes, erythropoietin deficiency.

Drug treatment: anticoagulants, anti-platelet agents, NSAIDs, β-lactam antibiotics, third generation cephalosporins.

Reproduced with permission from Galbusera M, et al. [23].

the test has poor reproducibility and accuracy and few centers continue to do bleeding time. In vitro tests of platelet function including platelet aggregation and platelet function analyzer (PFA-100®) have been investigated in uremic patients but need further validation for clinical application (see chapter 3 for details).

Renal Function Testing
Tests of renal function including glomerular filtration rate, serum creatinine and blood urea nitrogen are poor predictors of bleeding.

Management

Given the paucity of pediatric studies and guidelines, the following recommendations are based on adult studies and guidelines [23, 24].

Dialysis
Dialysis remains the cornerstone of management of renal failure, and may help prevent bleeding. Although heterogeneous in nature, most studies show that dialysis can improve platelet functional abnormalities and reduce the risk of hemorrhage. It is thought to work by removing uremic toxins from circulation. In patients with active bleeding, peritoneal dialysis may be preferable over hemodialysis as heparin administration is not required.

Desmopressin
DDAVP remains the most common modality of treatment of acute bleeds in uremic patients. It is thought to act by increasing plasma concentration of FVIII and VWF. It has a quick onset of action (1 h) and may be given subcutaneously or intravenously (0.3 μg/kg, maximum dose 20 μg). It may also be used intranasally (300 μg) in older patients. Major limitations of DDAVP remain tachyphylaxis with multiple doses, the need for water restriction and risk of hyponatremia and seizures.

Correction of Anemia
Correction of anemia either though transfusion of packed red blood cells (10–20 ml/kg) or the use of erythropoietin (50 U/kg × 3 times a week i.v. or s.c.) has shown to correct coagulation parameters in patients with CRF. In addition to correcting anemia, erythropoietin may be directly beneficial by increasing the number of reticulated platelets and improving platelet adhesion and aggregation.

Cryoprecipitate
In both prospective and retrospective studies, cryoprecipitate has been shown to improve coagulation parameters in uremic patients. It has a quick onset of action and may be beneficial in patients with acute bleeding. (The dose of cryoprecipitate is outlined in the appendix.)

Estrogen Therapy
Multiple adult studies have evaluated the role of estrogen in uremic bleeding, although there are no pediatric data available. While its exact mechanism remains unclear, conjugated estrogen (minimum dose of 0.6 mg/kg injected intravenously

over 30–40 min daily for 5 days) has been shown to improve clinical bleeding in uremic patients. Onset of action is within 24 h and duration is approximately 14–21 days. Given this, its use may be preferable for gastrointestinal bleeding and prior to major surgery.

Acquired Hemophilia

Acquired hemophilia is a rare but serious bleeding disorder characterized by the development of autoantibodies (inhibitors) against plasma coagulation factors, most commonly FVIII. It classically presents with the sudden onset of bleeding symptoms in a patient with no past or family history of bleeding disorder. It is thought to be exceedingly rare in the pediatric population with an estimated annual incidence to be 0.045 per million [25]. Pediatric acquired hemophilia has been described in association with autoimmune conditions, infections and antibiotics, most commonly penicillin or penicillin-like antibiotics [26].

Unlike classical hemophilia where hemarthrosis is the characteristic bleeding manifestation, most patients with acquired hemophilia present with bleeding into the skin, subcutaneous tissue and muscles, hematuria, hematemesis or melena and postoperative bleeding. Severe subcutaneous bleeds following venipuncture and intramuscular injections have been described.

Diagnosis
Acquired hemophilia should be suspected in any patient with a negative past and family history who presents with a sudden onset of subcutaneous or mucocutaneous bleeding. CBC shows a normal platelet count.

Coagulation Testing
Patients with acquired hemophilia have a prolonged aPTT and a normal PT (INR), and fibrinogen. Heparin contamination could be ruled out by performing an anti-Xa level, by neutralization of heparin with a heparinase (Hepzyme®) or by a TT and reptilase time (typically, heparin contamination results in a prolonged TT and a normal reptilase time). Mixing study helps differentiate between congenital factor deficiency and acquired antibodies. aPTT in congenital deficiency typically corrects after mixing the patient plasma in a 1:1 ratio with normal plasma. In case of acquired hemophilia and lupus anticoagulant, the aPTT remains prolonged after mixing. Note should be made that FVIII inhibitors are typically time and temperature sensitive and therefore incubated mixing studies must be performed (incubating the patient plasma in a 1:1 ratio with pooled plasma at 37°C for 1–2 h). Lupus anticoagulant must be excluded in patients who have a prolonged aPTT and an abnormal mixing study, as per criteria set forth by the ISTH [27].

Factor assays for FVIII, FIX, FXI and FXII should be done to identify specificity of inhibitor. In case of acquired FVIII inhibitors, the Bethesda assay and the Nijmegen modification of the Bethesda assay help quantify the inhibitor titer (see explanation in chapter 6).

Management
Given the rarity of acquired hemophilia in the pediatric population, there is little pediatric data to base recommendations. Management of acquired hemophilia entails avoiding nonurgent therapeutic and diagnostic interventions, management during acute bleeding episodes and eradication of inhibitors. Given the risk of life-threatening bleeds, these patients should be urgently referred to a comprehensive hemophilia center.

Management of Acute Bleeding Episode
Bypassing Agents
rFVIIa (Novoseven®) and aPCC (FEIBA®) have both been used in patients with acquired hemophilia. While there have been no prospective randomized studies comparing the 2 agents

in acquired hemophilia, retrospective studies suggest similar efficacy. Either rFVIIa (90 μg/kg/dose q2 h) or aPCC (50–100 U/kg/dose every 8–12 h; daily maximum 200 U/kg) may be used during acute bleeding episodes [28]. Both agents carry an increased risk of thrombosis and should be used with caution. There are no routine laboratory tests to monitor their efficacy, therefore clinical response and serial monitoring of hemoglobin may be used to monitor patients and assist in determining duration of therapy.

Plasma Derived or Recombinant FVIII

Plasma-derived or recombinant FVIII may be used in patients with low titer inhibitor (<5 BU). While there are no published dosing recommendations for FVIII in acquired hemophilia patients, large doses of 200 U/kg every 8–12 h have been recommended [28]. Response to FVIII is thought to be unpredictable and inferior to bypassing agents. Therefore, we recommend it as a second-line agent in patients with low titer inhibitor who have failed bypassing agents.

Desmopressin

DDAVP (0.3 μg/kg s.c./i.v., maximum dose 20 μg) may be used in patients with low titer inhibitors and minor bleeding symptoms. However, given the unpredictable response to DDAVP we recommend it be used as a third-line agent.

Inhibitor Eradication

Steroids and Cytotoxic Agents

Immunosuppression to eradicate inhibitors should be started as soon as the diagnosis of acquired hemophilia is made. We recommend starting treatment with oral prednisone alone (1 mg/kg/day). If the patient has no response after 4–6 weeks of therapy, oral cyclophosphamide (1–2 mg/kg/ day) may be considered.

Rituximab

Experience with the use of rituximab, a monoclonal anti-CD 20 antibody, in acquired hemophilia is restricted to case reports and case series, where the drug was either used alone or in combination with steroids and/or cyclophosphamide. In the absence of randomized control trials, we recommend that the use of rituximab (375 mg/m^2 weekly for 4 weeks) be restricted to patients who are nonresponsive to both steroids and cyclophosphamide.

Intravenous Immunoglobulin

Retrospective studies and case series have not documented any advantage of using IVIG alone or in combination with steroids and cyclophosphamide. Given the lack of evidence, we do not recommend using IVIG for acquired hemophilia.

Immunoadsorption

Extracorporeal immunoadsorption allows for removal of pathogenic antibodies in substantial amounts from the patient's circulation. While randomized trials are lacking, anecdotal evidence suggest that extracorporeal immunoadsorption may be a safe and potentially cost-effective alternative for inhibitor eradication particularly in patients with serious bleeds or prior to surgical interventions [29]. The procedure should be performed in specialized centers with experience in such interventions.

Immune Tolerance

Immune tolerance may be considered for patients with high titer inhibitors and serious bleeds.

Acquired von Willebrand Syndrome

While well-described in adults, AVWS is exceedingly rare in children with literature limited to case reports. In the pediatric population, AVWS has been described in association with Wilms' tumor, hypothyroidism, SLE, aortic stenosis and left ventricular assist device. This is distinct from adults where 50–60% of AVWS is seen in association with lymphoproliferative and myeloproliferative disorders. While the exact pathophysiology of AVWS remains unclear, five distinct mechanisms have been proposed – (1) decreased production of VWF, (2) increased clearance of the VWF-FVIII complex by circulating autoantibodies, (3) adsorption of VWF to tumor cells, (4) cell mediated or drug mediated destruction of VWF multimers, and (5) increased clearance of high-molecular-weight multimers in association with aortic valve stenosis (Heyde's syndrome) or defective aortic valve prosthesis [30]. Clinical manifestation of AVWS is identical to congenital VWD (see chapter 7 for details).

Diagnosis

In pediatric patients, the underlying etiology for AVWS is usually apparent. In the absence of a clear etiology for AVWS, it may be difficult to distinguish congenital VWD from AVWS. Absence of a past or family history of bleeding, and negative test results on parents may help. CBC is usually within the normal range.

Coagulation Testing

PT (INR) and fibrinogen are usually normal. aPTT may be slightly prolonged based on the FVIII procoagulant activity (FVIII:C). PFA-100® may show prolonged closure time with both collagen/epinephrine and collagen/ADP cartridges.

von Willebrand-specific testing typically reveals a low-to-normal VWF antigen (VWF:Ag) and FVIII:C. Functional assays of VWF, namely ristocetin cofactor activity (VWF:RCo) and collagen-binding activity (VWF:CBA) may show a more marked decrease. VWF multimer analysis typically shows decreased high molecular weight multimers. Presence of inhibitors can be evaluated by measuring ristocetin cofactor activity after incubating the patient's plasma in 1:1 ratio with normal plasma. However, unlike acquired hemophilia, anti VWF:FVIII inhibitors are rarely isolated in AVWS.

Management

Given the paucity of literature, evidence-based recommendations cannot be made for pediatric AVWS. Goals of management of AVWS include: (1) management of acute bleeding symptoms and prevention of bleeding with invasive procedures, and (2) treatment of the underlying disorder. Treatment of the underlying medical disorder, such as chemotherapy/surgery for Wilms' tumor, hormone replacement for hypothyroidism, immunosuppression (steroids/cytotoxic agents) for SLE and correction of a defective aortic valve or valvular stenosis, usually results in a rapid resolution of symptoms. Considerations for hemostatic and other immunomodulatory agents are as follows.

Desmopressin

DDAVP (0.3 μg/kg/dose, SC/IV, maximum dose 20 μg) results in a rapid increase in plasma VWF:Ag and may be used to treat minor bleeds. Response depends on the underlying medical condition, but its duration is usually shorter than the response to DDAVP in congenital VWD.

VWF Concentrates

Plasma-derived, viral-inactivated VWF:FVIII concentrates are available (Humate-P®, Wilate®) and may be used for more serious bleeding. It should be noted that patients with AVWS may require larger doses to overcome the antibodies or rapid clearance of the VWF:FVIII complex. A starting dose between 30 and 100 VWF:RCo U/kg can be used, depending on bleeding severity. Close laboratory monitoring of VWF is recommended.

Antifibrinolytic Agents

Antifibrinolytic agents such as tranexemic acid (10 mg/kg/dose i.v. q6–8 h; 25 mg/kg p.o. q8 h max dose 1,500 tid) and ε-aminocaproic acid (50 mg/kg/dose, q4–6 h; maximum daily dose 30 g) may be used in adjunct to VWF concentrates and/or DDAVP. These can be used orally or intravenously and are particularly useful in gastrointestinal bleeds.

Recombinant Factor VIIa

rFVIIa (Novoseven®) could be used for serious uncontrollable bleeds that does not respond to standard therapy. Risk of thrombosis needs to be considered.

Intravenous Immunoglobulin

IVIG (1 g/kg) is useful in AVWS associated with lymphoproliferative disorders, particularly monoclonal gammopathy of uncertain significance (MGUS-IgG). Its use has recently been reported in pediatric patients with acute lymphoblastic leukemia and biclonal IgM gammopathy.

Hypoprothrombinemia-Lupus Anticoagulant Syndrome

LAC is an acquired thrombophilia in which the risk of arterial and venous thrombosis is increased, particularly when the LAC is nontransient (see chapter 10 for details). HLAS is a rare condition where LAC is associated with a bleeding diathesis. This is thought to result from the presence of non-neutralizing antiprothrombin antibodies; the rapid clearance of prothrombin antigen-antibody complex eventually resulting in a prothrombin deficient state.

Case reports of HLAS typically describe a sudden onset of bleeding symptoms in a child with SLE or in a previously healthy child after a viral infection. Bleeding manifestations vary from mild mucocutaneous bleeds (epistaxis, gingival bleeding and petechiae) to life-threatening gastrointestinal bleeds and hemarthrosis. Laboratory findings in HLAS include prolonged PT (INR), prolonged aPTT with evidence of LAC, low prothrombin (FII) levels and evidence of antiprothrombin antibodies (FII IgG and IgM by ELISA). Since the antibodies are non-neutralizing, the mixing study for PT may be normal.

The rarity of HLAS makes it impossible to formulate evidence based guidelines. Patients with mild symptoms may not need any treatment. In patients with moderate-to-severe bleeding, FP, vitamin K and aPCC have been used. Concurrent immunosuppression with prednisone (1 mg/kg/day), IVIG and immunosuppressive agents (azathioprine and cyclophosphamide) have also been reported. In very severe life-threatening cases, plasmapheresis to remove antibodies may be warranted. It should be noted that case reports of thrombosis with aggressive hemostatic/prothrombotic management of HLAS have been described. If bleeding is controlled and/or non-life-threatening, steroids may be a reasonable as a first-line approach, with close monitoring of coagulation indices and clinical course.

Acquired Inhibitors after Bovine Thrombin Exposure

Topical preparations of bovine thrombin are used for surgical hemostasis after cardiovascular, neurosurgical and otolaryngologic procedures. These preparations are contaminated with coagulation proteins including fibrinogen, FV and FX. Repeated exposure to such preparations may elicit an immune response resulting in the formation of inhibitors, commonly directed against bovine FII and FV, with occasional cross-reactivity with human factors.

While common in adults, acquired inhibitors to FII and FV after bovine thrombin exposure are rare in children with few cases reported in the literature [31, 32]. These antibodies typically develop 7–10 days after exposure and may last for several weeks to months. While most patients are asymptomatic, hemorrhagic symptoms ranging from increased bruising to pulmonary, gastrointestinal and ICH have been described in up to 30% of the patients [32]. Laboratory manifestations typically include prolonged aPTT, INR and TT (with FII inhibitors) with minimal correction on mixing studies. In particular, TT may be markedly prolonged when bovine thrombin is used as the reagent. Plasma FV and FII levels are low and inhibitors can be confirmed using plasma mixing studies. Therapeutic interventions should be reserved for symptomatic patients and include bypassing agents (rFVIIa), steroids, IVIG, cytotoxic drugs and plasmapheresis. It is hypothesized that platelet transfusions may be more effective than FP, given that FV stored in the α-granules may be protected from the circulating antibody [31]. Use of purified, human plasma derived and/ or recombinant thrombin products may reduce the risk of inhibitor formation.

Conclusion

In summary, acquired bleeding disorders are a rare and heterogeneous group of disorders in children with symptoms ranging from mild mucocutaneous bleeding to life-threatening hemorrhage. A high index of suspicion and appropriate diagnostic tests are key to making a diagnosis and instituting appropriate therapy. There is little pediatric literature on management of these conditions and most recommendations have been extrapolated from adult literature. Bypassing agents such as rFVIIa and aPCC may be associated with an increased risk of thrombotic complications, and as such they should be used with caution.

Acknowledgment

The authors would like to express their appreciation for the thoughtful comments provided by Drs. Neil A. Goldenberg (St. Petersburg, Fla., USA), Georges E. Rivard (Montreal, Que., Canada), Christoph Male (Vienna, Austria), Simon C. Ling (Toronto, Ont., Canada) and Christoph Licht (Toronto, Ont., Canada) who reviewed this chapter.

References

1 Oren H, et al: Disseminated intravascular coagulation in pediatric patients: clinical and laboratory features and prognostic factors influencing the survival. Pediatr Hematol Oncol 2005;22:679–688.
2 Taylor FB Jr, et al: Towards definition, clinical and laboratory criteria and a scoring system for disseminated intravascular coagulation. Thromb Haemost 2001;86:1327–1330.
3 Khemani RG, et al: Disseminated intravascular coagulation score is associated with mortality for children with shock. Intensive Care Med 2009;35:327–333.
4 Shirahata A, Shirakawa Y, Murakami C: Diagnosis of DIC in very low birth weight infants. Semin Thromb Hemost 1998;24:467–471.
5 Levi M, et al: Guidelines for the diagnosis and management of disseminated intravascular coagulation. British Committee for Standards in Haematology. Br J Haematol 2009;145:24–33.
6 Franchini M, et al: Potential role of recombinant activated factor VII for the treatment of severe bleeding associated with disseminated intravascular coagulation: a systematic review. Blood Coagul Fibrinolysis 2007;18:589–593.
7 Goldstein B, et al: ENHANCE: results of a global open-label trial of drotrecogin alfa (activated) in children with severe sepsis. Pediatr Crit Care Med 2006;7:200–211.
8 Lynn RM, et al: Childhood hemolytic uremic syndrome, United Kingdom and Ireland. Emerg Infect Dis 2005;11:590–596.
9 Waters AM, Licht C: aHUS caused by complement dysregulation: new therapies on the horizon. Pediatr Nephrol 2011;26:41–57.
10 Noris M, Remuzzi G: Atypical hemolytic-uremic syndrome. N Engl J Med 2009;361:1676–1687.
11 Ariceta G, et al: Guideline for the investigation and initial therapy of diarrhea-negative hemolytic uremic syndrome. Pediatr Nephrol 2009;24:687–696.
12 Michael M, et al: Interventions for haemolytic uraemic syndrome and thrombotic thrombocytopenic purpura. Cochrane Database Syst Rev, 2009:p. CD003595.
13 George JN: How I treat patients with thrombotic thrombocytopenic purpura. Blood 2010;116:4060–4069.
14 Moake JL: Thrombotic microangiopathies. N Engl J Med 2002;347:589–600.
15 Fujimura Y, et al: Natural history of Upshaw-Schülman syndrome based on ADAMTS13 gene analysis in Japan. J Thromb Haemost 2011;9(suppl 1):283–301.
16 Bouw MC, et al: Thrombotic thrombocytopenic purpura in childhood. Pediatr Blood Cancer 2009;53:537–542.
17 Roberts LN, Patel RK, Arya R: Haemostasis and thrombosis in liver disease. Br J Haematol 2010;148:507–521.
18 Tripodi A, Mannucci PM: The coagulopathy of chronic liver disease. N Engl J Med 2010;365:147–156.
19 Wicklund BM: Bleeding and clotting disorders in pediatric liver disease. Hematology Am Soc Hematol Educ Program 2011, pp 170–177.
20 O'Shaughnessy DF, et al: Guidelines for the use of fresh-frozen plasma, cryoprecipitate and cryosupernatant. Br J Haematol 2004;126:11–28.
21 Chavez-Tapia NC, et al: Prophylactic activated recombinant factor VII in liver resection and liver transplantation: systematic review and meta-analysis. PLoS One 2011;6:e22581.

22 Liumbruno G, et al: Recommendations for the use of antithrombin concentrates and prothrombin complex concentrates. Blood Transf 2009;7:325–334.
23 Galbusera M, Remuzzi G, Boccardo P: Treatment of bleeding in dialysis patients. Semin Dial 2009;22:279–286.
24 Hedges SJ, et al: Evidence-based treatment recommendations for uremic bleeding. Nat Clin Pract Nephrol 2007;3:138–153.
25 Collins PW, et al: Acquired hemophilia A in the United Kingdom: a 2-year national surveillance study by the United Kingdom Haemophilia Centre Doctors' Organisation. Blood 2007;109:1870–1877.
26 Franchini M, Zaffanello M, Lippi G: Acquired hemophilia in pediatrics: a systematic review. Pediatr Blood Cancer 2011;55:606–611.
27 Pengo V, et al: Update of the guidelines for lupus anticoagulant detection. Subcommittee on Lupus Anticoagulant/Antiphospholipid Antibody of the Scientific and Standardisation Committee of the International Society on Thrombosis and Haemostasis. J Thromb Haemost 2009;7:1737–1740.
28 Collins PW: Management of acquired haemophilia A. J Thromb Haemost 2012;9(suppl 1):226–235.
29 Freedman J, et al: Immunoadsorption may provide a cost-effective approach to management of patients with inhibitors to FVIII. Transfusion 2003;43:1508–1513.
30 Franchini M, Lippi G: Acquired von Willebrand syndrome: an update. Am J Hematol 2007;82:368–375.
31 Bomgaars L, et al: Development of factor V and thrombin inhibitors in children following bovine thrombin exposure during cardiac surgery: a report of three cases. Congenit Heart Dis 2010; 5:303–308.
32 Savage WJ, Kickler TS, Takemoto CM: Acquired coagulation factor inhibitors in children after topical bovine thrombin exposure. Pediatr Blood Cancer 2007;49:1025–1029.

Abbreviations

ADAMTS13	A disintegrin and metalloproteinase with a thrombospondin type 1 motif, member 13
ADP	Adenosine 5′-diphospate
aHUS	Atypical hemolytic uremic syndrome
Anti-Xa	Anti-factor Xa
aPCC	Activated prothrombin complex concentrate
aPTT	Activated partial thromboplastin time
AVWS	Acquired von Willebrand syndrome
CBC	Complete blood count
CFB	Complement factor B
CFH	Complement factor H
CFHR	Complement factor H-related protein
CFI	Complement factor I
CLD	Chronic liver disease
CNS	Central nervous system
CRF	Chronic renal failure
DDAVP	1-Deamino-8-D-arginine vasopressin (desmopressin)
DIC	Disseminated intravascular coagulation
DVT	Deep vein thrombosis
FDPs	Fibrin degradation products
FP (FFP)	Frozen plasma (Fresh frozen plasma)
FII	Factor II (prothrombin)
FV	Factor V
FVII	Factor VII
FVIII	Factor VIII
FIX	Factor IX
FX	Factor X
FXI	Factor XI
FXIII	Factor XIII
HLAS	Hypoprothrombinemia-lupus anticoagulant syndrome
HSCT	Hemopoietic stem cell transplantation
HUS	Hemolytic uremic syndrome
ICH	Intracranial hemorrhage
INR	International normalized ratio
ISTH	International Society on Thrombosis and Haemostasis
IVH	Intraventricular hemorrhage
IVIG	Intravenous immunoglobulin
LAC	Lupus anticoagulant
LDH	Lactate dehydrogenase
LMWH	Low-molecular-weight heparin
MCP	Membrane cofactor protein
NSAIDs	Nonsteroidal anti-inflammatory drugs
PCC	Prothrombin complex concentrate
PCR	Polymerase chain reaction
PE	Pulmonary embolism
PFA-100®	Platelet function analyzer-100
PT	Prothrombin time
PVT	Portal vein thrombosis
rFVIIa	Recombinant activated factor VII
SLE	Systemic lupus erythematosus
TAFI	Thrombin-activatable fibrinolysis
TE	Thromboembolism/thromboembolic event
t-PA	Tissue-plasminogen activator
TT	Thrombin time
TTP	Thrombotic thrombocytopenic purpura
UFH	Unfractionated heparin
ULVWF	Unusually large von Willebrand factor
VWF	von Willebrand factor
VWF:CBA	VWF collagen binding activity
VWF:RCo	VWF activity (ristocetin cofactor assay)

Chapter 10

A Diagnostic Approach to a Child with Thrombosis

Mattia Rizzi
Chris Barnes

Introduction

The term 'thrombosis' refers to a clot in a blood vessel (arterial or venous) or in a chamber in the circulation (e.g. the atrium). In 1856, Rudolf Virchow postulated three factors that contribute to thrombosis: (1) impaired blood flow in vessels (stasis); (2) changes in the vessel wall (injury); (3) alterations in the constitution of the blood (hypercoagulability).

Compared to adults, TEs in children are relatively uncommon. Newborns and adolescents are the two age groups with the greatest incidence of VTEs [1–3]. Children <1 year of age represent the greatest risk group for ATEs [4]. The vast majority of children with TEs have associated underlying medical conditions. Increased awareness of thrombosis and continuing improvement of intensive care of critically ill children contribute to the increasing incidence of TEs in children [5].

TE in children is associated with a direct mortality rate of 1.5–2.2% and with significant morbidity, such as the development of PTS (see chapter 11), growth impairment of the involved limb or loss of organ function by arterial occlusion (see chapter 12) and neurological and neurocognitive deficits in the setting of stroke (see chapter 14).

The purpose of this chapter is to provide a clinical approach to the investigation of a child presenting with thrombosis. Assessment should start with a detailed personal and family history followed by a careful physical examination to determine the severity of the TE and to identify potential underlying conditions associated with an increased risk of thrombosis (table 1). Imaging studies such as DUS constitute determinant elements to confirm the diagnosis and to evaluate the extent and severity of the TE. Although no specific diagnostic laboratory tests for TE are available, measurement of coagulation parameters, a CBC and tests of renal and hepatic function are recommended as baseline investigations prior to initiating therapy. Investigation for an underlying hypercoagulable state, often referred to as a 'thrombophilia workup', may be part of the

Table 1. Clinical conditions associated with TEs in children

Age
Newborn > infant/child < adolescent
  Newborn-related risk factors
    Maternal conditions: diabetes mellitus, arterial hypertension, antiphospholipid syndrome
    Perinatal/neonatal risk factors: prematurity, asphyxia (including meconium aspiration), sepsis, congenital heart disease, congenital diaphragmatic hernia, polycythemia

Cancer
Tumor related (e.g. hyperleukocytosis, compression)
Drug related (e.g. steroids, L-asparaginase)
CVC related

Central venous/arterial catheter

Cardiac conditions
Congenital heart disease
Shunts (e.g. BT), surgical procedures (e.g. Fontan procedure)
Heart failure secondary to cardiomyopathy, myocarditis and/or arrhythmia
Mechanical valve
Endovascular stent
Extracorporeal device (e.g. ECMO)

Drugs
Oral contraceptive or hormone replacement
L-Asparaginase
Corticosteroids

Hematological disorders
Hyperviscosity syndrome (e.g. polycythemia vera)
Hemoglobinopathies (e.g. sickle cell disease, thalassemia)
Essential thrombocythemia
Paroxysmal nocturnal hemoglobinuria

Infections
Systemic (e.g. sepsis, HIV, varicella)
Localized (e.g. head/neck infection – Lemierre's syndrome, thrombophlebitis)

Inflammatory disorders
Autoimmune disorders (e.g. SLE, juvenile rheumatoid arthritis)
Vasculitis (e.g. Kawasaki disease)
Antiphospholipid syndrome
Inflammatory bowel diseases (ulcerative colitis, Crohn's disease)

Prolonged immobilization
Surgery
Trauma
Neurological diseases

Conditions with protein loss
Nephrotic syndrome
Protein-losing enteropathies
Chylothorax

Anatomical thrombophilia
Paget-Schroetter syndrome
May-Thurner syndrome

Others
Obesity
Previous thrombotic event

laboratory evaluation of a child with thrombosis. The indications for a thrombophilia workup will be discussed later in this chapter.

History

Risk Factors

TEs in children usually occur in the setting of acquired prothrombotic risk factors and frequently represent secondary complications of an underlying disease (table 1). Occasionally, TE may represent the primary manifestation of an unsuspected disorder, such as a tumor or a chronic inflammatory process.

The presence of a central venous and/or arterial catheter represents the single most important risk factor in the development of systemic ATE and VTE in the pediatric population and accounts for more than 90% of systemic TEs in newborn infants and more than half of TEs in all other age groups [3]. These 'foreign' devices are often essential for therapeutic and supportive care of critically ill children.

TEs occurring in the neonatal age group may be associated with maternal, perinatal and/or neonatal conditions (table 1). Purpura fulminans is a rare, life-threatening disorder affecting neonates and presents with cutaneous hemorrhage and necrosis resulting from microvascular thrombosis as a result of an inherited deficiency of protein C and/or protein S (see later) [6]. TEs in neonates may involve specific vessel sites, such as renal vein thrombosis and PVT, the latter frequently associated with the presence of an umbilical venous catheter (chapter 13). The setting of CSVT and AIS in the neonatal period is distinct from that occurring later in life (chapter 14).

VTEs or ATEs are less frequent in young children than in neonates and adolescents, and are generally associated with a combination of identifiable risk factors such as presence of a CVC, hematologic malignancy, congenital heart disease requiring cardiac catheterization or surgery, infection, or autoimmune disorders. Spontaneous TE in this age group is unusual and should raise the possibility of an undiagnosed disorder associated with an increased risk of TE.

TEs in adolescents are more common, and as with younger children, TE in adolescents may occur in association with an underlying disorder and/or its related treatment. Spontaneous (unprovoked) TEs occur more commonly in this age group and may be associated with the use of medications such as hormonal contraceptives and/or an underlying inherited prothrombotic trait such as the presence of FVL mutation [7].

Medical History

A detailed medical history should capture information about an underlying disease, ongoing treatments and medications (table 1). Past history of a TE including the type, location and presence (or absence) of associated risk factors is important and may have a direct impact on the management including the duration of anticoagulation. Finally, information on symptoms of bleeding or bruising and history of renal or hepatic problems should be obtained to assist in the assessment of risks of anticoagulation.

Family History

An accurate family history is important in assessing children presenting with TE. A positive family history of a TE is an independent risk factor for TEs. This risk increases with the number of relatives affected, younger age of a family member at the time of TE [8], and in the presence of a known thrombophilia trait [9]. A detailed family history should include information on VTE at any age, cardiovascular events such as myocardial infarction and AIS at a younger adult age, e.g. <40 years, and obstetric complications, particularly occurrence of recurrent miscarriage and/or known familial thrombophilia.

Even though no evidence suggests that children of any particular race are at higher risk of TE, information about ethnic origin may be helpful in estimating the risk of certain thrombophilic traits. For example, the presence of FVL mutation or prothrombin G20210A mutation are mostly found in Caucasians and are extremely rare in persons of Asian and African descent.

Physical Examination

Signs and symptoms of TE may be nonspecific, subtle or even absent. Clinical manifestations depend on a variety of factors, including type of blood vessel affected (arterial versus venous), the degree of vessel occlusion (occlusive versus nonocclusive), and site of organ affected (table 2). Many TEs are associated with nonspecific or absent symptoms/signs, and a high index of suspicion and awareness of the potential for TE and its related risk factors is important in order to make a timely diagnosis.

The physical examination should include an assessment of the affected body part, most often a limb, plus a general physical examination, in order to identify underlying disorders or conditions that may be associated with an increased risk of TE. The clinical examination of an affected limb should record skin discoloration (i.e. pale, cyanotic), skin temperature (cold in arterial and warm in venous occlusion), presence of swelling, tenderness, presence of collaterals and the degree of functional impairment. Presence of skin lesions may reflect the presence of a previous catheter or of localized inflammatory/infectious processes. Rapid onset of cutaneous purpuric lesions after

Table 2. Signs and symptoms in relation to the site of thrombosis and the suggested diagnostic imaging tests

Site of thrombosis	Sign(s) and symptom(s)	Suggested imaging	Detailed in
Limb (upper/lower) DVT	pain, swelling, discoloration, collaterals, tenderness, increased temperature, impaired function of involved limb; may be asymptomatic	DUS[1], CTV/MRV[2], venography[3]	chapter 11
Superior vena cava, intrathoracic and jugular DVT	neck/head pain and swelling, and/or with symptoms associated with upper limb DVT; may be asymptomatic	DUS (low sensitivity for intrathoracic)[1], CTV/MRV[2], venography (high sensitivity for intrathoracic)[3]	chapter 11
Inferior vena cava, common iliac vein DVT	back, buttock and/or abdominal pain, ±symptoms associated with lower limb DVT; may be asymptomatic	DUS[1], CTV/MRV[2], venography[3]	chapter 11
Right atrial thrombus	bradycardia, tachyarrhythmia, new heart murmur, heart failure, respiratory distress; may be asymptomatic	echocardiography	chapter 11
Pulmonary embolism	unexplained chest pain or shortness of breath with pleuretic chest pain, cough, hemoptysis, tachypnea, tachycardia, shock; may be asymptomatic	spiral CT (CTPA)[1], V/Q scan[2], MRI[3], pulmonary angiography[3]	chapter 11
Limb (upper/lower) arterial thrombosis	pain, pallor, reduced temperature, absent pulses or necrosis (late sign) of involved limb	DUS[1]	chapter 12
Portal/hepatic/mesenteric/splenic vein thrombosis	localized/diffuse abdominal pain, and/or hepato-splenomegaly; increased abdominal girth with or without ascites; may be asymptomatic	DUS[1], CTV/MRV[2]	chapter 13
Renal vein thrombosis	abdominal/flank pain, hematuria, oliguria, abdominal mass, thrombocytopenia	DUS[1]	chapter 13
Central nervous system TE Arterial ischemic stroke Sinus venous thrombosis	general neurologic symptoms: headache, altered level of consciousness, nausea, emesis, seizure (common in neonates) and/or focal neurologic deficit	MRA[1]/CTA[2] MRV[1]/CTV[2]	chapter 14

For details see diagnostic imaging in the specific chapter.
[1] Current practice.
[2] Second choice (if [1] non available or not conclusive).
[3] Third choice.

birth represents the clinical manifestation of purpura fulminans, a life-threatening condition requiring rapid treatment.

In VTE, the outflow of blood from the organ/body part is compromised causing progressive stasis of blood and fluid accumulation in the interstitial compartment leading to swelling. Acute onset of swelling and pain represent the most frequent clinical presentation of VTE affecting a limb. ATE may present with signs of absent or diminished peripheral pulses, cool and pale extremities or necrotic areas. Impaired arterial flow represents an urgent condition requiring rapid assessment and treatment.

Swelling may not always be apparent, and objective measurement of the circumference of the affected and non-affected limbs may help to quantify the degree of swelling. A number of specific clinical assessments used in adult patients may help in the assessment of older children suspected with lower limb TE. This includes calf pain induced either by dorsiflexion of the foot (Homan's sign), calf compression (May's sign) or sole pain induced by its compression (Payr's sign).

A Diagnostic Approach to a Child with Thrombosis

The presence of superficial collateral vessels, skin induration, increased skin pigmentation and ulcers are clinical signs of chronic venous stasis and PTS (discussed in chapter 11). Malfunctioning ('blocked') CVC, such as difficulty with infusion, flushing or getting blood return, or CVC-related infection may also suggest the presence of thrombosis.

A detailed neurological examination is required where there is suspicion of a cerebral TE (chapter 14).

Respiratory examination may help to identify whether the respiratory symptoms, such as dyspnea and/or chest pain, are due to an infective condition or other causes other than those associated with a PE.

Hepatosplenomegaly in the presence of an increased abdominal girth, with or without ascites, may reflect thrombosis occurring in the portal vein, in the hepatic, splenic and mesenteric veins or the IVC.

Diagnostic Imaging

The clinical suspicion of a TE should be followed by diagnostic imaging to confirm the presence of and extent of thrombosis. Knowledge of the different imaging techniques, their appropriate use and limitations, as well as an understanding of the normal vascular anatomy is important for the diagnosis of thrombosis in children.

Diagrams of the vascular anatomy for the upper and lower deep venous systems, major arteries and umbilical circulation are presented in figure 1. The cerebral venous sinus system and the cerebral arterial supply are further discussed in chapter 14.

Doppler Ultrasonography

Compression DUS is a noninvasive technique that is the preferred imaging option for the diagnosis of thrombosis in children. In vessels with thrombosis, Doppler signals are absent and the lumen cannot be compressed with direct pressure.

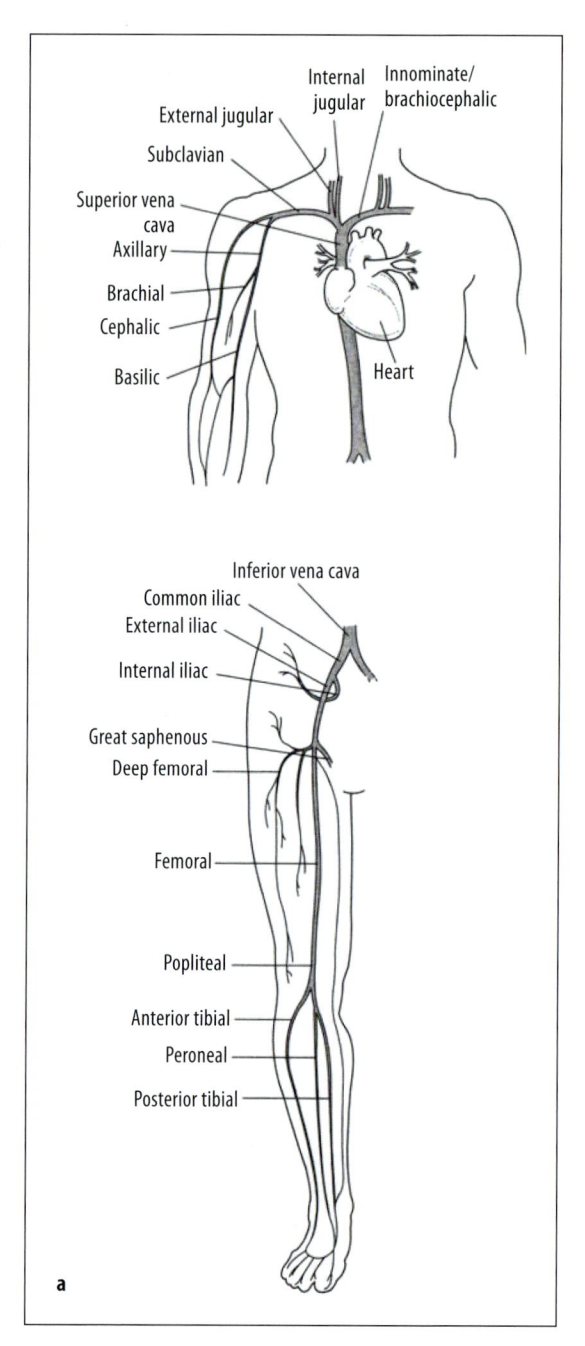

Figure 1a. Deep veins of the upper and lower venous systems. From *Andrew's Pediatric Thromboembolism and Stroke*, ed 3, Shelton, People's Medical Publishing Houses-USA, 2006.

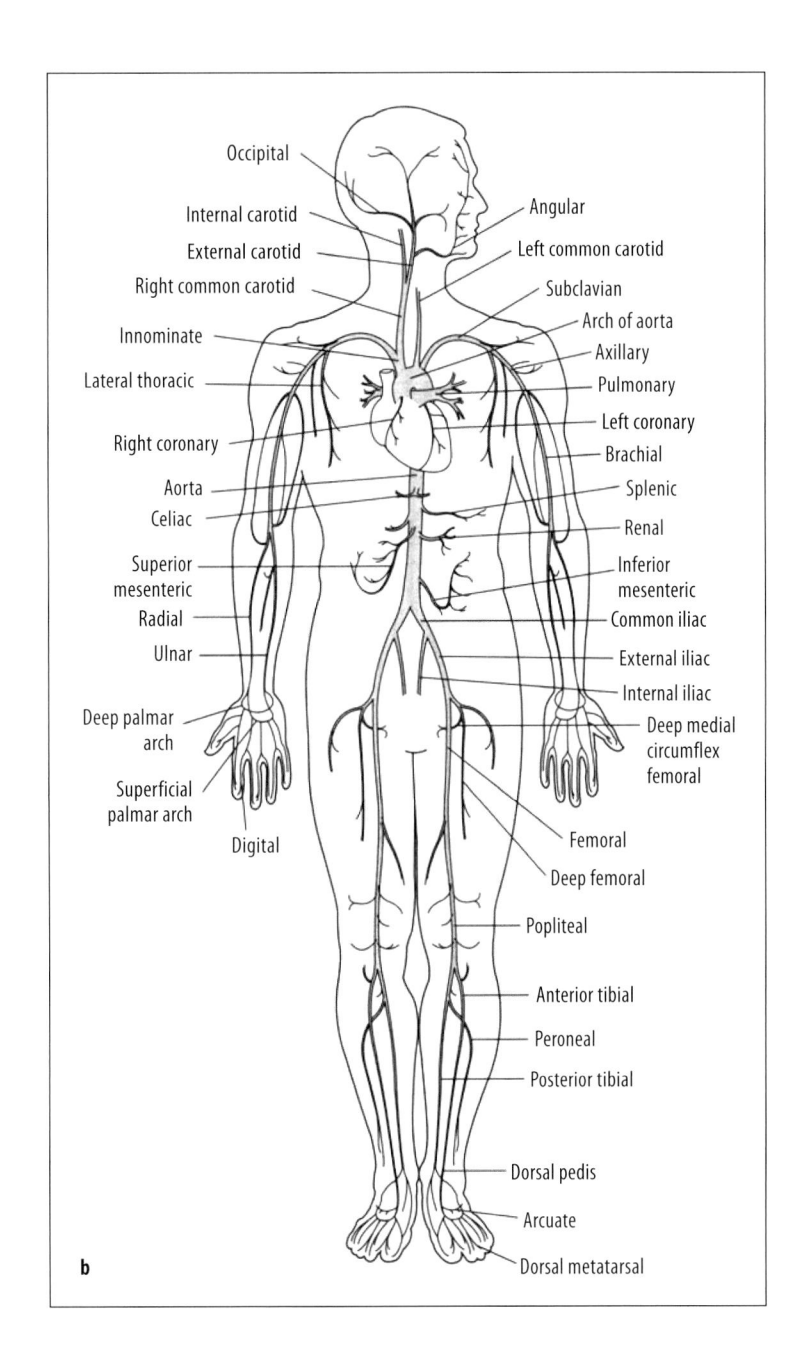

Figure 1 b. Major arteries. From *Andrew's Pediatric Thromboembolism and Stroke*, ed 3, Shelton, People's Medical Publishing Houses-USA, 2006.

Success of this technique is dependent on the experience of the examiner and on patient compliance. Its sensitivity in the assessment of the intrathoracic upper vessel system, including the proximal subclavian and innominate veins and the superior vena cava, is low because of the inability to compress the vessels [1]. Other factors that may interfere with DUS imaging in children include small-diameter vessels, low pulse pressure and the presence of a CVC that compromises the ability to

A Diagnostic Approach to a Child with Thrombosis

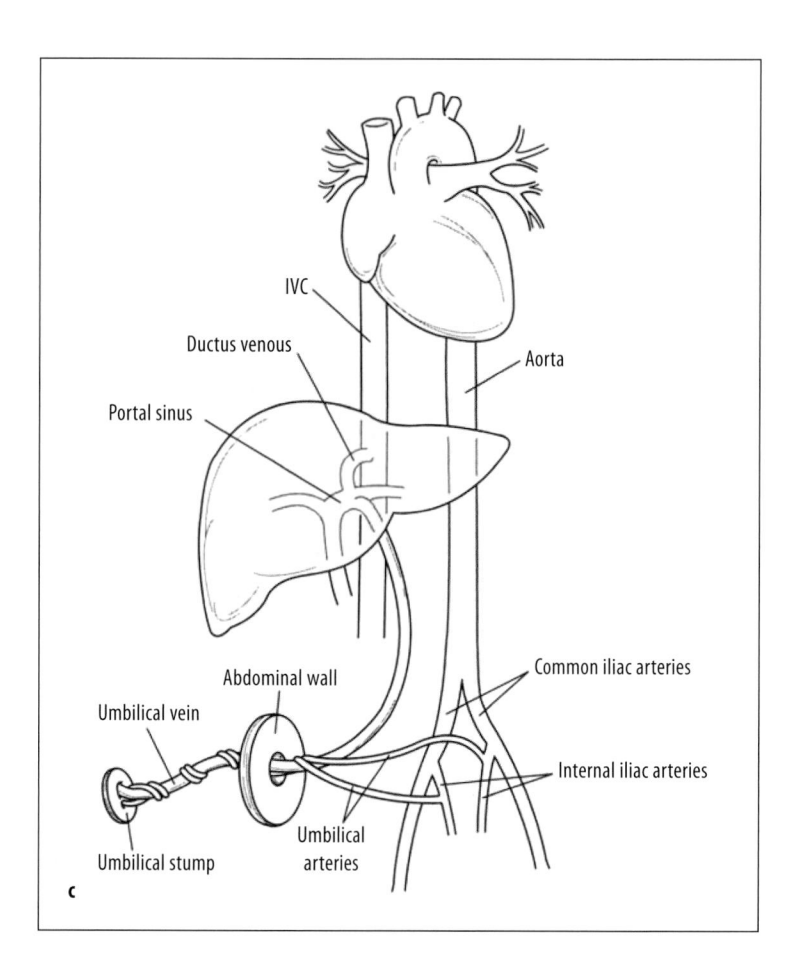

Figure 1 c. Umbilical circulation. From *Andrew's Pediatric Thromboembolism and Stroke*, ed 3, Shelton, People's Medical Publishing Houses-USA, 2006.

clearly compress the veins. Other techniques such as CTV or MRV may be used in difficult cases. Echocardiography is a valuable noninvasive modality for the diagnosis of a thrombus occurring in the heart.

Conventional Venography

Venography is a minimally invasive technique, where ionized dye is injected through a vein, thus enabling visualization of the vessels by X-ray. With the exception of the jugular veins, this technique enables the visualization of any portion of the venous system. Venography is considered the gold standard in the diagnosis of VTE in children; however, the need for good venous access, interventional radiologist and anesthesia support, as well the exposure to contrast and ionizing radiation makes this technique less suitable in children. In addition to a chest X-ray to visualize the line placement, a linogram (direct injection of contrast into the line of interest) and venography are occasionally used for the investigation of a malfunctioning CVC (chapter 11).

Computed Tomography

X-ray based CT with or without ionized contrast enables very rapid acquisition of images. CTPA, also termed spiral CT, is a noninvasive technique currently preferred in both pediatric and adult patients with clinically suspected PE (chapter 11). The most important disadvantages of CTPA are its use of ionizing radiation and its use in children with impaired renal function. CTA or CTV with contrast may be useful in the assessment of children presenting with stroke if other techniques are not available (chapter 14).

Magnetic Resonance Imaging

MRI with or without gadolinium-enhanced MRV or MRA is the preferred imaging technique for assessing children presenting with stroke and has the advantage of not exposing children to radiation (chapter 14). MRV may also have an important role for assessing thrombosis in the intrathoracic upper limb vessel system. Pulmonary contrast MRA should be considered as an alternative to CTPA for diagnosis of PE when ionized contrast injection or radiation is a significant consideration. A limitation of MRI in children is the time required to achieve adequate imaging plus the need for sedation and its potential related morbidity.

Ventilation/Perfusion Lung Scan

V/Q scan is a combination of scintigraphy with a radioisotope. In the ventilation phase, an aerosol form of the nuclide is inhaled and in the perfusion phase, a nuclide is injected intravenously. A gamma camera acquires the images required to determine the ventilation/perfusion rate. The V/Q scan is interpreted according to criteria adapted from adults (classified as low, moderate, or high PE probability according to the documented mismatch in the ventilation and perfusion; chapter 11). A high-probability scan results in a peripheral basal perfusion defect with normal ventilation. However, this technique is not always available, and requires a cooperative child (usually at least 5 years of age). Spiral CT has largely replaced V/Q scan in children with clinically suspected PE (see above).

Conventional Chest X-Ray

Conventional chest X-ray may help to identify or exclude alternative diagnoses, such as a pneumonia that occurs much more frequently than a PE. A chest X-ray should be performed to visualize the CVC position in cases with CVC dysfunction (chapter 11).

Laboratory Investigations

Laboratory Tests in the Acute Presentation

Specific diagnostic laboratory tests to confirm the presence of thrombosis are not available. Laboratory evaluation in the acute phase in a patient being assessed for TE may be helpful in assessing for other disorders or may be used to establish safety for a required treatment.

CBC (Blood Collected into EDTA)

A low platelet count may increase the risk of bleeding in patients who require antithrombotic therapy (see chapter 16 for details). Anemia and thrombocytopenia may suggest DIC. Thrombocytopenia associated with hematuria may suggest renal vein thrombosis (chapter 13).

PT/INR, aPTT (Blood Collected into Citrate)

Abnormal results may suggest factor deficiencies (see chapter 3 for details). Correction of factor deficiencies should be considered prior to initiation of antithrombotic therapy. A prolonged aPTT, if measured using an antiphospholipid sensitive assay, may suggest the presence of the APLA (see below). Shortened aPTT may reflect the presence of elevated FVIII secondary to inflammatory disorders (see below). A prolonged PT or aPTT and/or a low fibrinogen level with thrombocytopenia may suggest DIC.

D-Dimer Test (Blood Collected into Citrate)

D-dimers are degradation products of fibrin that are formed during fibrinolysis (chapter 2). Elevated D-dimer levels are associated with VTE (for normal values refer to the appendix). However, an elevated D-dimer level is often a nonspecific finding occurring in inflammation, sepsis, malignancy or other proinflammatory

Table 3. Prevalence and impact (expressed as pooled odds ratio) of laboratory thrombophilia in childhood TEs

Thrombophilia	Prevalence	First VTE odds ratio (95% CI)	Recurrent VTE odds ratio (95% CI)	First CSVT odds ratio (95% CI)	First AIS odds ratio (95% CI)
FV Leiden G1691A[1]	~1:20	3.8 (3–4.8)	0.6 (0.4–1.2)	2.7 (1.7–4.3)	3.7 (2.8–4.9)
Prothrombin G20210A[1]	~1:50	2.6 (1.6–4.4)	1.9 (1.0–3.5)	2.0 (0.9–4.1)	2.6 (1.7–4.1)
Protein C deficiency[1]	~1:500	7.7 (4.4–13.4)	2.4 (1.2–4.4)	6.3 (1.6–25.4)	11.0 (5.1–23.6)
Protein S deficiency[1]	~1:5,000	5.8 (3.0–11)	3.1 (1.5–6.5)	5.3 (1.5–18.2)	1.5 (0.3–6.9) (R)
Antithrombin deficiency[1]	~1:50,000	9.4 (3.3–26.7)	3.0 (1.4–6.3)	18.4 (3.3–104.3)	3.3 (0.7–15.5)
Lp(a)[1]	NA	4.5 (3.3–6.2)	0.8 (0.5–1.4)	NA	6.5 (4.5–9.6)
≥2 genetic traits[2]	NA	9.5 (4.9–18.4)	4.5 (2.9–6.9)	6.1 (0.9–43.1)	18.8 (6.5–54.1)
LAC/APLA	variable	4.9 (2.2–10.9)	NA	NA	7.0 (3.7–13.1)
FVIII:C	NA	5.5 (2.0–15.1)	NA	NA	NA
FVIII:Ag	NA	4.3 (1.5–12.1)	NA	NA	NA

Adapted from references [13–16]. FVIII:C = Activity (>90th percentiles); FVIII:Ag = antigen (>90th percentile); NA = not applicable; R = random effect model.
[1] Heterozygote trait.
[2] Including FV Leiden, Prothrombin G20210A mutation, Lp(a) (>30 mg/dl), antithrombin deficiency, protein C and/or protein S deficiency.

states. In adults, D-dimer levels have a good negative predictive value but poor positive predictive value; normal levels almost always rule out the diagnosis of VTE, whereas high levels are not necessarily diagnostic for VTE [10]. The negative predictive value of D-dimer was never validated in children; thus, D-dimer should be used cautiously in excluding VTE in adolescent patients and is not recommended to be used to exclude VTE in young children [11].

An elevated D-dimer plasma level at diagnosis and after 3–6 months of treatment has been shown to be associated with persistent VTE, recurrent VTE and/or development of PTS [12].

Evaluation of Renal and Liver Function (Blood Collected into Heparin)
Abnormal liver and/or renal function may lead to therapy adjustment in children with TE (see chapter 16 for details).

Laboratory Evaluation during Ongoing Anticoagulation

Effective and safe antithrombotic treatment requires appropriate monitoring (see chapter 16 for details).

Laboratory Thrombophilia

Thrombophilia is characterized by hypercoagulability and an increased tendency to develop thrombosis. A number of inherited and acquired laboratory thrombophilia markers have been identified; however, the interpretation of laboratory thrombophilia in individual clinical scenarios may be difficult. Age-dependent normal laboratory values for many laboratory thrombophilia markers are presented in the appendix. The inherited and acquired markers for thrombophilia are detailed below according to their mechanism of action. The impact of laboratory thrombophilia on primary systemic VTE, its recurrence and stroke is presented in table 3 [13–16].

Elevated Procoagulant Factors

Prothrombin (II) G20210A Mutation (Blood Collected into EDTA)
An elevated prothrombin (FII) level is caused by a point mutation (detected by PCR-based DNA mutation analysis) located on the noncoding region of the prothrombin gene (nucleotide 20210 G to A) leading to augmented thrombin

generation and potentially with an increased risk of thrombosis.

Elevated FVIII (Blood Collected into Citrate)

In adults as well as in children, persistent high levels of FVIII activity and antigen (both >90th percentiles) have been shown to be associated with TE, particularly in the onset of non-CVC-related VTE [14]. A persistent elevated plasma FVIII level, potentially reflecting a genetic trait, appears to be of more relevance as a risk factor for VTE than does an acute elevation of FVIII level (acute phase reaction). Therefore, measurement of FVIII is suggested after the resolution of the acute phase with assessment of inflammatory markers (usually 3–6 months after the event) as part of a thrombophilia workup. Moreover, measurement of FVIII plasma levels in the parents may be helpful. FVIII activity (FVIII:C) is usually measured by one-stage clotting assay (for normal values refer to the appendix).

Decreased Natural Anticoagulant Factors

Deficiencies of natural anticoagulants including protein C, protein S and antithrombin are uncommon, but represent a potent thrombotic risk. Levels are age specific and may be influenced by secondary conditions affecting their production, consumption or loss. Deficiencies of the three natural anticoagulants are inherited in an autosomal dominant manner. All diagnostic laboratories processing pediatric samples for natural anticoagulants should use and interpret results according to age-, analyzer- and reagent-specific reference ranges [17]. It should be emphasized that a single laboratory test result below the 95% confidence limit for age is not enough to define an inherited state. The diagnosis of inherited state should be based on the presence of compatible clinical phenotype, family history, and reproducible abnormal laboratory results.

Protein C and S Deficiency (Blood Collected into Citrate)

Both proteins are vitamin K-dependent natural anticoagulants and mainly produced in the liver. Protein C together with protein S forms a complex that inhibits activated FV and FVIII (chapter 2).

Protein C deficiency is classified into two types: type I (most frequent) is characterized by both a low activity and antigen level (quantitative deficiency), and type II by a low activity level but a normal antigen level (qualitative deficiency). First, protein C activity is measured (using a clotting assay) and, if abnormal, the protein C antigen level can be measured using an ELISA-based test (for normal values refer to the appendix).

Protein S circulates in plasma in two different forms: a free active form and an inactive form bound to C4b-free binding protein. Protein S deficiency is therefore classified into three different subtypes according to the amount of free or bound protein and its activity. Type I deficiency (quantitative) is defined by inadequate amount of both the free and total protein S (= bound and free protein S levels). Type III is also a quantitative deficiency characterized by a low free protein S antigen, but an overall normal amount of total protein S. Type II deficiency is defined by normal level of free and total protein S but reduced protein S activity (functional deficiency). Testing for protein S deficiency includes the measurement of free protein S antigen and, if abnormal, total protein S can be determined (both are measured using an ELISA-based test system; for normal values refer to the appendix). The distinction between type I and type III has no clinical implication. Functional protein S assays are difficult to perform and only rarely necessary as type II protein S deficiency is extremely rare.

Homozygous (or compound heterozygous) protein C or S cases generally present with neonatal purpura fulminans (separately addressed in this chapter) [6]. Acquired conditions with protein C and S deficiency reflect their increased consumption in sepsis- and non-sepsis-associated DIC, infections (typically varicella for protein S) or decreased production such as by vitamin K deficiency, liver disorders or medications (e.g. VKAs, oral contraceptives, asparaginase chemotherapy).

Antithrombin Deficiency (Blood Collected into Citrate)

Antithrombin is a natural anticoagulant that inactivates several coagulation factors such as FIIa, FXa, FIXa and FXIa (chapter 2). Antithrombin deficiency is classified into two types: type I (most frequent) is characterized by both a low activity and antigen level (quantitative deficiency); type II is characterized by a low activity, but a normal antigen level due to the production of a dysfunctional protein (qualitative defects). Antithrombin activity is measured by chromogenic assay and, if abnormal, antithrombin antigen may be tested using an ELISA-based test (for normal values refer to the appendix).

Homozygous deficiency is not considered compatible with life. Acquired antithrombin deficiency can occur in association with large protein losses (e.g. nephrotic syndrome), liver disease, sepsis and treatment with asparaginase chemotherapy (see chapter 11 for details). Patients with antithrombin deficiency may be heparin resistant (chapter 16).

Resistance to Intrinsic Anticoagulant Function

Activated Protein C Resistance (Blood Collected into Citrate) – FVL Mutation (Blood Collected into EDTA)

A point mutation in the FV gene (nucleotide 1691 A to G), also called the FVL mutation, is the most common genetic disorder associated with thrombosis in adults and in children, with a carrier rate of 5% in Caucasian populations. The mutation (detected by PCR-based DNA mutation analysis) leads to a change in FV conferring resistance to inactivation by protein C. The presence of a heterozygous mutation is associated with a low to mild risk of VTE and stroke in children [13, 15]. Patients with homozygous mutations are at much greater risk of thrombosis compared to heterozygous mutations. Acquired activated protein C resistance may occur in the setting of oral contraceptive use [7] or in association with high concentrations of coagulation FVIII.

Biochemical Mediators of Endothelial Damage

Lupus Anticoagulant (Blood Collected into Citrate)

LAC detection consists of three sequential laboratory steps [for details see 18]: (1) demonstration of an abnormal phospholipid-dependent coagulation screening test (using diluted Russell viper venom test and/or a lupus-sensitive aPTT); (2) a mixing study to ensure that the abnormality of the screening test is due to the presence of a circulating inhibitor; (3) a confirmatory test, which incorporates the addition of exogenous phospholipids to prove that the abnormality is phospholipid dependent. Assessment for the presence of an LAC may be helpful prior to initiation of anticoagulation since anticoagulation may affect the interpretation of LAC screens [18].

Anti-Cardiolipin Antibodies and Anti-β$_2$-Glycoprotein I Antibodies (Blood Collected into Clotted Blood Tube)

Both IgG and IgM ACLA and β$_2$-GPI are measured by immunoassay (ELISA) test (for normal values refer to the appendix).

APLA include LAC, ACLA and β$_2$-GPI. APLS is defined by the presence of vascular thrombosis or pregnancy loss with the persistent (two tests performed 12 weeks apart) presence of APLA including LAC or/and ACLA and/or β$_2$-GPI [19]. APLS is a common acquired condition associated with unprovoked VTEs and/or ATEs in childhood. Other abnormalities associated with APLA include thrombocytopenia, hemolytic anemia and renal dysfunction (thrombotic microangiopathy). APLA may be transient in the setting of acute infection, inflammation, malignancy and medications. APLA may also be transient in newborn infants with a positive maternal history for APLS but rarely cause neonatal TEs.

Children presenting with unprovoked TE should be assessed for the presence of APLA. Testing should be repeated 12 weeks following an initial positive test. Children with persistent APLA have a significant increased risk of recurrence, and prolonged (or long-term) anticoagulation may be considered [11, 16, 20].

Homocysteine (Blood Collected into Heparin)
Homocysteine is an amino acid that derives from dietary methionine. Elevated homocysteine may have an effect on endothelium conferring prothrombotic changes, and may be associated with an increased risk of VTE, spontaneous ATE and AIS in children [21]. No data are available on the significance of high homocysteine levels and the efficacy of lowering homocysteine levels to prevent thrombotic recurrence in children.

Hyperhomocysteinemia may arise from dietary conditions such as vitamin deficiency, e.g. vitamin B_6, vitamin B_{12} and folic acid, or increased dietary methionine intake, and has been linked to genetic defects, such as homocysteinuria, cobalamin C deficiency or polymorphisms in the MTHFR gene, such as MTHFR C677T mutation. Even in homozygotes, there is only a mild elevation of the homocysteine level usually only in the presence of a sub-therapeutic level of folic acid. MTHFR polymorphism independent of homocysteinemia does not increase the risk of TE. Therefore, an elevated level of homocysteine, rather than the presence of the MTHFR gene polymorphism may be a determinant for thrombotic risk [22]. Fasting homocysteine level can be measured in the plasma by electrospray tandem mass spectrometry (for normal values refer to the appendix).

Increased Antifibrinolytic Activity
Elevated Lipoprotein(a) (Blood Collected into EDTA)
Lp(a) is composed of a low-density lipid particle (LDL) and a polypeptide chain (apolipoprotein a). Lp(a) shares similar structural characteristics with plasminogen and t-PA and competes with plasminogen for its binding site to fibrin, leading to reduced fibrinolysis. Other thrombotic effects may be caused by the Lp(a)-induced secretion of plasminogen activator inhibitor (PAI-1) and by inducing atherosclerosis because of its (high) LDL cholesterol content. Plasma Lp(a) levels can be measured by high-performance affinity liquid chromatography (for normal values refer to the appendix).

Impact of Thrombophilia in Childhood Thrombosis
The reported prevalence of laboratory thrombophilic risk factors in different studies in children with thrombosis varies (13–79%) and mostly reflects differences in study design, and differences in the clinically and demographic characteristics of the study populations [22]. Previous analyses and more recently performed comprehensive studies in the form of systematic reviews, meta-analyses or observational studies enable us to understand the impact of thrombophilia specifically on the risk of developing primary VTE and its recurrence as well stroke in childhood, including CSVT and AIS (table 3) [13–16, 23]. These reviews, however, are limited by sample heterogeneity. The prevalence and impact of thrombophilia in non-cerebral ATE are even less clear [4].

Table 4. Laboratory thrombophilia testing in the pediatric population
a Proposal for laboratory thrombophilia testing in neonates, children and adolescents with VTEs and ATEs

Clinical scenario	Time	Testing	Tests included	Rationale
Purpura fulminans or non-sepsis DIC	Acute	Recommended	Protein C and S, antithrombin	Deficiency of protein S, protein C or antithrombin may warrant replacement therapy
Neonates/children/adolescents with unprovoked VTE	FU	Recommended	Thrombophilia workup	May help to determine the risk of recurrence, and to identify homozygous or combined defect. May allow screening of family members (if positive)
Children/adolescents with recurrent (non-catheter related) VTE	FU	Recommended	Thrombophilia workup	May help to determine the risk of recurrence, and to identify homozygous or combined defect. May allow screening of family members (if positive)
Children/adolescents with provoked (non-catheter related) VTE	FU	Suggest to discuss the utility with the patients/family	Thrombophilia workup	Insufficient data to recommend for or against
Neonates/children/adolescents with unprovoked, provoked (non-catheter related) or recurrent non-cerebral ATE	FU	Suggest to discuss the utility with the patients/family	Thrombophilia workup	Insufficient data to recommend for or against
Neonates/children/adolescents with catheter-related VTE/ATE	FU	Not suggested	–	Does not influence treatment strategy

b Proposal for laboratory thrombophilia testing in children and adolescents without personal history of TE

Clinical scenario	Testing	Test included	Rationale
Children/adolescents with family history of TE and known or unknown (not yet tested) thrombophilia trait	May be considered in selected patients: – to guide thromboprophylaxis in high-risk patient – concurrent exposure to other prothrombotic conditions (e.g. oral contraceptive, CVC insertion for acute lymphoblastic leukemia therapy, major surgery) – for research purpose	Proteins C and S, antithrombin; Prothrombin gene and FV Leiden gene or test according to known familial thrombophilia trait. If familial trait is unknown, consider testing the index family member with TE first	Current data suggest that one or more positive test results increase the likelihood to experience a TE in life. Testing needs to be discussed with the family for each individual situation
Children/adolescents without family history for TE and/or for thrombophilia trait in the setting of presence or potential exposure to acquired prothrombotic condition(s)	Not recommended	–	No clinical trial demonstrating efficacy and risk/benefit of thromboprophylaxis. No cost effectiveness

Acute = At the time of the event; FU = during follow-up. Thrombophilia workup, depending on clinician/center preferences and/or recommendations, may or may not include the following tests further addressed in the text: protein C activity, protein S free antigen level, antithrombin activity, activated protein C resistance, FVIII activity, Prothrombin gene mutation and FV Leiden gene mutation analysis, lupus anticoagulant test, anticardiolipin IgM and IgG antibodies, β_2-GPI IgM and IgG antibodies, fasting homocysteine level and Lp(a) plasma level.

Who and When and What Should Be Tested

Given the heterogeneity of patient populations and the multifactorial pathogenesis of TEs in the pediatric population, it is difficult to present definitive recommendations regarding laboratory testing for presence of a thrombophilic state. Diagnostic testing for thrombophilia in children should take into consideration the ethnic background of the subject and be discussed on an individual basis, at least for the symptomatic index patient. A tentative summary of circumstances in which testing for laboratory thrombophilia in children may be indicated is presented in table 4. Guidance for thrombophilia testing for children with VTE from the perinatal and pediatric Scientific and Standardization Committee of the ISTH was recently updated from the 2002 recommendations and is largely based on expert opinion [24].

In brief, diagnostic thrombophilia testing is recommended for neonates, children and adolescents with first unprovoked and recurrent VTE. For the first episode of provoked VTE, it is suggested to discuss the utility of diagnostic thrombophilia testing with patients and parents. Thrombophilia testing is not suggested for neonates, children or adolescents with asymptomatic or symptomatic CVC-related VTE.

The benefit of thrombophilia testing in neonates, children and adolescents in the setting of ATE is less clear, and no current definitive guideline is available. For AIS, a recent systematic review and meta-analysis of previous observational studies suggest an association between the presence of the laboratory thrombophilia (inherited as well acquired) and the onset of AIS (table 3) [13, 16]. However, there are insufficient data in the literature validating the utility of such testing, given the disparate setting in which AIS may occur (see chapter 14 for recommended testing). Non-cerebral ATE mainly occurs as a complication of catheter placement (see chapter 12). Thrombophilia testing is not suggested for neonates, children and adolescents with asymptomatic or symptomatic catheter-related ATE [4].

For unprovoked (non-catheter-related) non-cerebral ATE, only marginal data are available and do not enable a definitive recommendation [4].

It remains the responsibility of the involved physician to decide if, when and what tests are appropriate for the individual child, and in all cases testing should involve detailed discussion with the patient and family.

Thrombophilia testing rarely influences the acute management of a patient with a TE and the therapeutic treatment should be initiated independent of the laboratory thrombophilia results. Only in certain circumstances are selected laboratory thrombophilia tests required, e.g. neonates presenting with purpura fulminans. Decisions on extending anticoagulant therapy are individually based on the perceived risks of TE recurrence and anticoagulant-related bleeding. Whether long-term continuation of anticoagulant treatment or increased intensity should be considered after VTE in patients with a documented thrombophilia is still a matter of debate. In the current published pediatric VTE guidelines, it is recommended to manage children with VTE independent of the presence or absence of APLA or inherited thrombophilia [20].

Laboratory testing for thrombophilia in the acute TE phase may be difficult, and repeat testing is often required. In most cases, thrombophilia testing should be deferred for 3–6 months after the acute TE and after stopping the anticoagulant therapy. Testing of both parents should also be considered before concluding that an inherited deficiency of protein C, protein S or antithrombin is present.

Thrombophilia test results in children with TE may provide an estimate of the risk of recurrence and assist in a decision regarding anticoagulant prophylaxis, such as in situations where a child will be exposed to one or more risk situations for recurrent thrombosis, e.g. major surgery, need of a CVC, oral contraceptive medication and pregnancy. However, available evidence does not yet allow a definitive risk-based approach to be presented to patients and their families.

Comprehensive testing for laboratory thrombophilia in asymptomatic children on the basis of a positive family history for a TE remains controversial. Indeed, yet unknown inherited as well environmental thrombotic risk factors may occur and a normal thrombophilia workup may provide false reassurance.

A recent prospective cohort study showed that the risk of VTE in relatives of pediatric index cases with VTE was markedly increased in relatives with protein C, protein S or antithrombin deficiency. However, this was not the case for the more common thrombophilic traits, such as Prothrombin (II) gene mutation or FVL mutation [9]. A previous published large prospective study, The European Prospective Cohort on Thrombophilia, also showed that the risk of thrombosis in asymptomatic thrombophilia carriers was higher than for a control group; however, the risk did not exceeded the 1–3% annual risk of bleeding associated with long-term anticoagulation [22]. Therefore, screening for inherited thrombophilia in first-degree family members of pediatric VTE index cases with protein C, protein S or antithrombin deficiency or combined inherited thrombophilia may be considered, particularly when considering exposing them to further thrombophilic risk factors such as oral contraception [24].

The uses of prophylactic anticoagulation in children with positive thrombophilia trait in the presence of other TE risk factors remain controversial. It is recommended to counsel the family regarding the potential benefits and limitations prior to performing thrombophilia testing in children without a personal history of a TE only on the basis of a positive family history or the presence of a thrombophilic trait [22].

Testing of asymptomatic children or adolescents with a negative family history of thrombosis prior to surgery, oral contraceptive or CVC insertion is not recommended [24]. Depending on the specific treatment protocol used, individual patient counseling is suggested for thrombophilia testing of children with acute lymphoblastic leukemia prior to CVC insertion (chapter 11) [25].

Purpura Fulminans

Purpura fulminans is a rare, life-threatening condition characterized by progressive hemorrhagic skin necrosis that occurs in the first days of life mostly due to congenital severe (homozygous or compound heterozygous) protein C and/or S deficiency. Rarely, purpura fulminans may occur secondary to consumption or decreased synthesis associated with acquired conditions such as infection (sepsis), hepatic dysfunction or VKA therapy in older children and in adults [6]. Purpura fulminans is estimated to occur in 1/250,000–1/500,000 births, and the presentation is that of a DIC and with a rapid (within hours) onset of small ecchymotic lesions, rapidly increasing in size with the formation of bullae leading to necrotic and gangrenous tissue. Neonates and children with these lesions should be urgently tested for protein C and protein S deficiency and receive frozen plasma (10–20 ml/kg every 6–12 h) pending the results of these specialized tests [20]. For neonates with homozygous protein C or protein S deficiency, after initial stabilization, long-term treatment with VKA, LMWH, protein C replacement, frozen plasma (in case of protein S deficiency or when protein C concentrate is not available), or liver transplantation is recommended [20]. For dose of protein C concentrate see appendix. Initiation of VKA must always overlap replacement therapy and/or a rapid-acting anticoagulant (chapter 16).

Anatomical Thrombophilia

Certain anatomical conditions, though rare, may predispose to TEs, and should also be considered. In the upper extremities, the course of the subclavian and/or axillary veins at the thoracic inlet (between the clavicle and first costal rib) is at risk from repetitive activity of the upper extremity which may cause microtrauma of the vessel wall leading to thrombus formation. This is called activity-induced thrombosis or Paget-Schroetter syndrome [26]. In the lower extremity, a left-sided iliac vein outflow obstruction can result in an increased risk of VTE due to an intimal hypertrophy of the left common iliac vein as a consequence of its compression by the overlaying right common iliac artery, the so-called May-Thurner syndrome [1].

Conclusion

TEs in childhood, even if rare compared to adulthood, are increasingly diagnosed and recognized [5]. In most children, the TEs result from secondary complications of primary underlying diseases such as infection, cancer, congenital heart disease, inflammatory conditions or are related to therapeutic interventions such as central venous and/or arterial catheters. Idiopathic ('unprovoked') cases are rare. A detailed personal and family history and a careful physical examination are important steps to identify potential underlying conditions associated with an increased risk of thrombosis. Imaging studies and laboratory investigations are further determinants in the diagnostic approach to a child with thrombosis and will help in decisions about treatment options and counseling. The following chapters are specifically dedicated to different aspects of TEs in children.

Acknowledgment

The authors would like to express their appreciation for the thoughtful comments provided by Drs. Leslie J. Raffini (Philadelphia, Pa., USA), Gili Kenet (Tel Hashomer, Israel), Guy Young (Los Angeles, Calif., USA) and Margaret L. Rand (Toronto, Ont., Canada) who reviewed this chapter.

References

1 Macartney CA, Chan AK: Thrombosis in children. Semin Thromb Hemost 2011;37:763–761.
2 Yang JY, Chan AK: Neonatal systemic venous thrombosis. Thromb Res 2010;126:471–476.
3 Chalmers EA: Epidemiology of venous thromboembolism in neonates and children. Thromb Res 2006;118:3–12.
4 Price VE, Chan AK: Arterial thrombosis in children. Expert Rev Cardiovasc Ther 2008;6:419–428.
5 Raffini L, Huang YS, Witmer C, Feudtner C: Dramatic increase in venous thromboembolism in children's hospitals in the United States from 2001 to 2007. Pediatrics 2009;124:1001–1008.
6 Price VE, Ledingham DL, Krumpel A, Chan AK: Diagnosis and management of neonatal purpura fulminans. Semin Fetal Neonatal Med 2011;16:318–322.
7 Trenor CC 3rd, Chung RJ, Michelson AD, Neufeld EJ, Gordon CM, Laufer MR, et al: Hormonal contraception and thrombotic risk: a multidisciplinary approach. Pediatrics 2011;127:347–357.
8 Bezemer ID, van der Meer FJ, Eikenboom JC, Rosendaal FR, Doggen CJ: The value of family history as a risk indicator for venous thrombosis. Arch Intern Med 2009;169:610–615.
9 Holzhauer S, Goldenberg NA, Junker R, Heller C, Stoll M, Manner D, et al: Inherited thrombophilia in children with venous thromboembolism and the familial risk of thromboembolism: an observational study. Blood 2012;120:1510–1515.
10 Brandao LR, Labarque V, Diab Y, Williams S, Manson DE: Pulmonary embolism in children. Semin Thromb Hemost 2011;37:772–785.
11 Chalmers E, Ganesen V, Liesner R, Maroo S, Nokes T, Saunders D, et al: Guideline on the investigation, management and prevention of venous thrombosis in children. Br J Haematol 2011;154:196–207.
12 Goldenberg NA: Thrombophilia states and markers of coagulation activation in the prediction of pediatric venous thromboembolic outcomes: a comparative analysis with respect to adult evidence. Hematology Am Soc Hematol Educ Program 2008;2008:236–244.
13 Kenet G, Lutkhoff LK, Albisetti M, Bernard T, Bonduel M, Brandao L, et al: Impact of thrombophilia on risk of arterial ischemic stroke or cerebral sinovenous thrombosis in neonates and children: a systematic review and meta-analysis of observational studies. Circulation 2010;121:1838–1847.
14 Kreuz W, Stoll M, Junker R, Heinecke A, Schobess R, Kurnik K, et al: Familial elevated factor VIII in children with symptomatic venous thrombosis and post-thrombotic syndrome: results of a multicenter study. Arterioscler Thromb Vasc Biol 2006;26:1901–1906.
15 Young G, Albisetti M, Bonduel M, Brandao L, Chan A, Friedrichs F, et al: Impact of inherited thrombophilia on venous thromboembolism in children: a systematic review and meta-analysis of observational studies. Circulation 2008;118:1373–1382.
16 Kenet G, Aronis S, Berkun Y, Bonduel M, Chan A, Goldenberg NA, et al: Impact of persistent antiphospholipid antibodies on risk of incident symptomatic thromboembolism in children: a systematic review and meta-analysis. Semin Thromb Hemost 2011;37:802–809.
17 Ignjatovic V, Kenet G, Monagle P: Developmental hemostasis: recommendations for laboratories reporting pediatric samples. J Thromb Haemost 2012;10:298–300.

18 Pengo V, Tripodi A, Reber G, Rand JH, Ortel TL, Galli M, et al: Update of the guidelines for lupus anticoagulant detection. Subcommittee on Lupus Anticoagulant/Antiphospholipid Antibody of the Scientific and Standardisation Committee of the International Society on Thrombosis and Haemostasis. J Thromb Haemost 2009; 7:1737–1740.
19 Miyakis S, Lockshin MD, Atsumi T, Branch DW, Brey RL, Cervera R, et al: International consensus statement on an update of the classification criteria for definite antiphospholipid syndrome (APS). J Thromb Haemost 2006;4:295–306.
20 Monagle P, Chan AK, Goldenberg NA, Ichord RN, Journeycake JM, Nowak-Gottl U, et al: Antithrombotic therapy in neonates and children: Antithrombotic Therapy and Prevention of Thrombosis, 9th ed: American College of Chest Physicians Evidence-Based Clinical Practice Guidelines. Chest 2012;141:e737S–e801S.
21 Foy P, Moll S: Thrombophilia: 2009 update. Curr Treat Options Cardiovasc Med 2009;11:114–128.
22 Raffini L, Thornburg C: Testing children for inherited thrombophilia: more questions than answers. Br J Haematol 2009;147:277–288.
23 Nowak-Gottl U, Kurnik K, Manner D, Kenet G: Thrombophilia testing in neonates and infants with thrombosis. Semin Fetal Neonatal Med 2011;16:345–348.
24 Kenet G, Bonduel M, Chalmers EA, Chan A, Goldenberg NA, Journeycake J, et al: Venous thromboembolism in children: considerations for thrombophilia testing (update 2012) – guidance from the perinatal and pediatric SSC of the ISTH. J Thromb Haemost 2013, submitted.
25 Mitchell L, Lambers M, Flege S, Kenet G, Li-Thiao-Te V, Holzhauer S, et al: Validation of a predictive model for identifying an increased risk for thromboembolism in children with acute lymphoblastic leukemia: results of a multicenter cohort study. Blood 2010;115: 4999–5004.
26 Brandao LR, Williams S, Kahr WH, Ryan C, Temple M, Chan AK: Exercise-induced deep vein thrombosis of the upper extremity. 1. Literature review. Acta Haematol 2006;115:214–220.

Abbreviations

ACLA	Anticardiolipin antibodies
AIS	Arterial ischemic stroke
APLA	Antiphospholipid antibodies
APLS	Antiphospholipid syndrome
aPTT	Activated partial thromboplastin time
ATE	Arterial thromboembolism/thromboembolic event
β_2-GPI	Anti-β_2-glycoprotein antibody
BT shunt	Blalock-Taussig shunt
CBC	Complete blood count
CT	Computed tomography
CTA	Computed tomography angiography
CTPA	Computed tomography pulmonary angiography
CTV	Computed tomography venography
CSVT	Cerebral sinovenous thrombosis
CVC	Central venous catheter
DIC	Disseminated intravascular coagulation
DUS	Doppler ultrasonography
DVT	Deep vein thrombosis
ELISA	Enzyme-linked immunosorbent assay
EMCO	Extracorporeal membrane oxygenation
FII	Factor II (prothrombin)
FV	Factor V
FVIII	Factor VIII
FIX	Factor IX
FX	Factor X
FXI	Factor XI
FVL	Factor V Leiden
INR	International normalized ratio
ISTH	International Society on Thrombosis and Haemostasis
IVC	Inferior vena cava
LAC	Lupus anticoagulant
LMWH	Low-molecular-weight heparin
Lp(a)	Lipoprotein(a)
MRA	Magnetic resonance angiography
MRI	Magnetic resonance imaging
MRV	Magnetic resonance venography
MTHFR	Methylenetetrahydrofolate reductase
PCR	Polymerase chain reaction
PE	Pulmonary embolism
PT	Prothrombin time
PTS	Postthrombotic syndrome
PVT	Portal vein thrombosis
SLE	Systemic lupus erythematosus
TE	Thromboembolism/thromboembolic event
t-PA	Tissue-plasminogen activator
VKA	Vitamin K antagonist
VTE	Venous thromboembolism/thromboembolic event
V/Q scan	Ventilation-perfusion scan

Chapter 11 Venous Thrombosis

Victoria E. Price
Leonardo R. Brandão
Suzan Williams

Introduction

VTE is a rare complication in pediatric medicine. There has, however, been an increase in the frequency of VTE in childhood over the past two decades, likely due to a true increase in incidence and an increase in detection of previously undiagnosed VTE. This is largely a result of advances in medical expertise and technology leading to an increase in survival of children with previously fatal conditions and an increase in complications of complex conditions managed in tertiary care centers. The incidence of VTE in children is reported to be between 0.07 and 0.14 case per 10,000 children, and more recently 58 cases per 10,000 hospital admissions [1–3]. The incidence follows a bimodal pattern with a peak occurring in infants <1 year and adolescence [4]. In contrast to VTE in adults, idiopathic VTE is rare, and 95% of VTE in children are associated with predisposing risk factors including CVCs, cardiovascular disease, nephrotic syndrome, surgery, infection, malignancy and anatomic anomalies. The presence of a CVC is the single most important risk factor for VTE in childhood. The role of inherited thrombophilia in childhood VTE remains controversial and is discussed in chapter 10.

Deep Vein Thrombosis

Clinical Presentation

The clinical presentation of VTE depends on the anatomical location of the thrombus (see chapter 10). Symptoms of acute DVT in the upper and lower venous systems include localized area of pain, swelling, warmth, and discoloration of the overlying skin. Patients may present with complications of DVT, e.g. occlusion of CVC, superior vena cava syndrome, iliac compression syndrome, or PE (see below). Superior vena cava obstruction syndrome may present with swelling of the arms and face, dilation of veins on the skin surface, blue tinge to the skin, cough, chest pain, and/or hoarseness. Chronic signs of DVT include the presence of collateral circulation, chylothorax, chylopericardium, and PTS [1].

Diagnosis

The approach to diagnosis of DVT in children includes recognition of the clinical presentation and radiological investigations. Venography is considered the gold standard for diagnosis of DVT, but in children this is often not practical due to poor peripheral venous access and the concern for exposure to radiation. Doppler ultrasound has become the most common initial investigation. Advantages include that it is safe, painless, and portable. Doppler ultrasound is recommended to assess for DVT of the lower limb, peripheral upper limb, axillary, subclavian and internal jugular veins [5, 6]. The central intrathoracic venous system is contained within the bony thorax, making Doppler ultrasound a less sensitive tool for diagnosis of DVT in this anatomical location. If central intrathoracic DVT is clinically suspected, then proceed to venography, CTV, or MRV for assessment of central veins. For clinically suspected lower limb DVT with a normal Doppler ultrasound, consider performing venography (if high index of suspicion) or repeating the Doppler ultrasound after a week to assess for proximal progression of a calf vein thrombus. CTV or MRV should be considered in children with suspected proximal extension of femoral DVT. Echocardiography is used for the diagnosis of a right atrial thrombosis. The diagnosis of PE will be discussed later in this chapter.

Management

The aims of antithrombotic therapy in children with DVT are broadly similar to those for adults, i.e. reduce the risk of death due to thrombosis extension or embolization, reduce the incidence of recurrent thrombosis, reduce the incidence of PTS and maintain vessel patency, where clinically relevant [5]. The majority of children with DVT can be managed with anticoagulation therapy; however, there are indications for thrombolysis, thrombectomy, and the insertion of IVC filters (see below). Most of the recommendations detailed in this chapter are based on extrapolation from adults and based on expert's opinion [5, 7, 8].

Anticoagulation

In children with first DVT, initial anticoagulation with UFH or LMWH is recommended for at least 5 days [7]. For ongoing therapy, LMWH or VKA is recommended. Dosing and monitoring of UFH, LMWH and VKA therapy are detailed in chapter 16. The role of the new anticoagulant agents in children with VTE needs further study (see chapter 16).

The duration of anticoagulation in children with DVT depends on the clinical circumstance. Not all DVT have the same potential for progression or recurrence, and therapy may be based on risk factors for good or poor thrombotic outcome [8]. Children with idiopathic DVT should receive anticoagulant therapy for 6–12 months [7]. The decision to continue lifelong anticoagulation has to be weighed against the risk of bleeding and the impact on the quality of life of the child and family due to restrictions on certain activities. In the case of recurrent idiopathic DVT, indefinite therapeutic or prophylactic anticoagulation is recommended [7]. The implication of inherited or acquired thrombophilia on long-term management of DVT is discussed in chapter 10.

Children with secondary DVT in whom the risk factor has resolved should be treated with therapeutic anticoagulation for 3 months. If the risk factor for DVT is ongoing, for example asparaginase chemotherapy, active nephrotic syndrome, etc., anticoagulation therapy should continue in either therapeutic or prophylactic doses until the risk factor has resolved. In children with recurrent secondary DVT with an existing reversible risk, anticoagulation is recommended until resolution of the precipitating factor and for a minimum of 3 months.

For children with anatomic anomalies predisposing to DVT (thoracic outlet syndrome, interrupted duplex vena cava, etc.) percutaneous or surgical intervention may be needed in addition to anticoagulation [9]. For children with recurrent DVT secondary to structural venous abnormalities, it is recommended to treat with indefinite anticoagulation unless successful percutaneous or surgical intervention can be performed [7].

Complete or partial resolution of the DVT is expected in around 50% of children treated with anticoagulation, and is more common in non-occlusive DVT. Progression of DVT on anticoagulation is rare. If progression occurs on VKA therapy despite a therapeutic target INR range of 2.0–3.0, UFH or LMWH should be started and subsequently switched back to VKA using a higher therapeutic range of INR of 3.0–4.0 or addition of aspirin to VKA therapy [7]. If progression occurs on LMWH, increasing the dose of LMWH to a higher target anti-factor Xa level can be considered. Progression of an extensive lower limb despite anticoagulation therapy may be an indication for the insertion of IVC filter (see below).

Thrombolysis

The indication for thrombolysis is DVT threatening organ or limb function in the absence of contraindications. Thrombolysis therapy may be administered systemically or locally via catheter. Currently, there are no data to suggest routine use of catheter-directed thrombolysis over systemic thrombolysis. The use of catheter-directed local thrombolysis depends on institutional experience, technical feasibility, and absence of contraindications [10]. The theoretical advantages of catheter-directed thrombolysis, i.e. the ability to deliver lower doses of thrombolytic agent directly in to the thrombus, may be mitigated by the increased risk of local vessel injury in children with small vessel size. Local therapy may be used for catheter-related DVT when the catheter is already in situ. The suggested use of thrombolysis for occlusive thrombosis, especially in the IVC and ileofemoral location, in an attempt to reduce the long-term complication of PTS is controversial and deserves further investigation [5, 11]. If thrombolysis is used, t-PA rather than other thrombolytic agents is recommended [7]. Dosing, monitoring and relative contraindications of thrombolysis therapy are detailed in chapter 16.

Life-threatening DVT (e.g. in the immediate period after cardiac surgery) may warrant the consideration of thrombectomy, and this should be discussed with an experienced pediatric vascular surgeon.

Importantly, children with DVT requiring initial therapy with thrombolysis and/or thrombectomy need ongoing anticoagulant therapy. Type and duration of anticoagulation should follow previous recommendations.

Compression Stockings

In adults with lower limb DVT, daily use of graduated compression stockings for 2 years from the acute event is suggested to reduce the risk for PTS [12]. No data exist in children. There are specific limitations with elastic stockings use in children such as lack of compliance, need for replacement due to growth and difficulty in obtaining appropriately fit garments, particularly in young children. Still, the use of graduated compression stockings in older children with lower limb DVT should be considered on a case-to-case basis.

Historically, the practice has been to place patients with lower limb DVT on bed rest to reduce the risk of thrombus progression to PE. Current evidence suggests no harm associated with early ambulation in patients diagnosed with lower limb DVT. Considering the advantages of early ambulation, it should be considered in most cases.

Prophylaxis

The objective of prophylaxis is to prevent VTE in children who are at high risk for VTE. The indications and recommendations for thromboprophylaxis therapy are discussed in detail in chapter 16.

Catheter-Related Thrombosis

CVCs facilitate intravenous therapies in neonates, infants and older children with difficult venous access. The mechanisms of CVC-related VTE include endothelial damage during catheter insertion, disruption of blood flow, infusion of procoagulants and thrombogenic catheter material. CVC-related VTE is well described in children with cancer, hemophilia, cystic fibrosis, and children requiring total parenteral nutrition. The incidence of CVC-related VTE varies widely in the literature depending on whether or not asymptomatic VTE is included and what diagnostic modalities are used. The highest frequency occurs in children <1 year of age, and this likely reflects the increased ratio of catheter to vessel size, as well as challenging venous access at this age. The most common location of CVC-related VTE is the upper venous system, as this is the site most commonly used for CVC placement in children. CVC-related VTE is associated with mortality (secondary to PE) and morbidity including CVC infection, recurrence of VTE, PTS and loss of venous access.

The occurrence of CVC-related VTE in neonates and children is associated with host- and catheter-related risk factors. Host-related risk factors include sepsis, low birthweight, congenital heart disease. Catheter-related risk factors include CVC type (i.e. Hickman, Port-a-Cath, PICC), previous CVC infections and/or occlusions, insertion technique, CVC location, duration of CVC insertion, type of therapy infused (e.g. total parenteral nutrition and hyperosmolar fluids) and concomitant therapies (e.g. asparaginase, corticosteroids).

Clinical Presentation

A high index of suspicion is often required to investigate a child for CVC-related VTE as many of the signs of VTE can overlap with that of the underlying medical condition. Repeated mechanical occlusion and CVC-related infection may be the first sign of VTE. Neonates with CVC or UVC-related VTE may present with thrombocytopenia. Specific symptoms of superior vena cava occlusion include swelling of the head and neck, conjunctival edema, plethora, and pleural effusion. Occlusion of the IVC may present with lower extremity edema. There may be visible collateral vessels on the chest and/or abdominal wall. Right atrial thrombosis related to CVC may present with loss of CVC patency, respiratory distress, and/or arrhythmia. Asymptomatic right atrial thrombosis may be an incidental finding on echocardiography.

Diagnosis

Depending on the location of the catheter, various radiological techniques may be used to evaluate for the presence of VTE (see 'Deep Vein Thrombosis', 'Diagnosis'). Contrast lineogram may aid in the diagnosis of catheter occlusion due to a fibrin sheath at the tip of CVC, but is inadequate to diagnose or exclude CVC-related VTE [5]. Doppler ultrasound, conventional venography, CTV or MRV may be required to exclude large vessel thrombosis. Echocardiography can be used to detect right atrial thrombus. Flow problems, particularly soon after CVC placement, may be secondary to a catheter kink, malposition of the catheter tip, or a constricting suture. This may be diagnosed on a chest X-ray.

Management

Ideally, in children with CVC-related VTE, the catheter should be removed. However, this is not always possible if there is no alternate venous access. If the catheter can be removed or is not functioning, the recommendation is to administer anticoagulation for 3–5 days prior to catheter removal to reduce the risk of embolization at the time of removal [7]. Anticoagulation is suggested for 3 months. If after this period the CVC is still required, consider prophylactic anticoagulation until the CVC is removed. If recurrent VTE occurs while on prophylaxis, consider increasing the anticoagulation dose to a therapeutic dose until the CVC is removed and for a minimum of

Table 1. Initial management of blocked CVC

Chemical-related blockage	Blood-related blockage
Indications	
Infusion running then sudden unexplained occlusion	Blood sampling
	Blood administration
	Blood backup in infusion
Initial action	
1. Attempt to aspirate	1. Attempt to aspirate
2. Flush with 0.9% NaCl	2. Flush with 0.9% NaCl
3. Follow hydrochlorid acid local instillation guidelines (table 2)	3. Follow guidelines for t-PA local instillation (table 2)
If no blood return, follow guidelines for t-PA local instillation (table 2)	If unsuccessful clearing, a second attempt may be indicated
4. If able to flush the catheter but no blood return, proceed to diagnostic workup if clinically indicated	If able to flush the catheter but unable to get blood return, proceed to diagnostic workup, if clinically indicated
5. If unable to flush the catheter, proceed to diagnostic workup, if clinically indicated	4. If unable to flush the catheter, proceed to diagnostic workup, if clinically indicated

See text for the recommended diagnostic workup. Adapted from SickKids formulary.

3 months following the VTE. For neonates with CVC- or UVC-related VTE, refer to the section 'Venous Thrombosis in Neonates'.

For children with right atrial thrombosis related to CVC, risk stratification based on clot size and mobility is suggested [13]. Removal of the CVC is suggested, when possible, with or without anticoagulation depending on the individual risk factors [7]. For patients with high-risk features on echocardiography, such as atrial thrombus >2 cm in any dimension, mobile, pedunculated or snake-shaped thrombus, anticoagulation with appropriately timed CVC removal is recommended. Surgical thrombectomy or thrombolysis should be considered based on individualized risk-benefit assessment. Dosing and monitoring of anticoagulation and thrombolysis therapy is detailed in chapter 16.

Prophylaxis

The current recommendation is not to use prophylactic anticoagulation for the prevention of CVC-related VTE. The exception to this is in the case of long-term total parenteral nutrition administration where prophylaxis with VKA is recommended to maintain a target INR of 1.5–1.9 [7]. There has been much debate as to clinical significance of asymptomatic catheter-related VTE. Surveillance for asymptomatic VTE in children who have a CVC in place is currently not recommended.

Occlusion

Occlusion of a CVC may occur due to fibrin sheaths, intraluminal thrombus, VTE around the CVC, mechanical problems, or chemical precipitation. Catheter occlusion is associated with an increased risk of CVC-related infection and leads to increased need for CVC replacement. Flushing with normal saline, UFH or intermittent urokinase is recommended to prevent CVC occlusion [7]. The current available data do not recommend one option over the other. For blocked CVCs, t-PA or intermittent urokinase should be instilled in the catheter for 30 min, to be repeated once if the catheter remains occluded [7]. See tables 1 and 2 for suggested guidelines for the management of blocked CVCs.

Table 2. Guidelines for local installation for blocked CVC

Type of catheter	Chemical occlusion hydrochloric acid 0.1 M	Blood-related occlusion bodyweight	alteplase (t-PA)
Single lumen (e.g. Hickman, Cook Roko, PICC)	2 ml	>10 kg	1 mg/ml; use amount required to fill volume of line to maximum; 2 ml = 2 mg
		≤10 kg	1 mg diluted to 2 ml; 1 ml = 0.5 mg
Double lumen (e.g. Hickman, Cook, PICC, Quinton)	2 ml *per lumen*	>10 kg	1 mg/ml; use amount required to fill volume of line to maximum; 2 ml = 2 mg *per lumen*; treat one lumen at a time; second lumen may not need to be treated if catheter cleared
		≤10 kg	1 mg diluted to 2 ml *per lumen*; 1 ml = 0.5 mg
Subcutaneous ports (e.g. Port-A-Cath, PASport)	3 ml	>10 kg	2 mg diluted with NS to 3 ml; 1 ml = 0.65 mg *per lumen*; if double lumen port, treat one lumen at a time; second lumen may not need to be treated if port cleared
		≤10 kg	1.5 mg diluted with NS to 3 ml; 1 ml = 0.5 mg
Hemodialysis catheters[1]			
Small Quinton	1 ml	>10 kg	see guidelines above for single-lumen catheter
Large Quinton	1.5 ml	≤10 kg	0.75 mg diluted to 1.5 ml

After a minimum of 2-hour instillation of each drug, withdraw drug; if possible, flush the catheter with 0.9% NaCl; attempt to aspirate blood. Adapted from SickKids formulary.
[1] For *non*-nephrology patients, use double lumen guidelines.

If CVC remains blocked following two doses of local thrombolytic therapy, radiological imaging to rule out a CVC-related thrombosis is recommended [5, 7]. A chest X-ray is recommended to visualize the CVC position. A contrast lineogram is recommended to determine potential occlusion at the tip of the CVC, presence of retrograde flow and potential leak. Lineogram cannot rule out the presence of large-vessel VTE. Doppler US, conventional venography, CTV or contrast-enhanced MRV may be required to exclude large vessel VTE. Echocardiography can be used to detect right atrial thrombus.

Pulmonary Embolism

PE, although uncommon in children, is an increasingly recognized complication in children and can be a significant cause of morbidity and mortality. The incidence rate of PE in population-based studies has been age and gender specific, varying from no reported cases to several per 100,000 [1, 14]. Most cases of PE in children are secondary to underlying risk factors. The most common associated risk factor for PE is the presence of a CVC. Other risk factors include immobility, the use of the oral contraceptive pill, surgery, cancer, vascular malformations, nephrotic syndrome, long-term total parenteral nutrition, systemic lupus erythematosus, ventriculoatrial shunts, congenital and/or acquired thrombotic tendencies [14, 15]. About half of children with PE have evidence of acute DVT in the extremities. The diagnosis of PE in children requires an increased level of clinical suspicion to enable timely recognition and appropriate therapy.

Clinical Presentation

Clinical signs of PE are nonspecific in children and may be masked by underlying conditions. Shortness of breath, pleuritic pain, and dyspnea are possible findings, but it may be difficult to differentiate the overlapping signs of PE in a critically ill child. In adults, clinical prediction scores are used to identify those in whom PE can be ruled out by a negative D-dimer without further investigation. Currently, there are no data to support the use of these scores in children [16]. Children with PE were as likely as children without PE to have a D-dimer value within the normal range [16].

Diagnosis

The diagnosis of PE requires confirmatory diagnostic radiographic imaging. In a child with suspected PE, findings on echocardiogram, chest X-ray, echocardiography and D-dimer can be helpful.

Ventilation perfusion scanning (V/Q scan) is historically the first-line investigation for children with suspected PE and may still be appropriate for use in young women to avoid breast irradiation. It requires the child to be somewhat cooperative (older than 5–6 years of age). The V/Q scan in children is usually interpreted according to criteria adapted from adults (PIOPED or PISAPED), being classified as low, moderate, or high PE probability for PIOPED and normal, near normal, abnormal not consistent with PE and abnormal consistent with PE for PISAPED.

CTPA is being used increasingly in children, although there are no published studies on sensitivity or specificity. Currently, CTPA has become a noninvasive first-line imaging study in both pediatric and adult patients with clinically suspected PE. With young and uncooperative children, the risk of sedation or anesthetic to facilitate the investigation must be weighed against the benefit of identifying the PE. CTPA is contraindicated in patients with known or suspected allergy to contrast media, patients with renal failure, and requires precautions in patients who are pregnant or on metformin.

MRPA is an alternative to conventional pulmonary angiography in patients with suspected PE in whom CTPA is contraindicated. The experience with MRPA in children is limited.

Conventional catheter pulmonary angiography has been considered the 'gold standard' diagnostic test in both adults and children. Pulmonary angiography is expensive, invasive and requires expertise and sedation in children. Thus, it may not be readily available. Pulmonary angiography is considered when less invasive diagnostic tests are indeterminate.

Management

Treatment should be instituted promptly upon confirmation of the diagnosis of PE. Initiation of therapy may also be considered in selected unstable patients with high clinical suspicion while awaiting diagnostic confirmation.

As the clinical presentation of acute PE can be highly variable ranging from asymptomatic, nonspecific, or mild symptomatology to severe hypoxemia, right ventricular failure, shock, and even death, the treatment of pediatric patients should be guided by the risks associated with the individual clinical condition of the patient.

Anticoagulation is considered the main treatment in the majority of patients with PE. The choice of the initial and subsequent anticoagulant and guidelines for duration of anticoagulant therapy are similar to those of extremity DVT (see the section above).

In hemodynamically unstable patients, more aggressive therapy is warranted. Thrombolysis may be considered (see chapter 16 for details). Embolectomy performed percutaneously (using catheters) or surgically should be considered when systemic thrombolysis is contraindicated or unsuccessful. The choice of embolectomy technique depends on patient-related factors, availability of resources, and expertise at the local institution.

Chronic Thromboembolic Pulmonary Hypertension

CTPH is a potential rare long-term complication of acute or recurrent PE with considerable morbidity and mortality [17, 18]. CTPH is defined as mean pulmonary artery pressure >25 mm Hg that persists for 6 months after PE diagnosis.

Exercise intolerance, fatigue and dyspnea are the most commonly reported symptoms of CTPH, followed by chest discomfort, syncope, hemoptysis, light-headedness or peripheral leg edema. In the majority of patients, echocardiography, which detects the presence of elevated pulmonary artery pressure, provides the first indication of CTPH. Diagnosis is based on findings on CTPA or V/Q scan and confirmed with right heart catheterization and pulmonary angiography [18]. If left untreated, right heart failure and death are the inevitable end results. Pulmonary thromboendarterectomy surgery is well tolerated with improved functional status. Pulmonary vasodilators may contribute to increased survival among inoperable disease [18]. Due to high risk of recurrent thrombosis, children with CTPH need counseling about the need for strict, lifelong adherence to anticoagulation.

Venous Thrombosis in Neonates

Neonates are at highest risk of developing VTE among the childhood age group. Risk factors include sepsis, inflammation, hypotension, hypoxia, and the use of intravascular catheters in small-caliber and umbilical vessels [19, 20]. Renal vein thrombosis is the most common type of spontaneous VTE in neonates (see chapter 13). Purpura fulminans, due to homozygous protein C or protein S or compound heterozygous states, is an acute, life-threatening syndrome requiring specific management (see chapter 10).

The current guidelines for the management of neonatal VTE suggest considering treatment options based on site, extent, clinical consequences of the thrombosis, and the risk of bleeding associated with the use of anticoagulation or thrombolytic therapy [7]. The potential risk of hemorrhage versus the benefit of anticoagulation or thrombolysis needs to be carefully considered in the neonate. The risk of bleeding is associated with gestational age, birthweight, and comorbidities such as lung disease, necrotizing enterocolitis, sepsis and the presence of IVH. The incidence of recurrent VTE, PTS and other more specific complications of neonatal VTE, e.g. portal hypertension after UVC-related thrombosis, is unknown both in treated and untreated neonates. Thus, in neonates, management options include supportive care only, anticoagulant therapy, thrombolytic therapy, or surgery.

For neonatal VTE, initial anticoagulation or supportive care with radiologic monitoring for extension of thrombosis is recommended. If extension of the clot occurs, anticoagulation should be started. Initial anticoagulation may be with LMWH alone or UFH followed by LMWH for a total of 6 weeks to 3 months depending on presence of risk factors and VTE resolution [7]. For catheter-related VTE in neonates, removal of the catheter is suggested after 3–5 days of therapeutic anticoagulation. If thrombolysis is required, t-PA rather than other thrombolytic agents and plasminogen (frozen plasma) administration prior to or during therapy is recommended. Dosing and monitoring of anticoagulation and thrombolysis therapy in neonates are detailed in chapter 16.

Venous Thrombosis in Cancer Patients

The etiology of VTE in childhood cancer is multifactorial. The risk factors include increased thrombin generation related to disease (e.g. leukemia), age (highest risk during adolescence), the use of CVC, chemotherapy including asparaginase and corticosteroids, the use of total parenteral nutrition, and infection [21]. A scoring system for predicting the risk for thrombosis in children with acute lymphoblastic leukemia has been developed and validated [22]. According to current recommendations, the management of VTE in children with cancer should follow the general recommendations for management of VTE in children [7]. LMWH is the preferred anticoagulant in children with cancer because of the ease of maintaining the anticoagulation therapy around the usual frequent procedures [7].

As the presence of cancer presents a unique challenge in terms of balancing risk versus benefit, clinicians should consider these factors, and the decision to anticoagulate should be made on an individual basis [21]. For example, there are no evidence-based guidelines for anticoagulation in patients with VTE who develop chemotherapy-induced thrombocytopenia. Most experts recommend a platelet count of >50 × 10^9/l for full dose anticoagulation and of >30 × 10^9/l for prophylactic dose anticoagulation. In the presence of thrombocytopenia, whether to hold or reduce anticoagulation dose or to use platelet transfusions to maintain a platelet count at a higher level in order to give full dose anticoagulation should be decided on an individual basis (see chapter 16 for further discussion). For planned intrathecal chemotherapy, omission of LMWH for at least 24 h is suggested. For asparaginase-associated thrombotic complications, it is suggested that after a VTE, asparaginase can be restarted, after reimaging demonstrates clot stabilization or improvement, with closely monitored anticoagulation [23].

Inferior Vena Cava Filter

IVC interruption with an IVC filter is used to prevent PE. Its use in children has been limited to case reports and few published series [24]. Indications for placement of IVC filters in children with VTE are similar to adults including contraindication to anticoagulation (e.g. trauma patients with hemorrhagic risk) or progression of lower limb VTE despite adequate anticoagulation. The use of an IVC filter may be considered in children >10 kg bodyweight, and it should be inserted by an experienced interventional radiologist [7]. Complications of filter placement include filter migration or fracture, extension of existing thrombus to the filter, risk of PE during manipulation of the filter at insertion, perforation of blood vessels, and perforation of adjacent structures as the child grows. The IVC filter should be removed as soon as the contraindication to anticoagulation is resolved and the presence of thrombosis in the basket of the filter has been ruled out. The need to interrupt anticoagulation prior to IVC filter removal is not clear. Safe removal has been reported in patients receiving therapeutic anticoagulation. Anticoagulation should be continued after the removal of the filter as per previously stated guidelines [7].

Venous Stents

Endovascular balloon dilation is an interventional radiologic procedure to reestablish venous flow and relieve symptomatic venous obstructions secondary to benign disease, malignant disease, or radiotherapy. Stents are most commonly used for arterial disease, but have been used for venous stenosis or obstructions (e.g. May-Thurner syndrome).

Specific issues with the use of stents in the pediatric population include small patient sizes, the need to accommodate future vessel growth and increased risk for thrombosis in infants <1 year of age. Ideally, the stent should be reexpandable with the potential to achieve adequate size for an adult. The administration of UFH perioperatively is recommended [7].

Post-Thrombotic Syndrome

PTS is a syndrome of chronic venous insufficiency following DVT. The pathophysiology of PTS is thought to involve venous hypertension as a result of venous valvular reflux, thrombotic venous occlusion, or other causes of impaired venous return [12]. In a recent systematic review of the literature, the overall weighted mean frequency of PTS following upper or lower extremity DVT in children was 26% (95% CI: 23–28%) among a total of nearly 1,000 patients studied [25]. Younger age, obesity, lack of thrombus resolution, delayed initiation of anticoagulation, elevated D-dimer, and high FVIII levels are predictive of PTS in children [25].

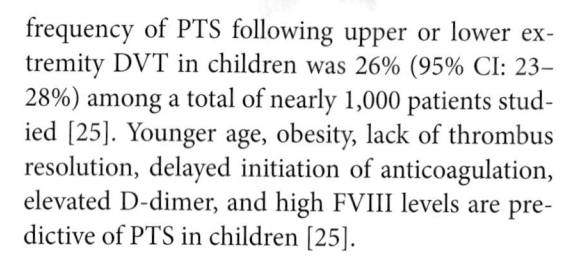

Clinical Presentation

PTS symptoms may be persistent or intermittent. Aching pain, heaviness, swelling, cramps, itching, or tingling in the affected limb as well as fatigue with exertion can occur. Symptoms in the lower extremities may be aggravated by standing or walking and improve with resting, leg elevation, and/or supine position. Physical findings of PTS in the lower limb include edema, dilated superficial collateral veins, perimalleolar or more extensive telangiectasia, secondary varicose veins, brownish pigmentation of stasis dermatitis, and venous eczema. Lipodermatosclerosis, brawny tender thickening of the subcutaneous tissues of the medial lower limb, may occur. In severe cases, venous leg ulcers may occur, which can be precipitated by minor trauma. These are generally chronic, painful, and slow to heal. In the upper extremity, there may be dilation of the superficial veins of the upper arm and chest wall and dependent cyanosis of the arm.

Diagnosis

There is no 'gold standard' diagnostic test. PTS is a clinical diagnosis based on the development of characteristic symptoms and signs in a patient with prior DVT. In some patients, it may take up to 3–6 months for resolution of the initial pain or swelling; therefore, the diagnosis of PTS should be deferred until after the acute phase.

There are two commonly used clinical scales for grading PTS in children, the modified Villalta Scale and the Manco-Johnson instrument [26] (table 3). In the modified Villalta Scale, individual symptoms and signs are graded on a scale of 0–2. The symptom and sign scores are added together to provide a final numerical score that is categorized as mild, moderate or severe PTS. The Manco-Johnson instrument includes physical examination findings and functional limitations, with the use of a Faces pain scale for pain assessment. Currently, there is insufficient justification to advocate for use of one measure over the other [26]. A training video has been developed for the administration of the Manco-Johnson instrument (at the Kids-DOTT clinical trial website [27]) and for the original Villalta score [28].

In a patient with previously documented DVT with symptoms and signs compatible with PTS, no further investigations are needed. In a patient with clinical manifestations compatible with PTS, with no prior history of DVT, further investigations such as compression ultrasound and contrast venography are useful to detect a previously undiagnosed DVT. Due to the cost, risks, radiation and contrast exposure, ultrasound is preferred over venography. Excluding a recurrent thrombotic event is warranted in the setting of progressive symptoms. An unequivocal change in the extent of thrombosis on the current ultrasound compared with the previous is considered to be indicative of new ipsilateral DVT.

Management

There are no controlled studies on the effectiveness of elastic bandages, lymphedema compression sleeves, elastic compression stockings, venoactive drugs, thrombolysis, or surgical therapies for treatment of PTS in children. These treatments are used in adults with some success [29]. However, as there may be symptomatic benefit, and unlikely harm, compression garments are a reasonable first-line approach. Other options should be considered on a case-by-case basis.

As severe PTS can be quite debilitating, multidisciplinary care may be required [29]. Venous ulcers are treated with compression therapy, skin care, and topical dressings. Wound care expertise

Table 3. Components of standardized outcome measures for PTS employed in pediatric studies

Modified Villalta Scale [30]	
Symptoms[1]	
Pain or abnormal use	1
Swelling	1
Signs	
Increased limb circumference[2]	1
Change in skin color	1
Pitting edema	1
Venous collaterals on skin	1
Pigmentation of skin	1
Tenderness on palpations of deep veins	1
Varicosities	1 moderate, 2 severe
Head swelling	1 moderate, 2 severe
Ulceration	9
Mild PTS	1–3
Moderate PTS	4–8
Severe	≥9
Manco-Johnson instrument [31]	
Signs	
Edema[3]	1
Dilated superficial collateral veins	1
Venous stasis dermatitis	1
Venous stasis ulcers	1
Symptoms	
Chronic lower-extremity pain	
Limiting aerobic activities	0–5
Limiting activities of daily living	0–5
At rest	0–5
PTS absent	0
Any PTS present	≥1
Physically and functionally significant PTS	signs ≥1 and symptoms ≥1

[1] Reported by patient, parent, caregiver or proxy.
[2] >3% compared with contralateral side.
[3] >1 cm increase in circumference in the affected extremity compared with the contralateral extremity.

should be utilized. More rapid pain relief and ulcer size reduction has been reported with the use of gauze pads with hyaluronic acid versus a neutral vehicle such as saline. Late thrombolysis strategies and venous stenting have been reported. Removal of the saphenous vein for lower extremity PTS in adults can be helpful in selected cases as the vessel may serve to transmit venous hypertension through reflux, rather than offering an effective alternative venous drainage route. Physiotherapy to maintain use of the affected limb, pain management and social support around adjustments for mobility and activity while at school are some of the ongoing services which may be required.

Prevention

Given the limited treatment options, prevention is important. As no prevention studies have been performed in children, the following recommendations are based on research in adults [29]. Primary prevention strategies can include judicious placement of CVCs and thromboprophylaxis in high risk patients. Once a DVT has occurred, prompt initiation of appropriate anticoagulation, use of thrombolysis in extensive lower limb DVT, prevention of recurrent ipsilateral DVT by appropriate intensity and duration of anticoagulation therapy could be protective. The use of knee-high elastic compression stockings (30–40 mm Hg) for up to 2 years after DVT was suggested to prevent PTS in adults [12]. The efficacy of graduated compression stockings for prevention of PTS in children with DVT has never been studied.

Conclusion

Although VTE is increasingly recognized in children, most data related to diagnosis and management are extrapolated from studies conducted in adults. For older children, this extrapolation is probably acceptable. However, differences in the hemostatic systems of neonates, infants and younger children compared to adults may limit the generalization of recommendations for adults with VTE, to children [30]. Until further studies are available, it is suggested to follow the American College of Chest Physicians guidelines for management of children with acute symptomatic VTE [7]. The clinical significance and management of asymptomatic VTE in children is still debated. Although a collaborative effort to improve standardization in the definition, measurement and reporting of PTS in children is underway [26], pediatric guidelines for prevention and management of PTS are lacking.

Acknowledgment

The authors would like to express their appreciation for the thoughtful comments provided by Drs. Paul Monagle (Melbourne, Vic., Australia) and Guy Young (Los Angeles, Calif., USA) who reviewed this chapter.

References

1 Andrew M, David M, Adams M, Ali K, Anderson R, Barnard D, et al: Venous thromboembolic complications (VTE) in children: first analyses of the Canadian Registry of VTE. Blood 1994;83:1251–1257.
2 van Ommen CH, Peters M: Venous thromboembolic disease in childhood. Semin Thromb Hemost 2003;29:391–404.
3 Raffini L, Huang YS, Witmer C, Feudtner C: Dramatic increase in venous thromboembolism in children's hospitals in the United States from 2001 to 2007. Pediatrics 2009;124:1001–1008.
4 Tuckuviene R, Christensen AL, Helgestad J, Johnsen SP, Kristensen SR: Pediatric venous and arterial noncerebral thromboembolism in Denmark: a nationwide population-based study. J Pediatr 2011;159:663–669.
5 Chalmers E, Ganesen V, Liesner R, Maroo S, Nokes T, Saunders D, et al: Guideline on the investigation, management and prevention of venous thrombosis in children. Br J Haematol 2011;154:196–207.
6 Macartney CA, Chan AK: Thrombosis in children. Semin Thromb Hemost 2011;37:763–761.
7 Monagle P, Chan AK, Goldenberg NA, Ichord RN, Journeycake JM, Nowak-Gottl U, et al: Antithrombotic therapy in neonates and children: Antithrombotic Therapy and Prevention of Thrombosis, 9th ed: American College of Chest Physicians Evidence-Based Clinical Practice Guidelines. Chest 2012;141(2 suppl):e737S–e801S.
8 Manco-Johnson MJ: How I treat venous thrombosis in children. Blood 2006;107:21–29.
9 Arthur LG, Teich S, Hogan M, Caniano DA, Smead W: Pediatric thoracic outlet syndrome: a disorder with serious vascular complications. J Pediatr Surg 2008;43:1089–1094.
10 Kukreja K, Vaidya S: Venous interventions in children. Tech Vasc Interv Radiol 2011;14:16–21.
11 Goldenberg NA, Branchford B, Wang M, Ray C Jr, Durham JD, Manco-Johnson MJ: Percutaneous mechanical and pharmacomechanical thrombolysis for occlusive deep vein thrombosis of the proximal limb in adolescent subjects: findings from an institution-based prospective inception cohort study of pediatric venous thromboembolism. J Vasc Interv Radiol 2011;22:121–132.
12 Kahn SR: The post-thrombotic syndrome. Hematology Am Soc Hematol Educ Program 2010;2010:216–220.
13 Yang JY, Williams S, Brandao LR, Chan AK: Neonatal and childhood right atrial thrombosis: recognition and a risk-stratified treatment approach. Blood Coagul Fibrinolysis 2010;21:301–307.
14 Biss TT, Brandao LR, Kahr WH, Chan AK, Williams S: Clinical features and outcome of pulmonary embolism in children. Br J Haematol 2008;142:808–818.
15 Lee EY, Tse SK, Zurakowski D, Johnson VM, Lee NJ, Tracy DA, et al: Children suspected of having pulmonary embolism: multidetector CT pulmonary angiography–thromboembolic risk factors and implications for appropriate use. Radiology 2012;262:242–251.
16 Biss TT, Brandao LR, Kahr WH, Chan AK, Williams S: Clinical probability score and D-dimer estimation lack utility in the diagnosis of childhood pulmonary embolism. J Thromb Haemost 2009;7:1633–1638.
17 Madani MM, Wittine LM, Auger WR, Fedullo PF, Kerr KM, Kim NH, et al: Chronic thromboembolic pulmonary hypertension in pediatric patients. J Thorac Cardiovasc Surg 2011;141:624–630.

18 Piazza G, Goldhaber SZ: Chronic thromboembolic pulmonary hypertension. N Engl J Med 2011;364:351–360.
19 Revel-Vilk S, Ergaz Z: Diagnosis and management of central-line-associated thrombosis in newborns and infants. Semin Fetal Neonatal Med 2011;16:340–344.
20 Yang JY, Chan AK: Neonatal systemic venous thrombosis. Thromb Res 2010;126:471–476.
21 Athale UH, Chan AK: Thromboembolic complications in pediatric hematologic malignancies. Semin Thromb Hemost 2007;33:416–426.
22 Mitchell L, Lambers M, Flege S, Kenet G, Li-Thiao-Te V, Holzhauer S, et al: Validation of a predictive model for identifying an increased risk for thromboembolism in children with acute lymphoblastic leukemia: results of a multicenter cohort study. Blood 2010;115:4999–5004.
23 Grace RF, Dahlberg SE, Neuberg D, Sallan SE, Connors JM, Neufeld EJ, et al: The frequency and management of asparaginase-related thrombosis in paediatric and adult patients with acute lymphoblastic leukaemia treated on Dana-Farber Cancer Institute consortium protocols. Br J Haematol 2011;152:452–459.
24 Kukreja KU, Gollamudi J, Patel MN, Johnson ND, Racadio JM: Inferior vena cava filters in children: our experience and suggested guidelines. J Pediatr Hematol Oncol 2011;33:334–338.
25 Goldenberg NA, Donadini MP, Kahn SR, Crowther M, Kenet G, Nowak-Gottl U, et al: Post-thrombotic syndrome in children: a systematic review of frequency of occurrence, validity of outcome measures, and prognostic factors. Haematologica 2010;95:1952–1959.
26 Goldenberg NA, Brandão L, Journeycake J, Kahn S, Monagle P, Revel-Vilk S, et al: Definition of post-thrombotic syndrome following lower extremity deep venous thrombosis and standardization of outcome measurement in pediatric clinical investigations. J Thromb Haemost 2012;10:477–480.
27 http://www.ucdenver.edu/academics/colleges/medicalschool/centers/HemophiliaThrombosis/research/kidsdott/Pages/KidsDOTT.aspx
28 http://medicine.utah.edu/internalmedicine/generalmedicine/Conferences/PTS/resources.htm.
29 Kahn SR: How I treat postthrombotic syndrome. Blood 2009;114:4624–4631.
30 Monagle P, Ignjatovic V, Savoia H: Hemostasis in neonates and children: pitfalls and dilemmas. Blood Rev 2010;24:63–68.

Abbreviations

CTPA	Computed tomography pulmonary angiography
CTPH	Chronic thromboembolic pulmonary hypertension
CTV	Computed tomography venography
CVC	Central venous catheter
DVT	Deep vein thrombosis
FVIII	Factor VIII
INR	International normalized ratio
IVC	Inferior vena cava
IVH	Intraventricular hemorrhage
LMWH	Low-molecular-weight heparin
MRPA	Magnetic resonance imaging pulmonary angiography
MRV	Magnetic resonance venography
NS	Normal saline
PE	Pulmonary embolism
PICC	Peripheral inserted central catheter
PIOPED	Prospective investigation of pulmonary embolism diagnosis
PISAPED	Prospective investigation study of acute pulmonary embolism diagnosis
PTS	Postthrombotic syndrome
t-PA	Tissue-plasminogen activator
UFH	Unfractionated heparin
UVC	Umbilical vein catheter
VKA	Vitamin K antagonist
VTE	Venous thromboembolism/thromboembolic event
V/Q scan	Ventilation-perfusion scan

Chapter 12 Arterial Thrombosis

Shoshana Revel-Vilk
Manuela Albisetti
M. Patricia Massicotte

Introduction

Arterial TEs in children are thought to be less common than venous TEs [1]. In a Danish nationwide pediatric population study, the incidence of arterial TE and venous TE was 0.29 and 2.09 per 100,000 person-years, respectively [2]. Analysis of an Australian prospective registry showed that the incidence of pediatric arterial TEs was 8.5/10,000 hospital admissions [3]. Most cases of non-CNS arterial TEs are catheter related [3, 4]. Arterial catheter-related TEs are more common in neonates treated in the intensive care unit while non-catheter-related arterial TEs are most common in older infants and children treated out of the intensive care setting.

Arterial Catheter-Related Thrombosis

Arterial catheters can be placed either peripherally or centrally. Peripheral arterial catheters are inserted to monitor blood pressure and oxygen saturation, and facilitate frequent blood sampling in critically ill children. In infants and older children, the preferred site is the radial artery. Alternative insertion sites include the ulnar, brachial, axillary, dorsalis pedis and tibialis posterior arteries (arterial vascular anatomy is described in chapter 10, figure 1b). Central arterial catheters are inserted if peripheral arterial access is not possible and usually involves cannulation of the more central femoral arteries. In addition, femoral artery cannulation occurs during cardiac catheterization. This invasive technique is used for the diagnosis and treatment of children with congenital or acquired heart disease (see chapter 15), as well as in children requiring ECMO, or in those that require cerebral angiography.

Arterial catheter-related TEs are thought to arise by several mechanisms. Firstly, there may be damage to the vascular endothelium by the catheter itself or by substances infused through the catheter. TEs may also be due to the disruption of blood flow, and/or by the effects of thrombogenic catheter materials.

The overall incidence of peripheral arterial catheter-related TEs has been reported as 3.25%

Table 1. Clinical classification of peripheral arterial TEs

Mild	Moderate	Severe
Early signs of threatened limb without risk for an irreversible limb/organ dysfunction (i.e. no evidence for moderate or severe state)	Capillary return >8 s for >24 h Absent SaO$_2$ pulse Damped Doppler wave Tight compartments	Complete limb ischemia Pregangrenous changes Paralyzed limb >24 h Doppler/angiogram obstruction with no distal flow >24 h Failure of reperfusion after 4 h of UFH ± thrombolysis

[4]. The relative incidence of arterial TE was 13% for femoral location, 9% in the brachial location, and 4% in the umbilical location [4]. Younger age was significantly associated with increased risk for femoral catheter-related arterial TEs [4]. In contrast, placement of the arterial catheter into the radial artery was found to be safe and not associated with increased risk of TE in children of all ages including young children [4]. Additional risk factors for arterial catheter-related TEs include longer duration of insertion, longer length and larger diameter of the catheter, the use of non-heparin-bonded arterial catheter, and conditions associated with poor perfusion such as severe sepsis or shock [1]. For cardiac catheterization, additional risk factors for TEs include balloon dilation, larger sheath size for a given weight and repeated catheter manipulation.

UFH is frequently used to maintain the patency of peripheral arterial catheters. Continuous infusion of UFH in a concentration of 0.5 U/ml at 1 ml/h is recommended to decrease the incidence of catheter occlusion and prolong the patency of peripheral artery catheters [5]. Intermittent flushes with UFH do not prevent the loss of catheter patency. For cardiac catheterization, a bolus dose of 100 U/kg UFH is recommended immediately after arterial puncture [5]. For prolonged procedures, further doses of UFH are recommended [5].

Clinical Presentation

The clinical presentation of arterial TEs varies according to the anatomical location and degree of occlusion of the artery involved. Accordingly, children show a spectrum of disease that ranges from asymptomatic to severely compromised with signs of a threatened limb or severe organ dysfunction. Signs of threatened limb may include absent palpable pulses, difference in blood pressure of over 10 mm Hg between legs, decreased skin temperature, skin discoloration (pale or cyanosed), and prolonged capillary refill time. Classification of arterial TEs may be based on the clinical signs and the risk for the related limb or organ (table 1).

Diagnosis

Diagnosis of catheter-related arterial TE can be made clinically (as previously described) or objectively. Objective tests for suspected arterial TE can be performed at the bedside including hand-held Doppler examination for absent pulses, a difference in blood pressure of >10 mm Hg between two limbs, and segmental plethysmography (pulse volume recording).

Doppler ultrasound can confirm the clinical diagnosis of arterial TE. Although the gold standard for diagnosis of arterial TE is contrast angiography, it is rarely done in this setting due to its invasiveness.

Differential Diagnosis

Catheterization of an artery can result in arterial spasm. The clinical signs and Doppler findings can be similar to arterial TEs; however, arterial spasm usually resolves approximately 6 h after catheterization. The use of 100 μg intravenous nitroglycerin in addition to UFH has been suggested for prevention of arterial spasm after cardiac catheterization [6]. Although not evidence based, hot compresses, subcutaneous nitroglycerin alone or in combination with 2% lidocaine have been used to resolve arterial spasm.

Management

If arterial occlusion is suspected, the catheter should be removed immediately [5]. If blood flow cannot be restored and arterial TE is diagnosed, anticoagulants should be strongly considered with or without thrombolysis or surgical thrombectomy, depending on the urgency to restore patency of the vessels [5].

An algorithm for the acute management of catheter-related arterial TE is presented (algorithm 1). The algorithm is based on expert opinion, as minimal evidence exists on the management of arterial TEs in children. The potential risk of hemorrhage versus the benefit of therapy, the local expertise, the surgical accessibility and the predicted time course need to be carefully considered in all cases, especially in neonates and in severely ill children who are more prone to hemorrhagic complications.

For arterial TE following cardiac catheterization, therapeutic UFH should be commenced as a continuous infusion without a bolus if <4 h have passed since the dose of UFH given immediately after cardiac catheterization [5]. LMWH may be a valuable option to UFH and used per algorithm 1. However, initiating therapy with UFH is preferred over LMWH in cases where interventional therapies, i.e. thrombolysis, surgical thrombectomy, might be needed (moderate and severe cases).

A follow-up Doppler ultrasound is usually done after 10–14 days of therapy. In the case of persistent complete or partial occlusion of the vessel, additional UFH/LMWH therapy may be considered for at least one month. It should be stated that the continuation of antithrombotic therapy after the first 10 days is not evidence based. If complete or partial occlusion persists after one month, the options are stopping anticoagulation, switching to antiplatelet therapy, i.e. ASA, or continuing anticoagulation therapy up to 3 months, but not longer. Currently, no evidence is available to recommend one of these therapeutic options over the other. A case to case decision considering the safety and efficacy of each option is recommended.

Dosing and monitoring details for anticoagulation, antiplatelet and thrombolytic therapy are outlined in detail in chapter 16. The role of thrombophilia testing in children with arterial thrombosis is discussed in chapter 10.

Umbilical Artery Catheter-Related Thrombosis

UAC is primarily used in newborns for monitoring of arterial blood pressure, monitoring of arterial blood gases and blood sampling. It may be used to give fluids, medications, and nutrition, if no other site is available. Systematic ultrasound screening identified UAC-related TEs in 17–32.3% of cases [7]. Most the cases were asymptomatic, occurring several days after the UAC was removed. Only 1–3% of cases were symptomatic [7].

Duration of UAC in situ was found to be associated with an increased risk of TEs. The adjusted odds ratio for developing arterial TE, for each additional day of using the UAC was 1.2 (95% CI: 1.1–1.3). Thus, it is strongly recommended to limit the use of UAC to as short a period as possible. Several other UAC-related risk factors for TEs were identified and are reviewed in a recent Cochrane review [7]. As more proximal placement of the UAC (defined as a position between T_6 and T_{10}) was associated with a lower incidence

▶

Algorithm 1. Acute management of catheter-related arterial thrombotic event. C/I = Contraindication. For additional therapy after 10 days, refer to text. Dosing and monitoring details for UFH, LMWH and thrombolytic therapy are outlined in chapter 16.

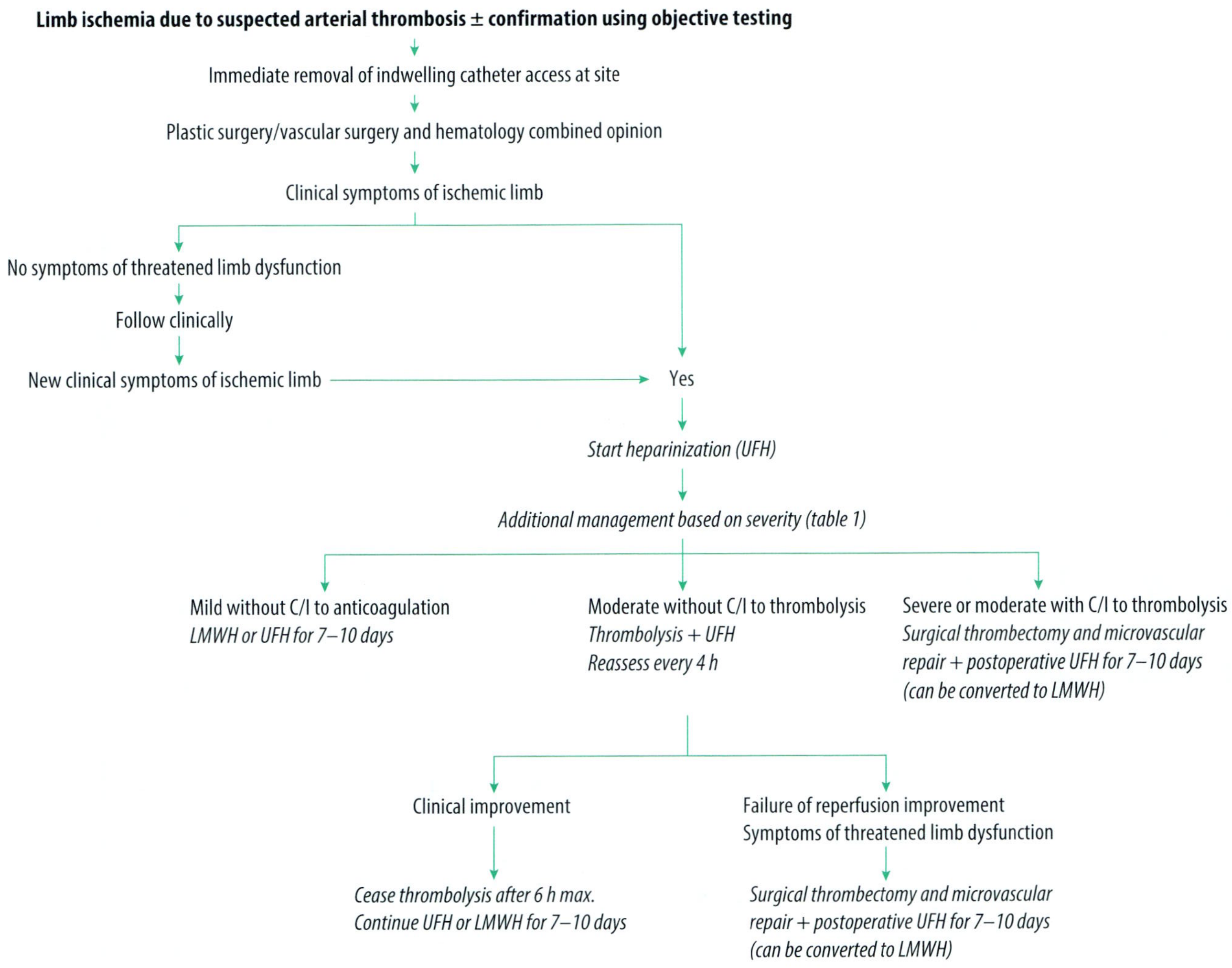

Limb ischemia due to suspected arterial thrombosis ± confirmation using objective testing

- Immediate removal of indwelling catheter access at site
- Plastic surgery/vascular surgery and hematology combined opinion
- Clinical symptoms of ischemic limb
  - No symptoms of threatened limb dysfunction → Follow clinically → New clinical symptoms of ischemic limb → Yes
  - → Start heparinization (UFH)
  - → *Additional management based on severity (table 1)*

- **Mild without C/I to anticoagulation**
  LMWH or UFH for 7–10 days

- **Moderate without C/I to thrombolysis**
  Thrombolysis + UFH
  Reassess every 4 h
  - Clinical improvement → *Cease thrombolysis after 6 h max. Continue UFH or LMWH for 7–10 days*
  - Failure of reperfusion improvement / Symptoms of threatened limb dysfunction → *Surgical thrombectomy and microvascular repair + postoperative UFH for 7–10 days (can be converted to LMWH)*

- **Severe or moderate with C/I to thrombolysis**
  Surgical thrombectomy and microvascular repair + postoperative UFH for 7–10 days (can be converted to LMWH)

Arterial Thrombosis

of clinical vascular complications, this positioning is preferred [5]. End hole catheters were associated with a significantly decreased risk of aortic TE compared to side hole catheters. Infusion of hyperosmolar solutions was associated with higher risk of TE. The use of heparin-bonded polyurethane catheters was not associated with a lower risk of TE. Inherited prothrombotic genetic mutations did not appear to increase the risk of UAC-associated TE [7]. Continuous infusion of low-dose UFH at a concentration of 0.25–1 U/ml (total UFH dose of 25–200 U/kg per day) is recommended to maintain patency of UAC [5].

Clinical Presentation

Aortic thrombosis is the most common vascular complication associated with the use of UAC (see below). Infants may be asymptomatic or show evidence of irritability, non-palpable lower limb pulses, decreased temperature of the extremities, and discoloration of the lower limbs or feet. Umbilical artery catheter-related TE affecting the aorta, the renal arteries or both is a common cause of hypertension observed in the typical neonatal intensive care unit. The onset of hypertension and narrowing of the pulse pressure may be early signs of UAC-related aortic thrombosis. Others signs may include catheter dysfunction, renal dysfunction, oliguria, hematuria, mesenteric ischemia, lower limb extremity signs of ischemia, and congestive heart failure.

Diagnosis

Doppler ultrasound is the diagnostic test of choice because it is noninvasive and can be performed at the bedside; however, its validity in the diagnosis of UAC-related TE has not been established.

Management

The management of UAC-related TE is largely dependent on the clinical scenario and the further requirement of the catheter. If possible, the UAC should be removed. The indication for anticoagulant depends on the extent of thrombosis. If there is no contraindication to anticoagulation therapy, therapy with UFH or LMWH is recommended for the duration of at least 5–7 days. The management of UAC-related aortic thrombosis is detailed in the next section. Dosing and monitoring details for UFH, LMWH and thrombolytic therapy in neonates are outlined in chapter 16. Intracranial ultrasound is recommended before a decision to treat a newborn with anticoagulation or thrombolytic therapy [8]. The potential risk of hemorrhage versus the benefit of anticoagulation needs to be carefully considered in the neonate, particularly in the presence of recent ICH. If the arterial TE will result in a potentially life-, organ-, or limb-threatening event, thrombolytic or surgical therapy should be considered.

The recommended management of radiographically detected asymptomatic UAC-related TE is less clear. If the UAC is no longer required, the catheter should be removed. As spontaneous resolution is reported in most cases, close clinical follow-up and administration of anticoagulation therapy only for symptomatic cases seems to be a reasonable option. Similar management should be applied in asymptomatic UAC-related TE that is radiographically detected after the catheter has been removed.

There are no consistent data to make a firm recommendation for thrombophilia screening for neonates with UAC-related TE (see chapter 10) [8, 9].

Aortic Thrombosis

Most cases of aortic thrombosis are catheter related, and spontaneous cases are extremely rare. The outcome is variable, but overall mortality appears to be relatively high. Aortic thrombosis can involve the thoracic aorta or the abdominal aorta.

Table 2. Clinical classification and therapeutic options of aortic thrombosis

	Mild	Moderate	Severe
Signs	Decreased femoral pulses Inability to withdraw blood Hypertension	Mild signs *plus* Absent femoral pulses Peripheral ischemia Congestive heart failure	Mild and moderate signs *plus* Severe limb-threatening ischemia Renal failure Visceral involvement Acidosis Sepsis
Therapeutic options	Anticoagulation (UFH or LMWH)	Thrombolysis + UFH. If contraindication to thrombolysis, consider surgical thrombectomy followed by postoperative UFH/LMWH	Surgical thrombectomy + followed by postoperative UFH/LMWH

Clinical Presentation

The presentation of aortic thrombosis is varied depending on the location and the extent of the clot (table 2). Clinical presentation can range from children who are asymptomatic to those presenting with severe irritability, poor feeding, paraplegia, or signs of congestive heart failure. Paraplegia presents classically with loss of lower limb motor function and bladder retention if the spinal artery of Adamkiewicz is involved. Children with aortic thrombosis can have clinical signs and symptoms mimicking congenital heart disease, and thus a high index of suspicion is needed to ensure accurate and timely diagnosis. For example, thoracic aortic thrombosis can present with signs mimicking coarctation such as poor peripheral perfusion, impaired left ventricular function, and diminished femoral pulses.

Diagnosis

Noninvasive ultrasound studies are usually used for the diagnosis of aortic thrombosis. However, false-negative ultrasound results have been reported in infants. Additional investigations include echocardiography, cardiac catheterization, CTA, MRA and contrast angiography.

Management

The classification of neonatal aortic thrombosis according to minor, moderate and major degree of thrombosis was developed in 1992 and can be used to provide a standardized description of thrombosis and for management decisions [8, 10] (table 2).

Similar to other arterial TEs, the therapeutic options include anticoagulation (LMWH or UFH), thrombolytic therapy and/or surgical thrombectomy. Therapeutic decisions may be based on the above-mentioned clinical classification [8] (table 2). A child with aortic thrombosis should be followed closely as severity could increase with time requiring a change in management. The therapeutic recommendations are based on expert opinion, as minimal evidence exists on the management of aortic thrombosis in children. The potential risk of hemorrhage versus the benefit of therapy, i.e. thrombolysis and anticoagulation, the local expertise, surgical accessibility and predicted time course, needs to be carefully considered in all cases, especially in neonates and in severely ill children who are more prone to hemorrhagic complications. The optimal duration of anticoagulation therapy for persistent complete or partial aortic thrombosis is not known. Dosing and monitoring details for anticoagulation and thrombolytic therapy are outlined in detail in chapter 16.

Arterial Stents – Non-Cardiac, Non-CNS

Endovascular arterial stents are used in children for the management of a variety of non-cardiac vascular disorders such as branch pulmonary artery stenosis, coarctation of the aorta, traumatic arterial injuries, arterial dissection, renovascular disease, anti-phospholipid antibodies syndrome and hepatic stenosis. The small vessel size in young children increases the risk of thrombosis. There are no studies assessing the role of anticoagulation or antiplatelet therapy to prevent stent occlusion in children. However, for children having endovascular stents inserted, administration of UFH at the time of insertion is suggested [5]. The dose of UFH is not specified in the recommendation; however, the common practice is to use a dose of UFH 100 U/kg. A common practice is to then continue with ASA therapy for 3–6 months.

Renal Artery Stents

Percutaneous transluminal renal angioplasty, with or without stenting, is a valuable treatment option in pediatric renal artery stenosis. This method is usually undertaken from a femoral arterial approach, with either a long vascular sheath or a guiding catheter. Angioplasty equipment designed for use in adult coronary arteries is ideal for the renal arteries of children and, in particular, in segmental arteries. Intra-arterial UFH (100 U/kg) is given before percutaneous transluminal renal angioplasty [11]. To further minimize the risk of thrombotic complications, LMWH or UFH (at 10 U/kg every hour for 12–24 h) can be given after the procedure [11]. ASA (1 mg/kg daily) is usually prescribed for 3–6 months [11].

Non-Catheter-Related Arterial Thrombosis

Non-catheter-related arterial TEs are rare events in children. Cases reported were associated with congenital or acquired disease including primary hyperlipidemia or hyperhomocysteinemia, organ transplantation, trauma, circumferential burns of the limbs, Kawasaki's disease, and Takayasu's arteritis, and likely develop in specific organ sites such as liver, kidney, heart and the CNS. Cardiac and CNS arterial TEs are discussed in chapter 15 and chapter 14, respectively. The clinical presentation and management of renal artery thrombosis and hepatic artery thrombosis are discussed in chapter 13.

Complications of Arterial Thrombosis

Children, like adults, may develop acute or chronic complications after an arterial TE. Reperfusion syndrome and limb and organ necrosis are significant acute complications of arterial TE. Chronic complications of arterial TE depend on the anatomical location of the thrombus, and may manifest as hypertension, renal function impairment, leg length discrepancies, muscle wasting, claudication, chronic pain, paraplegia and loss of arterial access.

In a retrospective study of arterial TE in ill children, about 30% of arterial TEs showed incomplete or no resolution on follow-up [12]. Although, the long-term implications of the occluded artery were not studied, the occluded artery likely increases the risk for leg length differences and claudication. The loss of arterial access in patients with complex congenital heart disease requiring repeated cardiac catheterizations is also a problem. The long-term morbidity of UAC-related TEs remains uncertain.

Children who develop peripheral arterial TE should be followed regularly for measurement of the extremity length and circumference, and for measurement of the systolic blood pressure in both extremities (ABI; see below). Some clinicians will follow with Doppler ultrasound imaging 3 and 6 months following the acute event. Subsequently, if imaging findings are stable, only clinical observation is continued. The clinical value and therapeutic consequence for follow-up Doppler ultrasound imaging in peripheral arterial TE is not clear. However, routine ultrasound imaging can objectively confirm clinical signs of no or partial resolution of thrombosis and can provide information on the flow in the collaterals.

Reperfusion Injury

Reperfusion injury occurs when blood supply returns to the tissue after a period of ischemia and results in inflammation and oxidative damage. Acute ischemia-reperfusion injury of the limbs is characterized by edema, compartment syndrome and neuromuscular dysfunction. Metabolic consequences of reperfusion injury can be variable, ranging from transient symptoms in the limb to systemic inflammation with multiple organ dysfunction [13]. Inflammatory mediators of the reperfusion injury can result in acute lung injury and rhabdomyolysis-induced acute renal failure. Prompt fasciotomy is necessary for reducing compartment pressure and limiting the degree of rhabdomyolysis. Treatment of rhabdomyolysis should focus on preventing life-threatening complications from hyperkalemia and preserving renal function. In adults, the use of hypertonic mannitol infusion has been suggested to decrease the need for fasciotomy and minimize neuromuscular dysfunction, but no data exist for pediatric patients.

Peripheral Arterial Insufficiency

The ABI is the first-line test for diagnosis of peripheral arterial insufficiency. The ABI is the ratio of the blood pressure in the ankle to the blood pressure in the arm (brachial); an index lower than 0.9 is diagnostic for peripheral arterial insufficiency. Values below 0.8 indicate moderate disease and below 0.5 imply severe arterial insufficiency. If the ABI is abnormal, the next steps for diagnosis are Doppler ultrasound examination, computerized tomography and/or angiography study.

Treatment of children with peripheral arterial insufficiency includes the elimination of other risk factors for arterial insufficiency, e.g. smoking, hypertension, hypercholesterolemia, etc. and instructions for regular exercise. No evidence supports the use of medical therapy for children with peripheral arterial insufficiency. If symptoms persist, consultation with a vascular surgeon is recommended for possible balloon angioplasty, stenting or bypass surgery.

Conclusion

Catheter-associated arterial TEs are serious iatrogenic complications seen mainly in the neonatal and pediatric intensive care units and following cardiac catheterizations. Treatment strategies vary widely depending on the clinical situation and can impact on short- and long-term outcomes. Data from pediatric cohorts suggest that early recognition and more aggressive therapeutic approaches, i.e. initiation of anticoagulation therapy in most patients and usage of interventional therapies in severe cases that do not respond to medical therapy, may result in improved short and long-term outcomes [3, 12].

Acknowledgment

The authors would like to express their appreciation for the thoughtful comments provided by Drs. Patrick McNamara (Toronto, Ont., Canada), Anne-Marie Guergerian (Toronto, Ont., Canada), Brian W. McCrindle (Toronto, Ont., Canada), Leonardo R. Brandão (Toronto, Ont., Canada), Yaser Diab (Washington, D.C., USA) and Paul Monagle (Melbourne, Vic., Australia) who reviewed this chapter.

References

1 Price VE, Chan AK: Arterial thrombosis in children. Expert Rev Cardiovasc Ther 2008;6:419.
2 Tuckuviene R, Christensen AL, Helgestad J, Johnsen SP, Kristensen SR: Pediatric venous and arterial noncerebral thromboembolism in Denmark: a nationwide population-based study. J Pediatr 2011; 159:663.
3 Monagle P, Newall F, Barnes C, Savoia H, Campbell J, Wallace T, Crock C: Arterial thromboembolic disease: a single-centre case series study. J Paediatr Child Health 2008;44:28.
4 Brotschi B, Hug MI, Latal B, Neuhaus D, Buerki C, Kroiss S, Spoerri C, Albisetti M: Incidence and predictors of indwelling arterial catheter-related thrombosis in children. J Thromb Haemost 2011;9: 1157.
5 Monagle P, Chan A, Goldenberg NA, Ichord R, Journeycake J, Nowak-Gottl U, Vesely SK: Antithrombotic therapy in neonates and children: American College of Chest Physicians Evidence-Based Clinical Practice Guidelines (9th Edition). Chest 2012;141: e737S.
6 Chen CW, Lin CL, Lin TK, Lin CD: A simple and effective regimen for prevention of radial artery spasm during coronary catheterization. Cardiology 2006;105:43.
7 Revel-Vilk S, Ergaz Z: Diagnosis and management of central-line-associated thrombosis in newborns and infants. Semin Fetal Neonatal Med 2011;16:340.
8 Nagel K, Tuckuviene R, Paes B, Chan AK: Neonatal aortic thrombosis: a comprehensive review. Klin Padiatr 2010;222:134.
9 Raffini L: Thrombophilia in children: who to test, how, when, and why? Hematology Am Soc Hematol Educ Program 2008;2008:228.
10 Colburn M, Gelabert JA, Quinones-Baldrich W: Neonatal aortic thrombosis. Surgery 1992;111:21.
11 Tullus K, Brennan E, Hamilton G, Lord R, McLaren CA, Marks SD, Roebuck DJ: Renovascular hypertension in children. Lancet 2008; 371:1453.
12 Albisetti M, Schmugge M, Haas R, Eckhardt BP, Bauersfeld U, Baenziger O, Hug MI: Arterial thromboembolic complications in critically ill children. J Crit Care 2005;20:296.
13 Eliason JL, Wakefield TW: Metabolic consequences of acute limb ischemia and their clinical implications. Semin Vasc Surg 2009;22: 29.

Abbreviations

ABI	Ankle-brachial index
ASA	Acetylsalicylic acid
CNS	Central nervous system
CTA	Computed tomography angiography
ECMO	Extracorporeal membrane oxygenation
ICH	Intracranial hemorrhage
LMWH	Low-molecular-weight heparin
MRA	Magnetic resonance angiography
SaO_2	Oxygen saturation
TE	Thromboembolism/thromboembolic event
UAC	Umbilical artery catheter
UFH	Unfractionated heparin

Chapter 13

Thromboembolic Events at Specific Organ Sites

Veerle Labarque
Anthony K.C. Chan
Suzan Williams

Introduction

TEs occur with and without underlying risk factors, most frequently in the deep venous, peripheral arterial and central nervous systems. Although rare, TEs may occur in the renal and hepatic veins and arteries, as well as other abdominal vessels such as portal, splenic and mesenteric veins or mesenteric arteries. These TEs may be clinically severe and challenging for the caregiver, with significant morbidity and mortality.

In this chapter, we describe TEs in the kidney, liver and splanchnic system with focus on clinical presentation, diagnosis and management. This chapter is mainly based on expert opinion and extrapolation from the literature on adults, as studies in children are lacking.

Kidney-Related Thromboembolic Events

Renal Vein Thrombosis

RVT is relatively uncommon and is predominantly a disease of children, primarily affecting newborns [1]. RVT accounts for 16–20% of all TEs in newborns and is the 3rd most prevalent non-catheter-related cause of TEs during the neonatal period, excluding AIS and CSVT [1]. Almost 80% of all RVT present within the first month of life, one third of which are diagnosed in the first week. Some cases develop in utero and are prenatally detected [1]. Males are more commonly affected than females (2:1 ratio). In approximately 70% of the cases, neonatal RVT is unilateral, with left-sided predominance. Extension of the thrombus into the IVC occurs in 40% of patients. Coexisting risk factors, other than the presence of a CVC, such as perinatal asphyxia, maternal diabetes, dehydration, infection, and cyanotic congenital heart disease, are found in up to 80% of the affected neonates [1] (table 1). Also in some children, a predisposing condition may be present (table 1).

Clinical Presentation
Neonates may be asymptomatic but most have at least one of the three cardinal signs at presentation: palpable flank mass (45%), hematuria (56%) and thrombocytopenia (48%) [1]. However, the

Table 1. Conditions frequently complicated by RVT

Neonates
- Umbilical venous catheter
- Perinatal asphyxia
- Infant of a diabetic mother
- Dehydration, shock
- Infection
- Prematurity
- Cyanotic congenital heart disease

Older children
- Dehydration, shock
- Acute blood loss
- Nephrotic syndrome
- Renal transplantation
- Consumptive coagulopathy
- Angiographic studies
- Corticosteroids

entire classic triad occurs only in less than a quarter of cases. Other possible presenting symptoms include vomiting, pallor, metabolic acidosis with electrolyte abnormalities, proteinuria, renal impairment, disseminated intravascular coagulation, and shock.

Diagnosis

Accurate and prompt diagnosis requires a high level of clinical suspicion. The diagnosis can be suspected on the basis of hematuria and renal masses in the presence of predisposing factors and can be confirmed on imaging.

Doppler ultrasonography has gained popularity over renal venography and has become the first-line investigation of choice because of its wide availability, practicality, sensitivity and lack of adverse effects [1]. The Doppler ultrasound findings vary according to the time of onset, the severity, the extent of the thrombus, and the development of collateral circulation. In addition to grey-scale ultrasound which demonstrates globular enlargement of the kidney, increased echogenicity and loss of corticomedullary boundary in the acute phase, color Doppler has also been shown to be very useful as it detects high arterial resistance and reversed diastolic flow. CTA and MRA have also been used but have no advantages over ultrasonography. With unclear initial imaging, renal venography may still be required.

Management

During the acute phase, a collaborative approach amongst subspecialists (neonatologists, hematologists, nephrologists, and radiologists) is essential. All children with RVT need urgent treatment of concurrent shock, sepsis, cyanosis and electrolyte imbalances. In severe cases, dialysis may be needed.

A review of retrospective case series reported no difference in renal outcomes irrespective of whether the infant received no therapy, UFH, or LMWH, as approximately 75% of the affected kidneys become atrophic regardless of the treatment [2]. However, prospective controlled trials are needed to give evidence-based recommendations on the treatment of RVT. Due to the lack of evidence of a clear benefit, the use of anticoagulant therapy in neonatal RVT remains controversial. In the absence of demonstrated efficacy of anticoagulation to improve outcome, one needs to balance the potential risk of the extension of the clot with conservative therapy to the risk imposed by using anticoagulation.

The decision to start anticoagulation in neonates should be influenced by the extent of the RVT (unilateral, bilateral, extension into the IVC) and presence or absence of renal impairment [3]. The presence or absence of thrombophilic abnormalities is not useful in determining initial therapy. Further details regarding the role of a prothrombotic work-up are outlined in chapter 10. The management of neonates with RVT is presented in algorithm 1. No guidelines are available for the acute management of unilateral RVT with renal impairment or for the rare case of bilateral RVT without renal impairment. For bilateral RVT with renal impairment, starting anticoagulation unless there is a contraindication (e.g. severe

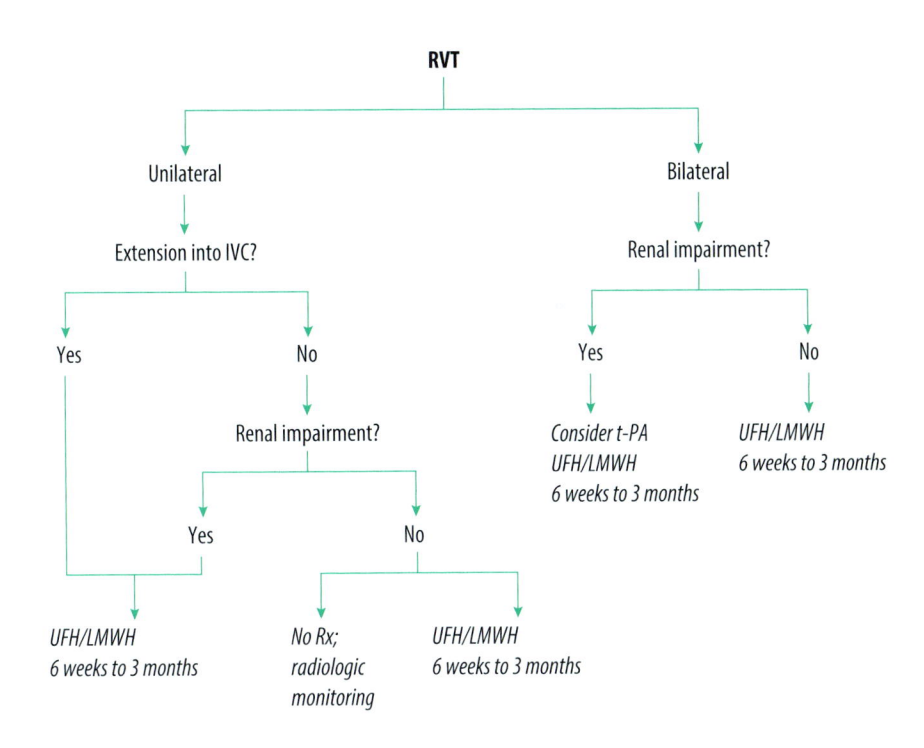

```
                              RVT
                               │
                ┌──────────────┴──────────────┐
            Unilateral                     Bilateral
                │                             │
         Extension into IVC?           Renal impairment?
            ┌───┴───┐                    ┌────┴────┐
           Yes     No                   Yes        No
            │      │                     │          │
            │  Renal impairment?    Consider t-PA  UFH/LMWH
            │   ┌──┴──┐              UFH/LMWH    6 weeks to 3 months
            │  Yes   No             6 weeks to 3 months
            │   │    │
        UFH/LMWH  No Rx;  UFH/LMWH
      6 weeks to  radiologic  6 weeks to
       3 months  monitoring   3 months
```

Algorithm 1. Proposed algorithm for the initiation of anticoagulant therapy in neonatal renal vein thrombosis. Rx = Anticoagulant therapy.

intraventricular hemorrhage) is suggested. In severe cases, thrombolysis followed by anticoagulation should also be considered. As LMWH may accumulate in the presence of renal impairment, it is preferable to start therapy with UFH in those patients or to reduce the dose of LMWH and adjust according to the anti-Xa level. Dosing and monitoring details for UFH, LMWH and thrombolytic therapy in neonates are outlined in chapter 16.

There are also no evidence-based recommendations for treatment of RVT in non-neonates (i.e. older than 1 month of age at time of presentation). Similar to treating adults with RVT, the main goal of therapy should be the preservation of renal parenchyma and prevention of embolic events. Therefore we suggest prompt initiation of anticoagulation with UFH or LMWH in the absence of contraindications. If a child presents with an acute onset of symptoms, thrombolysis followed by anticoagulation should also be considered. Although nephrectomy may eventually be required to control resulting hypertension, surgery has only limited usefulness in the acute treatment of RVT [1]. Dosing and monitoring details for UFH, LMWH and thrombolytic therapy in children are outlined in chapter 16.

Outcome

Although mortality rates are low, morbidity is considerable. In almost half of the neonates, RVT is associated with adrenal hemorrhage [2]. Other acute complications of RVT include AIS, PE, and CSVT [1]. Long-term outcomes depend on severity and laterality of kidneys affected and may vary from normal renal function to end stage renal disease. Atrophy of the affected kidney occurs in 75%

of cases. Approximately 20% of children develop hypertension on long-term follow-up and 3% of children develop end-stage chronic renal failure. Hence, children with a history of RVT warrant long-term close follow-up of growth, blood pressure, renal function and urinalysis and should be followed regularly by a nephrologist. Renal ultrasound with Doppler should also be performed at regular intervals to monitor the sizes of, and blood flow to, the affected kidney(s) [1].

Renal Artery Thrombosis

RAT is an infrequently encountered entity in children, with a paucity of informative literature available to aid clinical decisions. It is most commonly reported following renal transplantation but may also occur after blunt abdominal trauma. RAT can occur in the neonatal period; however, less commonly than RVT. In neonates, RAT is strongly associated with umbilical catheters and patent ductus arteriosus. Traumatic RAT is usually unilateral and the left side is involved more often, almost never occurs as an isolated event and indicates major associated injuries. RAT must be diagnosed and treated as soon as possible to avoid progressive, permanent loss of renal function.

Clinical Presentation

The clinical symptoms of acute RAT include steady, aching flank pain, abdominal pain, fever, nausea, vomiting and hematuria. Acute renal failure may develop. The presentation of chronic, progressive thrombosis is often silent, causing refractory hypertension and leading to chronic kidney disease. History of a kidney transplant or trauma to the back or abdomen may be helpful.

Diagnosis

Renal ultrasound findings can be minimal unless Doppler imaging is used. In the absence of renal failure, contrast-enhanced CT scan is the modality of choice for diagnosis, for prediction of the level of occlusion and follow-up of RAT. Angiography is equally useful for predicting the blockage, and can be relied upon if segmental obstruction to the blood flow is present. Unlike CT scan, angiography will not be helpful to delineate the extent of associated injuries. MRI is a promising alternative technique in the evaluation of vascular complications after renal transplantation.

Management

The optimal treatment for RAT is uncertain, given the absence of comparative studies. Conservative treatment with anticoagulation is reserved for unilateral cases [4]. For bilateral RAT and RAT in a solitary kidney, revascularization is usually indicated [4]. It can be performed either surgically or more preferably by less invasive percutaneous techniques which are directed to resolve the thrombosis or recanalize the involved vessel. In the setting of renal transplantation, prophylactic administration of low-dose LMWH may be effective to prevent RAT, as has been reported in adults.

Hemodialysis-Related Thrombosis

CVC and arteriovenous fistula are frequently used to obtain vascular access for hemodialysis in children. Both are associated with thrombotic complications. Failure of the vascular access can occur immediately and is caused by technical problems, whereas late dysfunction usually results from an intraluminal thrombus. TEs related to the use of CVC for hemodialysis may occur in the right atrium, on the vessel wall, or may completely occlude the vessel causing a DVT. Formation of a fibrin sheath that can elongate, cover the intake and outflow holes of the catheter, may lead to catheter dysfunction and shorter survival of the CVC (<1 year in most cases). Factors that increase the risk of CVC-related TEs include larger catheters relative to the size of the vessel and the fluid shifts occurring during intermittent dialysis. A thrombus in an arteriovenous fistula develops mainly as a consequence of venous stasis produced by stenotic lesions. Excessive vessel compression after needle withdrawal to avoid bleeding and dialysis-related hypotensive episodes are also important contributors to thrombus formation.

Clinical Presentation

A CVC-related TE in the setting of hemodialysis may be asymptomatic. It may present as a right atrial thrombosis, as a DVT or as an intraluminal thrombus, the most common thrombotic complication. The clinical presentation of CVC-related venous TEs is detailed in chapter 11. An intraluminal thrombus results in a blocked catheter (i.e. the catheter is unable to deliver the required blood flow).

Thrombosis of an arteriovenous fistula can present with absence of a thrill (vibration), discontinuous bruit, or edema distal to the fistula. Occasionally, thrombosis of the arteriovenous fistula may only be noted during the dialysis session due to difficulties with cannulation, aspiration of clots, inability to achieve the target dialysis blood flow, or prolonged bleeding from the needle puncture sites.

Diagnosis

CVC-related TE in the setting of hemodialysis is diagnosed with a similar approach as described for a CVC-related DVT and/or blocked CVC (see chapter 11 for details). Close monitoring of an arteriovenous fistula (presence of a thrill, growth of the fistula) and collaboration with a vascular surgeon is important to prevent complications. Abnormalities on physical examination of the arteriovenous fistula or problems during the dialysis session should prompt a fistulogram to diagnose a stenosis and/or thrombosis of the fistula.

Management

Management of a blocked CVC used for hemodialysis is similar to the management of a blocked CVC in nonhemodialysis patients (chapter 11). Similarly, management of DVT related to a CVC used for hemodialysis is similar to the management of DVT related to CVC in nonhemodialysis patients. The dose of LMWH should be reduced in renal insufficiency, as elimination happens primarily via the kidney. Close monitoring of the anti-Xa level is important, as accumulation may occur (see chapter 16 for details). There are no evidence-based guidelines to suggest whether LMWH should be administered prior to or after the hemodialysis session. As predicting long-term drug elimination may be challenging in the setting of hemodialysis, we suggest administration of the LMWH after the dialysis session.

Stenosis of an arteriovenous fistula may be managed by percutaneous transluminal angioplasty and stent placement but once thrombosis has occurred, urgent surgical revision usually is required.

Prophylaxis

The use of VKA or LMWH between hemodialysis sessions is recommended to prevent TEs of the arteriovenous fistula or the CVC used for hemodialysis [3]. It has been shown that a prophylactic dose of LMWH of 0.5 mg/kg/day is effective to prevent TEs in the majority of patients (anti-factor Xa levels: peak 0.25–0.5 U/ml). However, in patients at high risk for TEs, dosing at 1 mg/kg/day may be necessary (anti-factor Xa level: peak 0.5–1 U/ml) [5]. During hemodialysis, anticoagulation with LMWH or UFH is recommended to prevent thrombosis within the artificial circuit, independent of the type of vascular access used [3]. Clinical practice varies from dosing according to body weight to empirical dosing, even in children. Most authors recommend calculating the appropriate dose based on body weight (LMWH: 0.5–1 mg/kg; UFH: a loading dose of 50 U/kg, followed by a maintenance infusion at 25 U/kg/h or a loading dose of 50 U/kg followed by a second bolus of 25 U/kg halfway through the dialysis session) [6]. Adjustments can be based on clinical signs and/or laboratory monitoring (i.e. ACT or aPTT; see chapter 16 for details). Although rare, HIT has been reported in children as a complication of exposure to UFH during hemodialysis. The diagnosis and management of HIT is detailed in chapter 16. Although nonheparin anticoagulant options are available and used in children needing hemodialysis treatment, their use should probably be restricted to children with a high risk for hemorrhage and children who developed a heparin allergy or HIT [6]. The most frequently used nonheparin anticoagulant is citrate (hypertonic sodium citrate or 3% acid citrate dextrose). As the half-life of citrate is minutes, this anticoagulant offers the potential to anticoagulate the circuit but not the patient. The ACT test can be used to monitor the anticoagulant effect of citrate.

Nephrotic Syndrome-Associated Thrombosis

Thrombotic complications are not rare in children with nephrotic syndrome. In a large cohort study of 326 children with nephrotic syndrome, almost 10% of children had experienced at least one TE. The overall incidence was 20.4 patients with TEs/1,000 patient-years [7]. The incidence seems greater in the first presentation of nephrotic syndrome, but TEs were also reported to occur when nephrotic syndrome relapses. Thromboembolic events more commonly occur in children with congenital nephrotic syndrome, minimal change disease, and focal segmental glomerulosclerosis.

The pathophysiology of nephrotic syndrome-associated TEs is thought to be multifactorial including acquired thrombophilia, hyperlipidemia, diuretics and hemoconcentration [7]. Acquired thrombophilia occurs as a result of increased procoagulant activity (i.e. increased production of fibrinogen, FV and FVIII by the liver), reduced anticoagulant activity (i.e. urinary loss of antithrombin, proteins C and S), reduced fibrinolytic system and increased platelet activation and aggregability [7]. Inherited thrombophilia seems to be only a weak risk factor for TEs in children with nephrotic syndrome [7].

Both venous and arterial TEs have been described. The majority of the events (76.3%) are DVT [7] and the most commonly affected vessels are the deep leg veins, followed by the IVC. VTEs are most frequently associated with the use of CVC. PE has been found in up to 28% of children. RVT, a well-known complication in adults with nephrotic syndrome, occurs rarely in children, with the exception of infants with congenital nephrotic syndrome. Involvement of cerebral vessels has also been reported and has probably been underdiagnosed in the past. Peripheral artery thrombosis in children with nephrotic syndrome is usually secondary to arterial punctures or arterial catheters.

Clinical Presentation

Symptoms of TEs in children with nephrotic syndrome are the same as those of children without nephrotic syndrome and are described in the relevant chapters (chapters 11 (DVT or PE), 12 (arterial TE), and 14 (arterial and venous stroke)). However, TEs in children with nephrotic syndrome may be subclinical [7].

Diagnosis

Diagnostic measures in children with nephrotic syndrome do not differ from the methods used in children without nephrotic syndrome and are described in chapters 11, 12 and 14.

Management

The initial treatment of TEs in children with nephrotic syndrome is similar to children without nephrotic syndrome as discussed in the relevant chapters (chapters 11, 12 and 14). It is recommended to continue anticoagulation therapy until the resolution of active nephrotic syndrome. As antithrombin levels are low in these patients, they are preferably treated with LMWH. Prophylactic anticoagulation at times of active nephrotic syndrome recurrence is recommended for children with a previous history of a venous TE [3]. What to do in children with a previous catheter-related TE and who have no CVC at the time of nephrotic syndrome recurrence remains an unanswered question. According to the current practice at SickKids, all children with a history of nephrotic syndrome-associated TE are started on anticoagulation as soon as recurrent prominent proteinuria occurs. As children with severe congenital nephrotic syndrome are at high risk for TE, they receive full dose anticoagulation at times of active disease even in the absence of a previous TE.

Liver-Related Thromboembolic Events

Portal Vein Thrombosis

PVT with cavernous transformation is a major cause of extrahepatic portal hypertension and an important cause of variceal bleeding in children. Although the thrombosis might date back to infancy or the newborn period, presentation is often later. PVT is a well-known vascular complication of liver transplantation in children, associated with the difficult reconstitution of the portal vein, especially in living donor liver transplantation. Intra-abdominal sepsis, umbilical venous catheterization in the newborn period, prothrombotic abnormalities, and cirrhosis are the most frequent risk factors in nontransplanted children. Other possible risk factors include splenectomy and sickle cell anemia. An underlying etiology is not identified in approximately 50% of children with PVT [8].

Clinical Presentation

In most cases, PVT is diagnosed in children as part of the investigation for pancytopenia, splenomegaly or upper gastrointestinal bleeding. The acute occurrence of PVT in neonates and children is usually asymptomatic. In neonates, thrombocytopenia may be seen at the time of diagnosis, but this is usually secondary to other concomitant conditions [8]. In children, mild elevation of alanine aminotransferase may be seen. Liver function is usually normal. Transient ascites may be seen in acute PVT, but in chronic PVT ascites is rarely seen even in the presence of significant portal hypertension, unless the PVT is a complication of already-established cirrhosis.

Diagnosis

Abdominal ultrasound with color Doppler remains the imaging modality of choice to diagnose PVT. Typical findings in chronic PVT include loss of visualization of the main portal vein for at least part of its length, associated cavernous transformation around the portal vein at the porta hepatis, splenomegaly and the presence of portosystemic collaterals, for example at the splenic hilum or around the stomach and esophagus. In acute PVT, findings may be limited to the loss of flow in the portal vein, evidence of progressive splenomegaly and, occasionally, ascites. However, the accuracy of ultrasound depends on technical factors such as the skills of the sonographer, patient cooperation, and the presence of abdominal gas and anatomic variations, which may preclude the visualization of the portal vein and its collaterals. Other investigations (such as CT scan, MRI and angiography) may also identify PVT, with MRI performing at least as well or better than CT [8]. However, those modalities have limited utility due to their disadvantages, including the use of ionizing radiation, need for sedation, and/or invasiveness.

Management

There are no evidence-based guidelines for the treatment of acute PVT in children. Differences in etiology and pathophysiology reduce the usefulness of extrapolation of the guidelines for management of adults with PVT to children.

If the PVT is identified in the acute phase (within approximately 2–4 weeks of its likely occurrence for neonatal PVT, or while the underlying condition is still present for non-neonatal PVT), therapeutic options include conventional anticoagulant therapy, short term anticoagulation, or close monitoring of the thrombus with Doppler ultrasound and the use of anticoagulation if thrombus extension occurs. Thrombolysis should be used with caution and only considered in non-neonates if the acute PVT is progressive and signs of mesenteric ischemia are present [9]. The choice of therapy will depend upon the age of the thrombus, its location (main portal vein versus left or right portal venous branch), its extent (occlusive versus non-occlusive, single versus multiple), patient age and comorbidities. Separate algorithms for the management in neonates (algorithm 2) and older children (algorithm 3) are proposed by expert hematologists at SickKids but these are not the only potential strategies. Importantly, thrombocytopenia, coagulopathy and renal dysfunction should be ruled out prior to the start of anticoagulation. In neonates, a head ultrasound should also be performed and removal of an umbilical venous catheter should be strongly considered.

Most often, PVT in children is diagnosed long after its original occurrence, with evidence of complete occlusion and well-established cavernous transformation and portal hypertension. In these circumstances, anticoagulation is not indicated. Management of chronic PVT is focused on the complications of portal hypertension (e.g. esophageal varices, hypersplenism) and portosystemic shunting (e.g. minimal hepatic encephalopathy and hepatopulmonary syndrome). Involvement of a pediatric hepatologist and pediatric surgeon is important when planning appropriate care. The advent of a surgical procedure to create a conduit from mesenteric vein to left portal vein (so called 'meso-Rex bypass') has enabled restitution of portal venous flow and resolution of complications of portal hypertension and portosystemic shunting for many affected children [10].

The optimal management of partial PVT in children with cirrhosis and portal hypertension is unclear. It is desirable to prevent progression to complete occlusion because this may adversely affect the options for surgical treatment including transplantation. However, because of the potential risk of fatal variceal bleeding, many physicians are reluctant to offer anticoagulation.

The need for primary thromboprophylaxis in children undergoing splenectomy is still under debate. Currently, it is suggested that thromboprophylaxis should not be used routinely in children undergoing splenectomy. Yet, it could be considered for those with an underlying inherited and acquired prothrombotic risk factor, including children with thalassemia. Careful observation and prompt investigation of all children with abdominal symptoms postsplenectomy for the possibility of PVT is recommended.

Hepatic Artery Thrombosis

HAT is also rare in children. It is most often seen as a complication of liver transplantation, where it occurs more frequently in children than in adults, with a reported incidence that varies widely, ranging from 5 to 20% [11]. Children at high risk are those younger than 3 years, who weigh less than 10 kg and have a graft with multiple arteries, or a hepatic artery diameter <2 mm. Surgical risk factors include an abnormal arterial anatomy in the graft requiring reconstruction and a delay in arterial reperfusion.

Clinical Presentation

HAT can present early (<1 month post-transplantation) or late (>1 month post-transplantation). While early HAT is associated with an aggressive course, a high rate of allograft loss, and increased patient mortality, late HAT may follow a more benign course.

In children, early HAT may present with fulminant hepatic necrosis and graft failure, sepsis and liver abscesses or worsening of graft function. Late HAT, on the other hand, may be asymptomatic or have a milder clinical course. Acute presentations may include fever, right upper quadrant pain, jaundice, or hepatic abscesses. Chronic HAT may lead to ischemic cholangiopathy, which typically presents with biliary strictures, due to

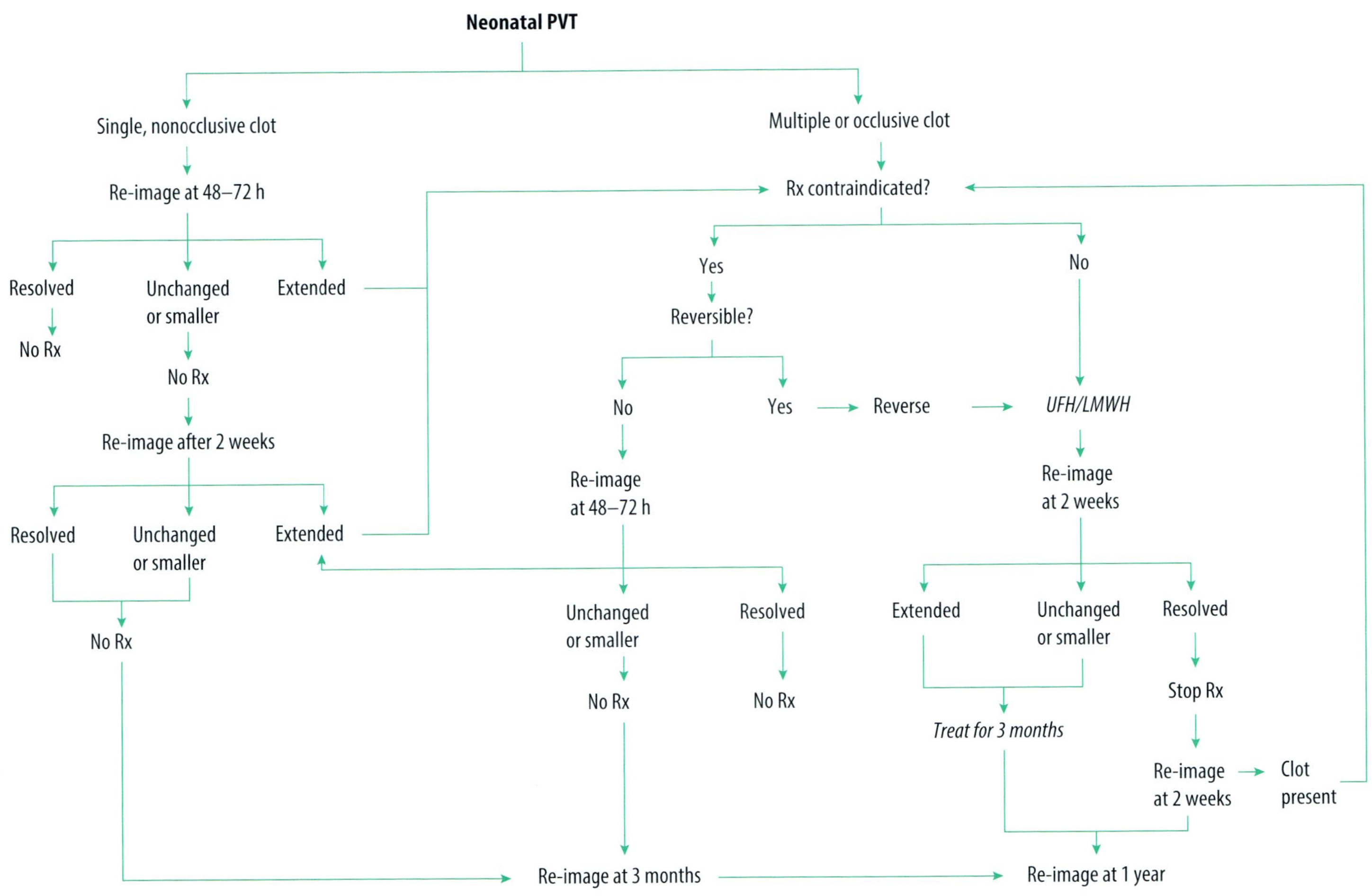

Algorithm 2. Proposed algorithm for management of neonatal portal vein thrombosis. Rx = Anticoagulant therapy.

Thromboembolic Events at Specific Organ Sites

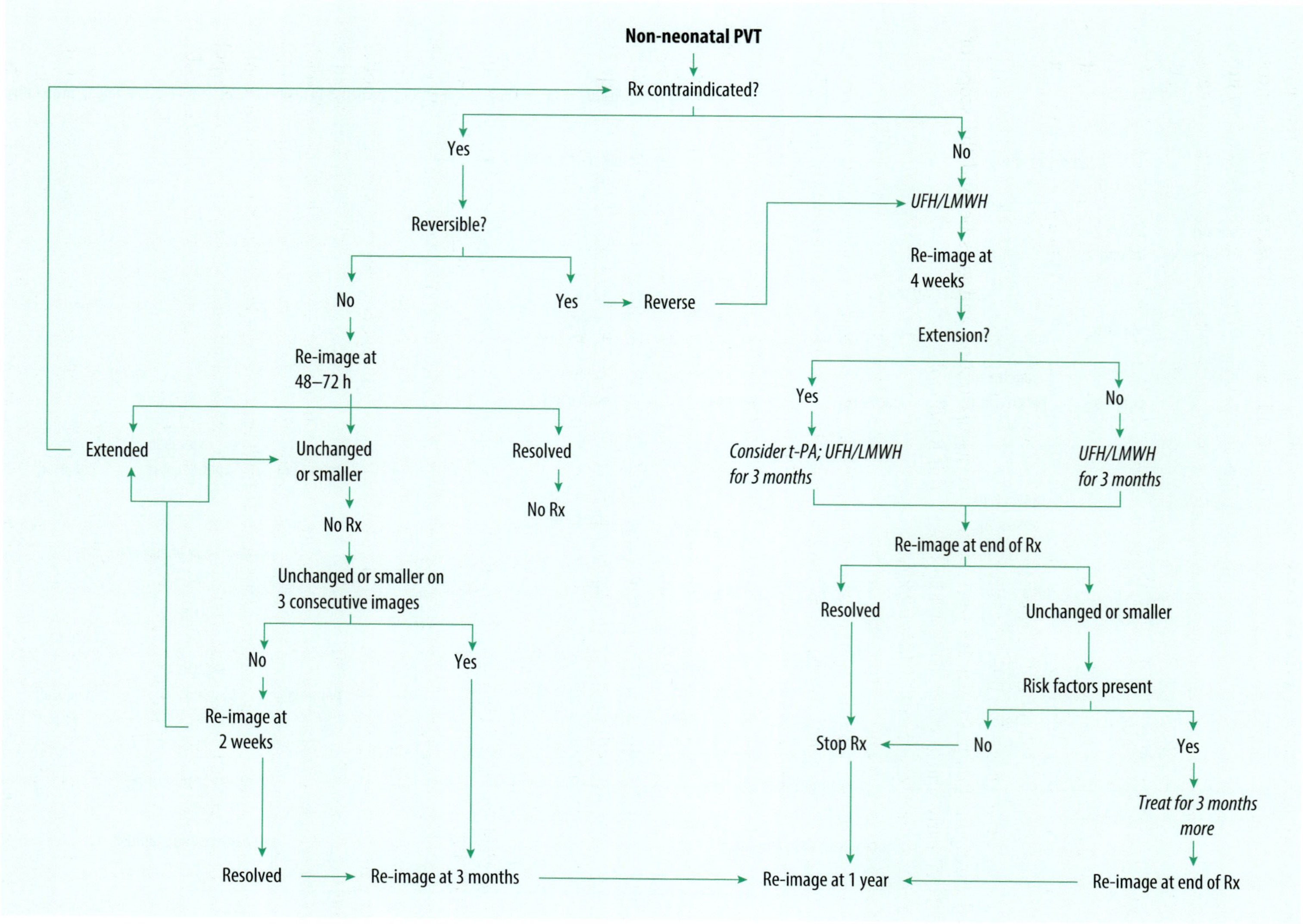

Algorithm 3. Proposed algorithm for management of non-neonatal portal vein thrombosis. Rx = Anticoagulant therapy.

the HAT providing the sole source of blood for the bile ducts.

Diagnosis

Doppler ultrasonography is a sensitive radiologic investigation to detect HAT. Microbubble ultrasound has also been used. It is critical that a clear arterial waveform is seen well within the liver parenchyma. CTA is sometimes required to confirm or refute suspicion of HAT. The role of MRI remains to be determined. Serial testing is recommended during the first postoperative week to diagnose HAT early and prevent irreversible liver damage. According to current SickKids practice, a single routine Doppler ultrasound on postoperative day 1 and further scanning only if problems are noted (e.g. coagulopathy, rising liver enzymes) is an alternative approach.

Management

The risks and benefits of prophylactic LMWH and antiplatelet drugs are unproven. Published data suggest prophylactic antiplatelet drugs, such as ASA, might prevent late HAT but the role in prevention of early HAT is more controversial. The current liver transplantation protocols at SickKids include the initial intravenous administration of UFH and dipyridamole, replaced by enteral ASA as soon as enteral feeds are tolerated. The dosages used are dipyramidole 3 mg/h with UFH 50 U/h in children less than 20 kg, and dipyramidole 6 mg/h with UFH 100 U/h in children greater than 20 kg, ASA 3–5 mg/kg/day.

Identification of early HAT is an indication for immediate return to the operating room to attempt surgical reconstruction of the arterial anastomosis. Surgical revascularization has been associated with improved graft salvage: a 20-year graft survival rate of almost 80% was reported in children who had undergone successful revascularization compared to 24% when revascularization was not attempted or failed [12]. Outside the immediate postoperative period and when recipients are mildly symptomatic, nonsurgical interventions such as transcatheter arterial thrombolysis, balloon angioplasty, or intraluminal stenting can also be attempted. Anticoagulant therapy alone is not effective. Repeat liver transplantation is the appropriate therapeutic choice in the setting of either acute hepatic decompensation, or chronic problems with ischemic cholangiopathy with cholestasis, progressive fibrosis and recurrent biliary sepsis.

The management of late HAT is not based on revascularization and goes beyond the scope of this handbook.

Sinusoidal Obstruction Syndrome

SOS was formerly called hepatic veno-occlusive disease and is a serious complication of HSCT [13]. In addition, several case reports describe SOS occurring postirradiation, after the administration of some chemotherapeutic agents, or after ingestion of certain herbal toxins (e.g. pyrrolizidine alkaloids contained in bush teas). SOS is most likely due to sinusoidal endothelial cell damage, loss of sinusoidal integrity and consequent obstruction of the hepatic sinusoids.

Clinical Presentation

Clinical symptoms of SOS usually begin within the first 3 weeks after HSCT and include jaundice, unexplained fluid retention (manifesting as weight gain, edema and ascites), and painful hepatomegaly with right upper quadrant pain. Mild, moderate and severe SOS can be distinguished based on the Bearman model (serum bilirubin and weight gain). Children with severe SOS often develop multiorgan failure including renal failure, confusion or disorientation, bleeding, and cardiopulmonary failure. Severe SOS has an almost 100% mortality rate.

Diagnosis

The diagnosis of SOS is made based on clinical symptoms using the Seattle or Baltimore criteria (table 2). Ultrasonography may help

Table 2. Baltimore and Seattle criteria to diagnose sinusoidal obstruction syndrome

Seattle criteria [22]
Presence of ≥2 of the following in the first 20 days after HSCT
  Bilirubin >2 mg/dl (34.2 µmol/l)
  Hepatomegaly or RUQ pain
  Weight gain (>2% from basal weight)

Baltimore criteria [23]
Presence of bilirubin >2 mg/dl (34.2 µmol/l) in the first 21 days after HSCT plus ≥2 of the following
  Painful hepatomegaly
  Ascites
  Weight gain (>5% from basal weight)

RUQ = Right upper quadrant.

but none of the abnormalities are diagnostic for SOS. Reversal of flow in the portal vein on Doppler ultrasound is the most suggestive sign, yet the sensitivity is low. Other ultrasonography findings include the presence of ascites, a hepatic artery resistance index greater than 0.75, and marked thickening of the gallbladder wall. Flow in the hepatic veins is present on Doppler ultrasound.

Management

The mainstay of the management of SOS consists of prevention and supportive care. Whenever possible, HSCT should be delayed if acute hepatitis exists or a reduced-intensity conditioning regimen should be considered. Recently, the use of treosulfan compared to busulfan was associated with a reduced incidence of SOS. Studies on pharmacological prevention are most convincing for the use of ursodeoxycholic acid, a synthetic bile acid (10 mg/kg, 3 times per day). More conflicting data or limited experience exists regarding the prophylactic use of low dose UFH, LMWH or N-acetylcysteine. Currently, no evidence-based recommendations can be made for the use of these therapies for SOS prophylaxis.

Symptomatic measures should be initiated first to treat established SOS and these will most probably suffice for mild and moderate SOS. These measures include analgesia, diuretics and salt and fluid restriction. Hepatotoxic or nephrotoxic medications should be avoided. Preservation of the intravascular volume and renal perfusion using albumin or transfusions (keeping hematocrit ≥30%) is essential. Platelet transfusions and correction of coagulopathy using FP may also be necessary.

Specific measures must be reserved for more severe cases. The use of t-PA or UFH/LMWH is discouraged, as they have shown only modest efficacy but clearly increase the risk of bleeding. The safety and efficacy of defibrotide is now well established and it has been used in children without significant toxicity. A dose of 6.25 mg/kg in a 2-hour infusion, given intravenously every 6 h for at least 14 days, is as effective as the higher dose of 10 mg/kg [14]. Although defibrotide has a relatively mild anticoagulant activity, it should be used cautiously in patients with high bleeding risk. It is contraindicated in patients receiving systemic thrombolysis or systemic anticoagulation and in children with clinically significant uncontrolled bleeding. Anticoagulation for CVC maintenance is not contraindicated. During therapy, wherever possible, platelet count should be kept ≥20,000 × 10^9/l.

Budd-Chiari Syndrome

BCS is caused by obstruction of the hepatic venous outflow anywhere between the small branch hepatic veins to the suprahepatic IVC and right atrium [15]. BCS is rare in children and is usually associated with congenital or acquired webs of the hepatic venous outflow tract, an underlying malignancy or myeloproliferative disorder, inflammatory processes or inherited or acquired thrombophilia [15]. In adults, approximately half of the patients with primary BCS are affected with a myeloproliferative disease with the JAK2 mutation.

Clinical Presentation

The acute symptoms of BCS clinically resemble those of the sinusoidal obstruction syndrome: hepatic dysfunction associated with abdominal pain, jaundice, ascites and hepatosplenomegaly. The presentation may be fulminant, acute or chronic. The slower onset form can be painless and may progress silently to cirrhosis, presenting ultimately with manifestations of portal hypertension or liver failure.

Diagnosis

Doppler ultrasonography is the most useful diagnostic test to screen for the presence of BCS. In cases in whom the results are negative or nondiagnostic but there is a strong clinical suspicion, venography of the hepatic veins should be performed. CT or MRI are generally not as sensitive, but may provide useful complementary information in challenging cases. Genetic testing for a JAK2 mutation may be performed in children with suspected underlying myeloproliferative disorder. For laboratory thrombophilia screening refer to chapter 10.

Management

There are no guidelines available for the management of pediatric BCS. However, the common approaches used in adults have been extrapolated for use in children [16]. The management of BCS should follow a step-by-step strategy [17]. The first-line treatment consists of medical therapy including anticoagulation, treatment of the underlying disease, and symptomatic therapy of complications of portal hypertension (ascites, varices and encephalopathy). Clinical experience in adults suggests that angioplasty with or without local thrombolysis and stenting may be successful in certain patients with short-length stenoses who do not respond to medical therapy, although studies do not yet provide a clear understanding of the risk/benefit ratio. Transjugular intrahepatic portosystemic shunt or surgical portosystemic shunt are indicated when medical therapy fails and angioplasty and stenting are not possible or not successful. Liver transplantation may be required in children who fail to improve following the above therapies, in those with fulminant liver failure or in those with decompensated end-stage cirrhosis at presentation or during follow-up.

Mesenteric Vascular Thrombosis

Thrombosis into the mesenteric vein and/or artery primarily occurs in adults and is a highly lethal condition. Although extremely rare, this entity may also be encountered in childhood but only case reports and small case series of children with mesenteric VT have been published.

Idiopathic or primary mesenteric VT has been described in otherwise healthy children. Mesenteric VT occurs more frequently in association with a broad spectrum of predisposing diseases (systemic vasculitis, abdominal infection, paroxysmal nocturnal hemoglobinuria, inherited or acquired prothrombotic risk factors) [18].

Clinical Presentation

The onset of a mesenteric VT is characterized by acute abdominal pain in the vast majority of patients. Other common symptoms include diarrhea, nausea, vomiting and lower gastrointestinal bleeding [18]. Acute thrombosis of either the mesenteric vein or artery result in bowel infarction but a chronic presentation of thrombosis in the mesenteric vein with protracted symptoms of recurrent abdominal pain and growth failure has been described.

Diagnosis

Diagnosis by ultrasonography is often limited by overlying bowel gas. Therefore, a CT scan should be considered the primary diagnostic technique for patients who may have a mesenteric VT. CT scan can show signs of infarcted or ischemic bowel and it may be diagnostic for venous thrombosis. In cases of arterial thrombosis selective angiography is more specific [18].

Management

There are no evidence-based guidelines for the treatment of mesenteric VT in children. Therapeutic options are extrapolated from adult literature. Immediate surgical exploration to evaluate bowel viability and anticoagulation are the mainstay of the management of acute mesenteric VT in adults and should be carried out without delay. The optimal long-term approach remains a matter of debate [19]. Prolonged anticoagulant therapy seems not to be justified by the relatively low rate of recurrence and considerable rate of major hemorrhage. Nevertheless, the mortality rate from mesenteric VT is significantly higher as compared to the mortality rate from bleeding in these patients. On the basis of these results, experts recommend anticoagulation for all patients during the acute phase, but the duration of therapy must be individualized. In cases of arterial thrombosis or when it is important to rapidly resolve the venous thrombosis (e.g. when infarction of the bowel is imminent), thrombolysis may also be considered and has been reported successful [19].

Splenic Vein Thrombosis

SpVT is extremely rare. It usually accompanies a PVT or mesenteric VT but isolated SpVT has also been reported. Isolated SpVT in children has been described as a complication of umbilical vein catheterization and post-liver transplantation. Pancreatic pathologies represent the most common risk factors in adults [20].

Clinical Presentation

Many patients with isolated SpVT remain asymptomatic. The most frequent presenting symptom is gastrointestinal bleeding due to gastric or gastroesophageal varices. Splenomegaly is usually present and may be accompanied by thrombocytopenia.

Diagnosis

Despite limited accuracy, ultrasound sonography is noninvasive and should therefore be the initial test. Sensitivity is improved if the ultrasonographer is asked to specifically look for this entity. A venous phase angiography is the gold standard confirmatory test. The diagnosis of SpVT may be challenging, even with angiography, and SpVT should be considered in patients with gastrointestinal bleeding and unexplained splenomegaly but normal liver function [20].

Management

Endoscopic management of gastric or esophageal varices may be sufficient. Splenectomy is the management of choice for children with recurrent variceal hemorrhage or problematic hypersplenism. Splenic arterial embolization has been reported in the management of SpVT, provoking splenic necrosis with the need for control of significant symptoms including pain and fevers in the week or so thereafter, achieving loss of the spleen without the need for surgery. The role for splenectomy in asymptomatic patients remains controversial. Anticoagulant therapy has not been described in management of isolated SpVT [20]. Children following splenic arterial embolization and splenectomy are at increased risk of life-threatening infections due to encapsulated bacteria. They should receive pneumococcal, *Haemophilus influenzae*, meningococcal and influenza vaccines as well as prophylactic antibiotics, with oral penicillin being the drug of choice in areas with low rates of penicillin resistant pneumococcus.

Long-Term Complications

PTS is a well-known long-term complication of DVT (see chapter 11 for details). However, the assessment and study of incidence and risk factors for PTS in children with TEs in specific organs is limited by the absence of assessment tools. The two existing scales measuring severity of PTS in children cannot be applied to nonextremity TEs. Therefore, Rajpurkar et al. [21] have recently suggested the establishment and validation of a new PTS scale for use in children with nonextremity TEs. Four aspects will need to be considered, while developing such a scale: venous hypertension, severity, pain, and quality of life.

Conclusion

Apart from the well-known thromboembolic events in the deep venous, peripheral arterial, and central nervous system, children may also develop thromboses in specific organs. Most of these events occur in specific circumstances but need to be recognized early as they are usually associated with high rates of morbidity and mortality. General principles of TEs management apply in most cases, but a specific approach may be necessary. As very few guidelines are available, further studies are required to improve care for affected children.

Acknowledgment

The authors would like to express their appreciation for the thoughtful comments provided by Drs. David Grant (Toronto, Ont., Canada), Christoph Licht (Toronto, Ont., Canada), Guy Young (Los Angeles, Calif., USA) and Leonardo R. Brandão (Toronto, Ont., Canada) who reviewed this chapter.

References

1 Brandão LR, Simpson EA, Lau KK: Neonatal renal vein thrombosis. Semin Fetal Neonatal Med 2011;16:323–328.
2 Lau KK, Stoffman JM, Williams S, McCusker P, Brandão L, Patel S, Chan AK, Canadian Pediatric Thrombosis and Hemostasis Network: Neonatal renal vein thrombosis: review of the English-language literature between 1992 and 2006. Pediatrics 2007;120:e1278–e1284.
3 Monagle P, Chan AK, Goldenberg NA, Ichord RN, Journeycake JM, Nowak-Göttl U, Vesely SK: Antithrombotic Therapy in Neonates and Children: Antithrombotic Therapy and Prevention of Thrombosis, ed 9. American College of Chest Physicians Evidence-Based Clinical Practice Guidelines. Chest 2012;141(suppl):e737S–e801S.
4 Singh O, Gupta SS, Sharma D, Lahoti BK, Mathur RK: Isolated renal artery thrombosis because of blunt trauma abdomen: report of a case with review of the literature. Urol Int 2011;86:233–238.
5 Sharathkumar A, Hirschl R, Pipe S, Crandell C, Adams B, Lin JJ: Primary thromboprophylaxis with heparins for arteriovenous fistula failure in pediatric patients. J Vasc Access 2007;8:235–244.
6 Davenport A: Alternatives to standard unfractionated heparin for pediatric hemodialysis treatments. Pediatr Nephrol 2012;27:1869–1879.
7 Kerlin BA, Blatt NB, Fuh B, Zhao S, Lehman A, Blanchong C, Mahan JD, Smoyer WE: Epidemiology and risk factors for thromboembolic complications of childhood nephrotic syndrome: a Midwest Pediatric Nephrology Consortium (MWPNC) study. J Pediatr 2009;155:105–110.
8 Williams S, Chan AK: Neonatal portal vein thrombosis: diagnosis and management. Semin Fetal Neonatal Med 2011;16:329–339.
9 Hall TC, Garcea G, Metcalfe M, Bilku D, Dennison AR: Management of acute non-cirrhotic and non-malignant portal vein thrombosis: a systematic review. World J Surg 2011;35:2510–2520.
10 Shneider BL, Bosch J, de Franchis R, Emre SH, Groszmann RJ, Ling SC, Lorenz JM, Squires RH, Superina RA, Thompson AE, Mazariegos GV: Portal hypertension in children: expert pediatric opinion on the report of the Baveno v Consensus Workshop on Methodology of Diagnosis and Therapy in Portal Hypertension. Pediatr Transplant 2012;16:426–437.
11 Sevmis S, Karakayali H, Tutar NU, Boyvat F, Ozcay F, Torgay A, Haberal M: Management of early hepatic arterial thrombosis after pediatric living-donor liver transplantation. Transplant Proc 2011;43:605–608.
12 Ackermann O, Branchereau S, Franchi-Abella S, Pariente D, Chevret L, Debray D, Jacquemin E, Gauthier F, Hill C, Bernard O: The long-term outcome of hepatic artery thrombosis after liver transplantation in children: role of urgent revascularisation. Am J Transplant 2012;12:1496–1503.
13 Gharib MI, Bulley SR, Doyle JJ, Wynn RF: Venous occlusive disease in children. Thromb Res 2006;118:27–38.

14 Richardson PG, Soiffer RJ, Antin JH, Uno H, Jin Z, Kurtzberg J, Martin PL, Steinbach G, Murray KF, Vogelsang GB, Chen AR, Krishnan A, Kernan NA, Avigan DE, Spitzer TR, Shulman HM, Di Salvo DN, Revta C, Warren D, Momtaz P, Bradwin G, Wei LJ, Iacobelli M, McDonald GB, Guinan EC: Defibrotide for the treatment of severe hepatic veno-occlusive disease and multiorgan failure after stem cell transplantation: a multicenter, randomized, dose-finding trial. Biol Blood Marrow Transplant 2010;16:1005–1017.

15 Cauchi JA, Oliff S, Baumann U, Mirza D, Kelly DA, Hewitson J, Rode H, McCulloch M, Spearman W, Millar AJW: The Budd-Chiari syndrome in children: the spectrum of management. J Pediatr Surg 2006;41:1919–1923.

16 DeLeve LD, Valla DC, Garcia-Tsao G, American Association for the Study Liver Diseases: Vascular disorders of the liver. Hepatology 2009;49:1729–1764.

17 Mancuso A: Budd-Chiari syndrome management: lights and shadows. World J Hepatol 2011;3:262–264.

18 Oğuzkurt P, Şenocak ME, Ciftci AO, Tanyel FC, Büyükoalukçu N: Mesenteric vascular occlusion resulting in intestinal necrosis in children. J Pediatr Surg 2000;35:1161–1164.

19 Bergqvist D, Svensson PJ: Treatment of mesenteric vein thrombosis. Semin Vasc Surg 2010;23:65–68.

20 Köklü S, Köksal A, Yolcu ÖF, Bayram G, Sakaoğullan Z, Arda K, Şahin B: Isolated splenic vein thrombosis: an unusual cause and review of the literature. Can J Gastroenerol 2004;18:173–174.

21 Rajpurkar M, Monagle P, Massicotte P, Chan A: Need for a new paediatric post thrombotic sequelae outcome measure for non-extremity thrombosis. Thromb Haemost 2011;105:1105–1106.

Abbreviations

ACT	Activated clotting time
AIS	Arterial ischemic stroke
Anti-Xa	Anti-factor Xa
aPTT	Activated partial thromboplastin time
ASA	Acetylsalicylic acid
BCS	Budd-Chiari syndrome
CSVT	Cerebral sinovenous thrombosis
CT	Computed tomography
CTA	Computed tomography angiography
CVC	Central venous catheter
DVT	Deep vein thrombosis
FP (FFP)	Frozen plasma (Fresh frozen plasma)
FV	Factor V
FVIII	Factor VIII
HAT	Hepatic artery thrombosis
HIT	Heparin-induced thrombocytopenia
HSCT	Hematopoietic stem cell transplantation
IVC	Inferior vena cava
LMWH	Low-molecular-weight heparin
MRA	Magnetic resonance angiography
MRI	Magnetic resonance imaging
PE	Pulmonary embolism
PTS	Postthrombotic syndrome
PVT	Portal vein thrombosis
RAT	Renal artery thrombosis
RVT	Renal vein thrombosis
SOS	Sinusoidal obstruction syndrome
SpVT	Splenic vein thrombosis
TE	Thromboembolism/thromboembolic event
t-PA	Tissue-plasminogen activator
UFH	Unfractionated heparin
VKA	Vitamin K antagonist
VT	Vascular thrombosis
VTE	Venous thromboembolism/thromboembolic event

Chapter 14 Pediatric Stroke

Andrea Andrade
Rebecca Ichord
Nomazulu Dlamini
Suzan Williams
Gabrielle deVeber

Introduction

Cerebrovascular diseases involving thrombosis or thromboembolism in children are well-recognized entities, and can be divided in two main categories: AIS, and CSVT. Both conditions can affect newborns to adolescents. Early recognition allows prompt initiation of treatment that may prevent clot propagation, infarct expansion, or stroke recurrence, thereby improving long-term functional outcome.

Arterial Ischemic Stroke

AIS is defined as an acute neurologic syndrome manifest as an acute neurologic deficit with a corresponding acute focal infarction conforming to an arterial territory on neuroimaging. This may be caused by thromboembolic occlusion or critical focal hypoperfusion due to stenosis in the involved artery. Thromboembolic occlusion affects large- or small-vessel territories, while critical hypoperfusion more commonly affects those areas of the brain that are located in the border zones between two different arterial territories. These border zone infarcts, also referred to as watershed infarcts, most commonly affect the border zone between the anterior cerebral and the MCA territories, in the setting of intracranial carotid steno-occlusive disease (figure 1).

The incidence of pediatric AIS in North America has been estimated as 2.4/100,000/year [1]. There is a male predominance [2]. Neonates comprise 25% of pediatric patients with AIS, with an estimated prevalence of 1 per 3,500 live term births [1, 2]. AIS in the perinatal period is now estimated to be as frequent as large vessel AIS in adults. Incidence of neonatal AIS is 17 times higher than the incidence of AIS during childhood. The reported incidence rates of pediatric AIS have increased probably due to an increasing awareness of the condition and to improved imaging techniques [3]. AIS is one of the top ten causes of death in the pediatric population. Approximately 10–50% of children with initial AIS occurring after

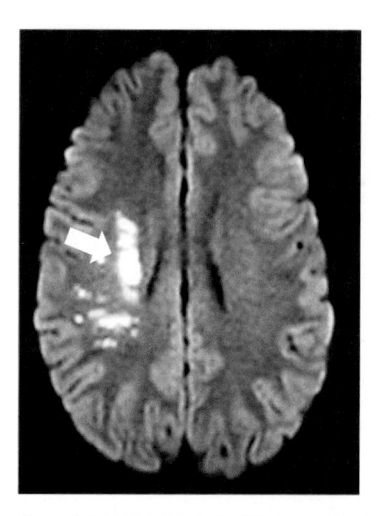

Figure 1. Axial MRI of the brain, diffusion weighted sequence showing a right watershed distribution (ACA/MCA) ischemic infarct. 11-year-old boy with no identifiable risk factors for stroke.

the newborn period experience recurrent AIS or TIAs. Increased rates generally reflect children with no antithrombotic treatment or those affected with an underlying arteriopathy [4, 5].

Most older infants and children with AIS have a preexisting condition predisposing them to AIS. After completion of a diagnostic work-up, approximately two thirds of these children have an arteriopathy discovered on vascular imaging. Congenital or acquired heart disease and SCD are common causes of AIS in children. Heart disease is responsible for 20–25% of AIS in children [6]. Additional acute or chronic systemic risk factors including infection, dehydration, iron deficiency anemia, prothrombotic disorders, or other chronic diseases are frequently found. Individual children frequently have multiple converging risk factors for AIS. No etiology is found in up to a third of neonates and approximately 10% of older infants and children, even after extensive diagnostic investigations [7].

Clinical Presentation

The clinical presentation varies among age groups. In the newborn period (0–28 days), the most common clinical presentation is acute encephalopathy with altered mental status and focal seizures typically with onset beyond 12 h after delivery. Less common presentations in this age group are unexplained irritability and focal neurological motor deficits [7].

A separate category of perinatal AIS termed presumed perinatal ischemic stroke is recognized in children who present in the 4- to 12-month age period with an emerging hemiparesis or early hand dominance. These children have imaging findings of a remote vaso-occlusive pattern of AIS, presumed to have occurred in utero or silently in the early neonatal period [7].

The relevant information in the history and physical examination of neonates and older children with suspected AIS are described in table 1 [8, 9].

Diagnosis

The 'gold standard' test to confirm a clinical diagnosis of AIS in the acute setting is by MRI/MRA of the brain and the vessels of the head and neck. The most useful sequences in the 'stroke protocol' MRI/MRA would include: diffusion-weighted images, and apparent diffusion coefficient, to evaluate the presence of cytotoxic edema as a result of acute ischemic injury (figures 2, 3). CT scans are frequently normal up to 12 h after symptom onset in childhood AIS. In patients with larger infarcts involving complete large vessel territories, or in those whose symptoms started in the prior 24 h, CT may show large areas of hypodensity, involving specific vascular territories. The importance of MRA or CTA, as a part of the initial screen, is to evaluate the integrity of the anterior and posterior circulation of the brain. Additionally, the presence of a filling defect in a major artery may be indicative of the presence of a thrombus, and requires further investigation. Both thrombotic occlusions and arteriopathies (FCA, moya moya, and dissection) are detected by MRA or CTA.

Initial blood work should include: aPTT, PT/INR, fibrinogen and CBC. Normal results on

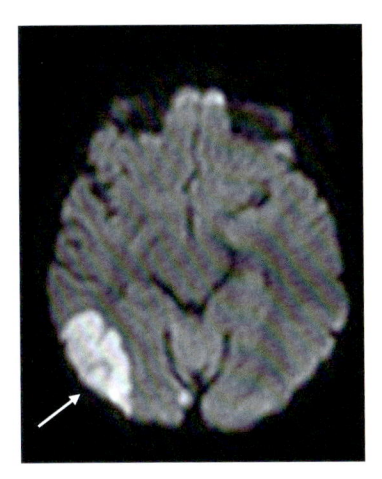

Figure 2. MRI of the brain in an axial view on diffusion-weighted sequence, the arrow demonstrates an area of restricted diffusion involving the inferior branch of the right MCA, indicative of an acute ischemic infarct.

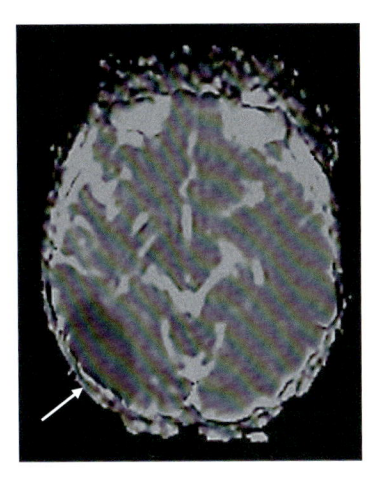

Figure 3. Same patient, the arrow shows the counterpart apparent diffusion coefficient map sequence with hypointense signal in the same vascular territory.

Table 1. Relevant history and physical exam in suspected AIS by age group

Neonates	
Clinical presentation	acute focal motor seizures after the first 12 h of life
Past medical history	maternal thrombosis, gestational/obstetric disorders
Physical examination	gaze preference, asymmetric limb tone and movements, subtle seizures – heart murmur suggests possible congenital heart disease
Older infant or child	
Clinical presentation	acute focal neurological deficit usually abrupt onset, can be self-resolving, including hemiparesis, hemisensory deficit, visual field deficit, aphasia, facial weakness, other cranial nerve deficits, unilateral ataxia
Past medical history	recent head or neck trauma, head or neck irradiation, migraine headaches, varicella infection or vaccination (in the past 12 months), use of oral contraceptives, use of illicit drugs such as cocaine or amphetamines
Family history	hyperlipidemia, migraines, thrombotic events (age < 55 with stroke, myocardial infarction, deep venous thrombosis, maternal recurrent fetal loss)
Physical examination	carotid/head bruits, skin lesions of neurocutaneous disease (NF1, PHACE, Sturge Weber), cardiac murmur if febrile search for physical stigmata of infectious endocarditis baseline neurological exam should very clearly define severity of deficits

NF1 = Neurofibromatosis type 1; PHACE = posterior fossa brain malformations, hemangiomas, arterial anomalies, coarctation of aorta and cardiac defects and eye abnormalities.

screening coagulation parameters and platelet count should be confirmed before giving any antithrombotic treatment for acute AIS. It is reasonable and common practice to obtain a complete profile of studies for hypercoagulable states in all cases of confirmed acute AIS, regardless of a known risk factor such as heart disease or cervical arterial dissection. As initial treatment considerations are not related to laboratory hypercoagulable state, blood tests can be sent after starting therapy and might include:

(1) An initial screen usually done during the acute stage: fibrinogen, protein C, protein S, antithrombin, APLA screening (chapter 10).

(2) Additional tests can be done acutely or, for small infants to preserve blood volume, at any

time up to 3–6 months after the stroke: activated protein C-resistant, FVL mutation, prothrombin gene mutation, lipoprotein (a), homocysteine, and factor VIII (chapter 10).

The stroke work up should include an echocardiogram, to evaluate for a cardiac source of thrombus including cardiac malformations and other right to left shunt lesions, e.g. PFO.

Further testing should be considered on a case-by-case basis and may include conventional angiogram, vasculitis work up (erythrocyte sedimentation rate, C3 and C4, rheumatoid factor, antinuclear antibody and C-reactive protein), cerebrospinal fluid tests for vasculitis or infection and other blood testing (varicella titers, metabolic work up, formal eye examination and sickle cell testing) [8, 9].

In neonates and children whose initial symptom is a focal seizure, and in those whose level of consciousness is compromised, an EEG may be helpful to evaluate and treat the presence of subclinical seizures [9].

Management

The treatment of patients with AIS can be divided into different types and different stages. The initial treatment is based on early institution of neuroprotective measures and initial antithrombotic therapy (antiplatelet or anticoagulant). It should be noted that none of these therapies has been evaluated in clinical trials in children, and therefore they are based on expert opinion consensus and adaptation from the adult stroke literature [8, 10].

Neuroprotective Measures

Neuroprotective measures aim to minimize the extent of neuronal damage and should include measures to reduce cerebral metabolic demands and increase blood supply to the brain:
- aggressive treatment to prevent and reverse fever
- anti-seizure medication to treat seizures
- maintenance of normoglycemia
- avoidance of relative hypotension with maintenance of blood pressure at minimum 50th percentile for age.

Antithrombotic Therapy

Antithrombotic therapy aims to reduce the risk of recurrent thrombotic occlusion of cerebral arteries in children with AIS and in neonates with cardioembolic AIS.

Antithrombotic Recommendations for Children (Non-Neonate) with AIS

For children with AIS, the current recommendation is to begin antithrombotic therapy promptly, provided that initial imaging shows no ICH. Initial therapy may be with UFH, LMWH or ASA (1–5 mg/kg) and should be given with or without confirming the presence of thrombophilia while awaiting results of diagnostic studies aimed at defining stroke mechanism and risk factors [10]. A recent study reported the safety of anticoagulant treatment in children with AIS, with a 4% risk of symptomatic ICH [11]. For children with AIS, once dissection and cardioembolic causes are excluded, daily ASA prophylaxis for a minimum of 2 years is recommended. For children with recurrent AIS while on ASA therapy, it is reasonable to change to clopidogrel (1 mg/kg) or to anticoagulant therapy with LMWH or VKA [10]. For children with AIS secondary to cardioembolic cause, anticoagulation with LMWH or VKA is recommended for at least 3 months [10]. For management of children with AIS secondary to dissection, see below. Dosing and monitoring of UFH, LMWH, VKA and ASA therapy are detailed in chapter 16.

If there is hemorrhagic conversion, if the patient is severely hypertensive, or if there are other risks for bleeding, anticoagulation treatment in patients with AIS may not be feasible. In patients with large territorial infarctions (for example >2/3 of the MCA territory), it is common practice to postpone beginning anticoagulation to later than 48–72 h after stroke onset in hopes of minimizing the risk of hemorrhagic conversion. However, the risk benefit ratio must be considered in each case and management approach individualized. A close follow-up brain imaging (CT or MRI) can be a reasonable strategy and may lead to cessation of antithrombotic therapy if hemorrhagic conversion occurs [8, 10, 12].

Treatment of Pediatric AIS: Special Considerations

AIS in the Neonatal Period

The mortality rate following AIS in newborns is less than 10%. Neurologic deficits are detected in about two thirds of survivors in young childhood. Lesions that involve the motor cortex, internal capsule, and basal ganglia together are associated with increased motor disability compared with lesions limited to the cortex or the basal ganglia alone. A seizure disorder is present in up to 15% of children. The diagnostic investigations in neonatal stroke include: MRI/MRA of the brain, prothrombotic work up, and an EEG if there is suspicion of subclinical seizures.

In contrast to older infants and children, fewer than 5% of newborns with AIS have recurrent systemic or cerebral thrombosis. Thus, for neonates with non-cardiogenic AIS, the use of anticoagulation or ASA is not recommended [10]. For neonates with a first cardioembolic AIS, anticoagulation should be considered with either UFH or LMWH for 3 to 6 months, followed by ASA if the cardiac defect has not been fully repaired, since they have a 14% risk of recurrent AIS [10, 13]. For neonates with recurrent AIS, anticoagulation or ASA therapy for an indefinite time may be considered. Dosing and monitoring of UFH, LMWH, VKA and ASA therapy in neonates are detailed in chapter 16.

Cardiogenic AIS

AIS can be attributed to emboli arising from the heart or systemic venous circulation with shunting via a septal defect, PFO or other right-to-left shunt in up to 20–25% of children. Approximately one third to one half of these are procedure-related AISs, occurring in the setting of cardiac surgery or catheter-based interventions (chapter 15) [13, 14]. AIS is most common in children with uncorrected heart lesions and with congestive heart failure. Surgical repair of the defect significantly lowers the risk of stroke; however the risk remains substantial [13, 14]. In children with AIS with a PFO associated with demonstrable right to left shunt, surgical closure of the defect is controversial although adult studies indicate possible benefit [10]. Other cardiac diseases such as rheumatic fever and mitral stenosis, prosthetic valves, cardiomyopathy, can also promote cerebral embolism in children. For recommended thromboprophylaxis of AIS in children with cardiac disease see chapter 15.

AIS Due to Arterial Dissection

CCAD is probably an underrecognized cause of AIS in the pediatric patients, accounting for 7.5% of incident non-neonatal AIS in one cohort study [3]. The International Pediatric Stroke Study (IPSS) defines CCAD as: (1) angiographic evidence of double lumen, intimal flap, or pseudoaneurysm or axial T1 fat saturation MRI images consisting of a 'bright crescent sign' in the arterial wall; (2) cervical or cranial trauma, or neck pain, less than 6 weeks preceding angiographic findings of segmental arterial narrowing (or occlusion) located in the cervical arteries, and (3) angiographic segmental narrowing (or occlusion) of the vertebral artery at the level of the C2 vertebral body, even without known traumatic history [3]. The pathophysiology of CCAD is explained by the separation between the intimal layer of the vessel wall that creates an area of damaged endothelium with exposure of collagen, activated tissue factor, and exposed VWF. These factors generate secondary fibrin and platelet adhesion, leading to thrombus propagation. Once a clot has formed, ischemia occurs from vessel occlusion at the site of the dissection or from artery-to-artery clot embolization downstream. Aneurysmal dilatation can occur secondary to impaired integrity of the vessel wall and persistent arterial pressure occlusion frequently appears in the C1–C2 vertebral circulation in children.

AIS can occur immediately after CCAD. Stroke can also occur up to several months later, probably because of delayed artery-to-artery emboli from the dissection site. In the absence of an effective agent to limit the damage from an acute infarction, therapy for CCAD aims to prevent stroke due to delayed embolism until the dissection site has healed or recanalized. The risk of recurrent AIS or TIA in children with CCAD is around 12%. Recurrence appears to be reduced by antithrombotic treatment, but is still observed during anticoagulation or antiplatelet treatment [3].

There are two types of CCAD in children, extracranial and intracranial dissection. These entities have different risk factors and management. Extracranial dissection accounts for 5–25% of childhood-onset AIS, and is often preceded by trauma. Typically, extracranial dissection affecting the anterior circulation (specially the distal segment of the internal carotid artery) presents with focal neurological symptoms such as hemiparesis and aphasia. Posterior circulation dissection (affecting mainly the vertebral arteries) is more challenging and symptoms can vary from dizziness and vertigo to coma. Clues to the diagnosis include recent history of trauma and/or cranial nerve abnormalities. CCAD can occur spontaneously or after blunt or penetrating trauma or high velocity head flexion/extension/rotation with stretch injury of the arterial wall. Intraoral trauma is a well-recognized cause of internal carotid artery dissection. When children present with spontaneous CCAD it is important to investigate for an underlying defect of the affected artery, such as collagen defects like Ehlers-Danlos syndrome, that weaken the artery wall, and can make the child more prone to dissection with minor or no trauma.

Intracranial arterial dissection is considered to be a rare event in children. There are few cases reported in the literature, and the majority of these have been confirmed postmortem in an autopsy. The most common presentation is headache, followed by focal deficit. The arteries most commonly affected are the distal segment of the internal carotid artery, and the proximal segments of the MCA and ACA. It comprises one cause for FCA. Features that distinguish intracranial dissection from inflammatory FCA (or transient cerebral arteriopathy) include the findings on angiography of double lumen and intimal flap in the artery. On wall imaging MRI, the presence of wall hematoma is highly suggestive of intracranial dissection. Some authors suggest that children with an intracranial dissection should probably avoid anticoagulation due to an increased risk of subarachnoid hemorrhage. However, the treatment of these patients is controversial, because the concern for increased risk of ICH is only based on anecdotal and sporadic cases [3].

Treatment of AIS secondary to extracranial dissection with anticoagulation (LMWH or VKA) for at least 6 weeks is an acceptable and widely used approach [10]. Treatment with ASA alone (or other antiplatelet agent) is also reasonable, as there are no data from clinical trials in children evaluating the effectiveness of anticoagulation compared to ASA. If the patient requires an invasive procedure such as a cerebral angiogram, it is reasonable to start treatment with UFH, which is more easily stopped temporarily for a procedure. Duration of treatment with LMWH or VKA is typically guided by clinical and radiologic status at regularly scheduled follow-up intervals. It is reasonable and common practice for children with CCAD to receive LMWH or VKA for a minimum of 3 months, followed by transition to ASA, which is commonly continued for a minimum period of 2 years after the incident AIS. This duration of treatment is based on the concern for risk of further recurrent AIS from pseudoaneurysm or other vascular abnormalities at the site of prior dissection [3].

In the cases of suspected intracranial dissections, the differentiation from FCA is usually very challenging [15]. As there are no data to support the superiority in efficacy or safety of anticoagulation compared to ASA, either approach is reasonable, pending results of more definitive vascular imaging such as catheter angiogram. Further evolution of the clinical picture (e.g. recurrent clinical events), follow-up imaging, and results of thrombophilia testing are all important in contributing to the decisions regarding long-term antithrombotic therapy. As with extracranial CCAD, it is common practice and reasonable to treat with some form of antithrombotic treatment for a minimum of 2 years after incident AIS.

Moyamoya Disease

Moyamoya disease is characterized by progressive stenosis of the distal internal carotid arteries with formation of secondary distal collateral vessels. Other cranial arteries may be affected as well. When moyamoya occurs in isolation it is classified as moyamoya disease, while patients with recognized risk factors have a moyamoya syndrome. The clinical conditions commonly associated with moyamoya syndrome include: cranial radiotherapy, neurofibromatosis type I, SCD, trisomy 21 syndrome and other genetic syndromes [3]. Moyamoya disease is most commonly seen in Asian population, but has been also described in other ethnicities. The incidence of moyamoya disease is high in countries in East Asia, such as Japan and Korea. In Japan the annual prevalence and incidence have been estimated to be 3.16–10.5 and 0.35–0.94 per 100,000. The annual incidence in the USA and Europe has been reported to be about 10% of that in Japan [3].

Moyamoya disease has a bimodal age distribution of clinical presentation, with one peak in the first decade and a second peak in adults 30–40 years of age. Affected family members can be identified in 6–20% of cases and an autosomal-dominant inheritance with variable expression has been proposed. Moyamoya disease is genetically heterogeneous, and has been linked to 3p24.2–26,17q25, and other genetic sites.

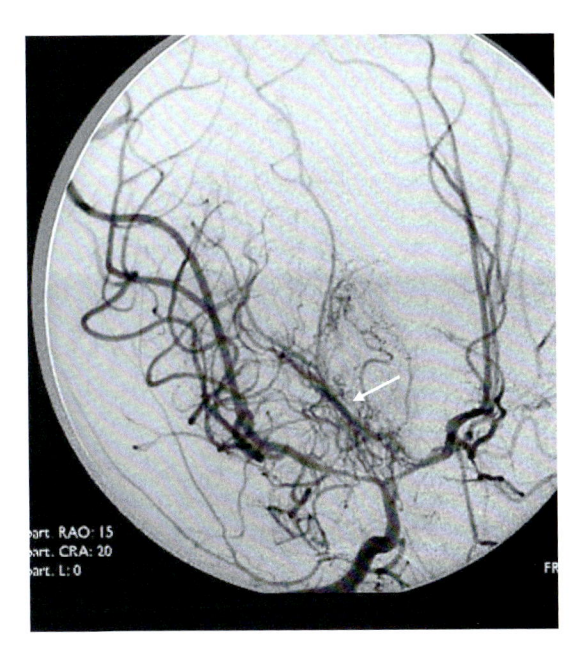

Figure 4. Conventional cerebral angiography on a coronal view of a child with moyamoya disease. The arrow shows the collateral moyamoya vessels arising from the lenticulostriatal branches of the stenosed proximal right middle cerebral artery.

The most common clinical features in patients with moyamoya syndrome/disease include recurrent TIA or AIS, cognitive decline (around 50% of children, especially in those who developed the disease prior the age of 4 years), headaches and recurrent seizures (20–30%). The diagnosis can usually be confirmed with noninvasive vascular imaging (e.g. 3T MRI/MRA) (fig. 4). Evaluation with a conventional angiogram is needed for surgical planning. Measurement of cerebral perfusion with gadolinium-contrast or arterial spin label techniques, and assessment of blood flow reserve with acetazolamide challenge may contribute to the evaluation and follow-up of individuals with moyamoya disease. TCD is sometimes used to evaluate and follow up children with moyamoya due to SCD [8].

Various surgical revascularization techniques are used for moyamoya disease, including direct bypass procedures and indirect encephaloduroarteriosynangiosis. Direct bypass procedures are typically used in selected older children where the superficial temporal artery is sutured to the MCA. Encephaloduroarteriosynangiosis implants an extracranial artery intracranially resulting in the growth of new collateral branches into the underperfused cerebral territories over time. Two large long-term follow up studies have indicated that surgical treatment of moyamoya is reasonably safe (4% risk of stroke within 30 days of surgery per hemisphere) and effective (96% probability of remaining stroke free over a 5-year follow-up period) [8].

ASA may be useful in preventing moyamoya-related AIS [8].

Anticoagulants are rarely recommended because of the risk of ICH. Low-dose LMWH has been used in patients with rapid progression, before they undergo surgical treatment.

Moyamoya patients are at additional risk of ischemic symptoms during the perioperative period. Hyperventilation related to crying can lower the $PaCO_2$ and induce ischemia secondary to cerebral vasoconstriction. Adequate intraoperative blood pressure maintenance and postoperative pain control and procedures to reduce the discomfort and anxiety related to dressing changes, suture removal, etc., may reduce the risk of ischemic symptoms and shorten the hospitalization [8].

Sickle Cell Disease

AIS occurs in 11% of children with SCD by age 20 years, with the peak age of onset being 2–5 years. The postulated mechanism is proliferation of vascular intima, leading to progressive stenosis of intracranial portions of the internal carotid, middle and anterior cerebral arteries. Silent cerebral infarcts, defined as foci of T2 hyperintensiity with no history or physical findings of focal neurologic deficit, are the most common neurologic injury in SCD. Silent cerebral infarcts occur in 22% by age 14 years. Unlike overt AISs located in the cortex and deep white matter, silent cerebral infarcts are typically in the deep white matter in the frontal, parietal and temporal lobes. Silent cerebral infarcts are recognized as a cause of school problems and neurocognitive deficits. After abnormal TCD velocities, the presence of silent cerebral infarcts is the greatest risk factor for overt AIS in patients with SCD [16].

The use of antithrombotic therapy in primary and secondary AIS prevention in patients with SCD is controversial, due to the complex pathophysiology of stroke in SCD, and the perceived increased risk of hemorrhage in patients with Moyamoya-type vasculopathy.

The basic principle for SCD stroke treatment is to improve oxygen delivery to the brain. In addition to the general neuroprotective measures for AIS, supportive measures include oxygen and RBC transfusion. Exchange RBC transfusion is generally the preferred option. Because of the time involved to arrange an exchange transfusion, and associated risks of fluctuating blood pressure, if the initial hemoglobin is less than 100 g/l, a simple RBC transfusion may be considered while arranging an exchange transfusion. In addition to oxygen and RBC transfusion, a septic work-up should be completed and empiric antibiotics administered in the setting of fever [17].

Following the initial exchange transfusion, a long-term chronic transfusion program is generally recommended after the first AIS in SCD, given the high recurrence rates. Fifty percent will have a second stroke within 2 years. However, transfusion therapy is not completely effective; 20% of children will have recurrent AIS despite transfusion therapy [18]. The transfusion interval and volumes are tailored to the transfusion targets of a hemoglobin S less than 30% and hemoglobin nadir of 80–100 g/l. An example of a chronic transfusion program would be transfusion interval of 3–4 weeks with volume of 15 ml/kg. The National Institutes of Health recommends that all SCD patients older than 6 months should have extensive antigenic phenotyping: ABO, Rh, Kell, Duffy, Kidd, Lewis, Lutheran, P, and MNS blood groups, to minimize the risk of allo-immunization with transfusion

[19]. Despite the complications of a chronic RBC transfusion program, a practical alternative has not been yet identified [20]. Clinical trials for alternative therapies to prevent AIS recurrence in patients with SCD are still ongoing.

A long-term chronic RBC transfusion program is also recommended to prevent AIS in children with SCD identified as high risk for stroke [17]. TCD velocities are tested on an annual basis from age 2–16 years in children with SCD. Children with 'abnormal' TCD velocities, defined as greater than 200 cm/s in the large cerebral vessels, have a 40% stroke risk within 3 years. Significant reduction in the risk for AIS was found by chronic RBC transfusion to decrease hemoglobin S levels to <30%. As rebound increased risk of AIS following discontinuation of chronic RBC transfusion program was found [21], the current recommendations are to continue the chronic RBC transfusion program for primary and secondary prophylaxis of stroke in SCD.

Hematopoietic stem cell transplant with an HLA-matched, sibling donor may offer secondary stroke prevention.

Thrombolysis in Hyperacute AIS

Although t-PA has revolutionized the treatment of AIS in the adult population, no acute interventional trials have been completed in the pediatric patients. Children increasingly reach tertiary centers within the 3- to 6-hour window required for t-PA administration. However, there are limited data on t-PA safety and dosing in children [22]. Data on safety and dosing in children are needed to guide therapy because immature fibrinolytic and coagulation systems are different than those in adults. A safety and dose-finding trial for t-PA in childhood has been designed and is underway – Thrombolysis in Pediatric Stroke Study [8]. As per the American Heart Association guidelines and others, t-PA is not recommended for stroke in children outside of a study setting [8]; however, in young adults (adolescents, teenagers) no consensus against its use was established.

Other Endovascular Treatment

Adults are frequently treated with endovascular clot retrieval devices during the first 12 h after stroke onset and balloon angioplasty or stenting in later time frames. There are no data to support safety in children and considerable concern about risks. Until definitive clinical trial evidence supports these approaches in adults, and safety data are available in children, they should not be applied except in rare cases in consultation with pediatric neurologists expert in stroke.

Cerebral Sinovenous Thrombosis

CSVT is thrombosis with or without infarction of the cerebral sinovenous system [23, 24]. The incidence of CSVT is approximately 0.4 to 0.7 per 100,000 children per year. Around 40% of cases occurring during the neonatal period, giving an incidence in newborns of 1 to 12 per 100,000 per year [23, 24].

Venous sinuses and veins are located within the subarachnoid space. Arachnoid villi project into the venous sinuses of the dura and are concentrated in the superior sagittal sinus, which is important for absorption and drainage of cerebrospinal fluid [23]. The cerebral venous system is divided into two major networks of veins and sinuses (figures 5, 6). The superficial system includes: (a) the superficial cortical veins; (b) the superior sagittal vein; (c) the confluence of the sinuses; (d) the transverse sinuses; (e) the sigmoid sinuses, and (f) the internal jugular veins. The deep system is formed by: (1) the basal veins that are responsible for the drainage from the basal ganglia and, in preterm newborns, the germinal matrix; (2) the galenic system which is composed of the two internal cerebral veins and the vein of Galen; (3) the straight sinus; (4) the basal vein of Rosenthal, and (5) the torcula.

CSVT in children is usually multifactorial, with a predisposing comorbid condition identified in up to 95% of children (table 2). The two

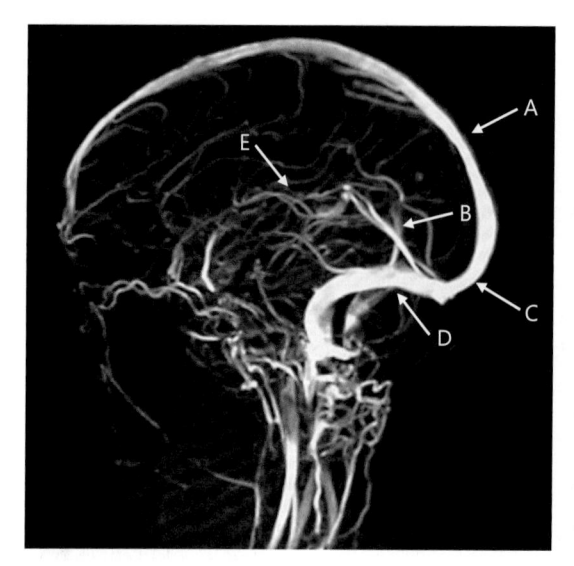

Figure 5. MRV (sagittal view), demonstrating normal cerebral venous anatomy: A = superior sagittal sinus; B = straight sinus; C = torcula; D = left transverse sinus; E = internal cerebral veins.

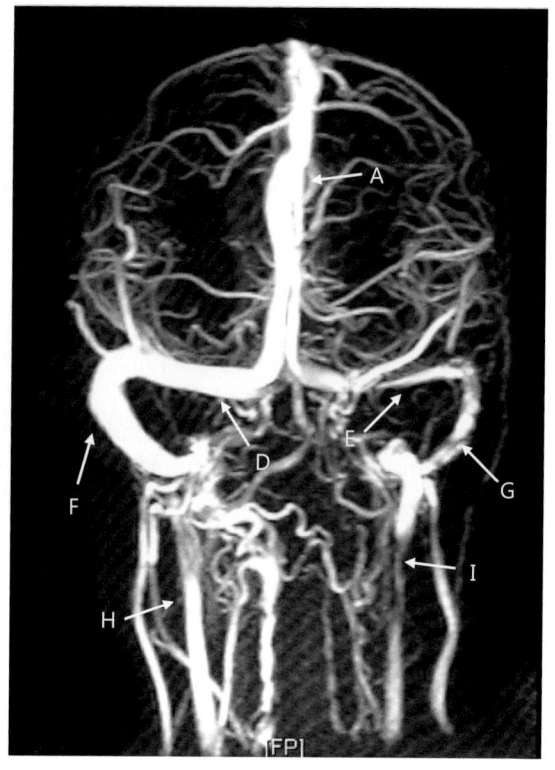

Figure 6. MRV, coronal view, showing the normal anatomy of the cerebral sinuses: A = superior sagittal sinus; D = right transverse sinus; E = left transverse sinus (nondominant); F = right sigmoid sinus; G = left sigmoid sinus; H = right internal jugular vein; I = left internal jugular vein.

main mechanisms implicated in the physiopathology of CSVT are venous congestion and parenchymal ischemic lesions. Thrombosis within the venous system results in outflow obstruction, venous congestion, and a consequent increase in capillary hydrostatic pressure, driving fluid into the interstitial space and producing edema, and ultimately infarction [25]. In the majority of cases, infarction is hemorrhagic. In term and preterm newborns there is an association between IVH and CSVT. Positioning of the neonate has a major influence on venous outflow. Neck flexion and compression of the superior sagittal sinus by the occipital bone in supine lying have been implicated in venous stasis and thrombosis, and further study of these associations are ongoing [25].

Clinical Presentation

The clinical picture of children with CSVT can be nonspecific and subtle, and may include seizures (focal or generalized), altered level of consciousness and encephalopathy, nausea, vomiting, headache, visual impairment, papilledema, hemiparesis, hemisensory loss, ataxia, speech impairment, cranial nerves palsies (specially VI nerve palsy) and acute psychiatric symptoms [23].

Diagnosis

Unenhanced CT scans may detect CSVT as hyperintensity in the expected locations of the superficial deep sinuses. However, these findings are not specific and may have a similar appearance in cases of generalized hemoconcentration as is common in neonates. Addition of contrast may disclose a filling defect, referred to as the 'empty delta sign' in the posterior part of the sagittal sinus. While simple CT scan with contrast misses the diagnosis of CSVT in up to 40% of patients, dedicated CTV confirms the diagnosis reliably. Diffusion and perfusion MRI

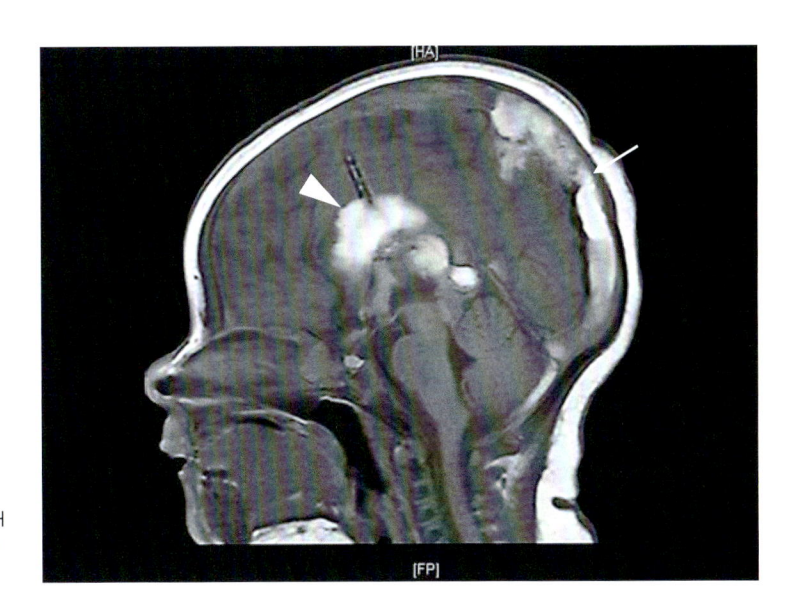

Figure 7. MRV with contrast on a sagittal view of a neonate with extensive CSVT involving the superior sagittal sinus (arrow) and associated IVH (arrowhead) due to involvements of the internal cerebral veins.

Table 2. Relevant history and physical examination in suspected CSVT by age group

Neonates	
Clinical presentation	acute seizures after the first 12 h of life, hydrocephalus, altered mental status
Past medical history	maternal factors: chorioamniotis, gestational diabetes, maternal hypertension
	perinatal factors: meconium aspiration, hypoxic-ischemic encephalopathy, polycythemia and neonatal infection
Physical examination	increased head circumference, hypotonia; focal motor deficit
Older infant or child	
Clinical presentation	headache, vision problems (blurred vision, double vision), less frequent seizures and focal deficits
Past medical history	*acute illness:* head and neck infection (otitis media, mastoiditis), dehydration, trauma, CNS tumors, recent intracranial surgery, anemia (iron deficiency)
	chronic conditions: congenital heart disease, nephritic syndrome, systemic lupus erythematosus and malignancies
	drugs: L-asparaginase, oral contraceptives, steroids, epoetin-alpha
Family history	thrombotic events (age <55 with stroke, myocardial infarction, deep venous thrombosis, maternal recurrent fetal loss)
Physical examination	*general examination*: signs of ear infection or trauma, nausea and vomiting
	neurological examination: papilledema, pupil asymmetries, ocular palsies (specially cranial nerve VI), facial sensory deficits hemiparesis, hemisensory deficit, psychiatric symptoms

may play a role in detecting venous congestion in CSVT, and in the differentiation of cytotoxic and vasogenic edema, but does not differentiate venous from arterial infarction. MRV can present false-positive findings suggesting CSVT including flow gaps in the left transverse sinus. MRV or CTV to confirm are now the methods of choice for diagnosing CSVT (fig. 7). The diagnosis is established by demonstrating a lack of flow in the cerebral veins with or without brain infarction.

The superficial venous system is more frequently involved than the deep system, and the most common sites of CSVT are the transverse, superior sagittal, sigmoid and straight sinuses. Between one and two thirds of children with CSVT may have parenchymal brain lesions such as venous infarction and hemorrhage.

Management

Anticoagulation is usually used for children with CSVT, based on the current adult recommendations. Other risk factors such as hypertension, comorbid bleeding diathesis, or other risks of bleeding such as head trauma or recent surgery, may impact the decision to treat with anticoagulation [23]. If anticoagulation is started, follow-up imaging within 2–5 days may be needed if the patient worsens or fails to improve clinically in order to assess for hemorrhage or clot propagation. In rare cases of catastrophic and life-threatening thrombosis failing to respond to systemic anticoagulation, it may be reasonable to consider endovascular thrombolysis [23].

Additional supportive interventions are commonly needed. These include correcting fluid and electrolyte disturbances, treating infection especially of the head and neck, optimizing hemoglobin and platelet counts, and monitoring and treating seizures. In cases where an associated disease condition exists, it is important to optimize treatment of the comorbid disease such as exchange transfusion in SCD, mastoidectomy and abscess drainage for mastoiditis, and immune modulation for autoimmune-mediated thrombophilia (e.g. Behcet's, inflammatory bowel disease).

CSVT in the Neonatal Period

Over 90% of newborns will survive their CSVT. In the Canadian registry, the outcomes at a mean of 1.6 years' follow-up were normal in 59%, neurological deficits in 22% including seizures and 8% had recurrent thrombosis [23]. However, recent studies applying standardized outcome measures found unfavorable outcome (death or neurological deficit) in 37/63 (59%) [26].

The current data indicate that the presence of venous infarction is associated with worse outcome [25].

For neonates with CSVT that have no evidence of ICH or large parenchymal infarct, it is reasonable to treat with anticoagulation using LMWH, or UFH followed by LMWH, for 6 weeks to 3 months [10]. For neonates who have CSVT with radiological evidence of significant ICH or large ischemic infarct, it is reasonable to hold anticoagulation, to repeat neuroimaging early (2–5 days) with CT/CTV or MRI/MRV, and start anticoagulation if progression of the thrombus is observed [10, 23].

CSVT in Older Infants and Children

About 90% of older children with CSVT survive the acute thrombosis event. In the Canadian Registry, the outcome was evaluated in 82 older infants and children at a mean interval from thrombosis to the last follow-up visit of 1.6 (range 0.05–5.2) years. There were 42 (51%) with a normal outcome, 32 (39%) with neurological deficits, and 8 (10%) deaths as a result of CSVT. Other complications included seizures in 11% and recurrent thromboembolic events in 17% [23]. Standardized outcome studies demonstrate unfavorable outcome (death or neurological deficit) in 25/68 (37%) [26].

For children with CSVT without significant ICH, anticoagulation initially with UFH or LMWH and subsequently with LMWH or VKA for a minimum of 3 months is recommended [10, 23]. In children who after 3 months of therapy still experience occlusion of CSVT or ongoing symptoms, it is reasonable to treat a further 3 months with anticoagulation [10]. For children with CSVT with associated significant hemorrhagic parenchymal venous infarction, an extended discussion with the parents about the risks and benefits of anticoagulation is necessary. In cases of extensive and rapidly progressive thrombosis and infarction, the risk of mortality if anticoagulation is withheld is high, and anticoagulation may be the only, and life-saving, treatment available. In less severe cases of CSVT with ICH, it may be reasonable to repeat radiologic monitoring of the thrombosis at 3–5 days, and consider anticoagulation if thrombus extension is noted at that time, and if the ICH is stable or resolving [10].

In children with severe progressive CSVT that is unresponsive to a trial of therapeutic anticoagulation other alternatives could include thrombolysis or surgical decompression [10]. Surgical or endovascular thrombectomy has been used in seriously ill patients, including children, usually in coma and with extensive thrombosis of superficial and deep venous structures and no response to anticoagulation [10]. In children with a history of CSVT who are at risk of recurrence, such as nephrotic syndrome, asparginase chemotherapy, etc., prophylactic anticoagulation may be considered when the patient is exposed to the inciting agent (e.g. asparaginase) or has an exacerbation of the underlying provoking disease condition [10].

Transient Ischemic Attack

TIA in general, refers to a transient episode of neurological dysfunction caused by a focal brain, spinal cord, or retinal ischemia, without evidence of infarction. TIAs are frequent in the adult population and are usually associated with atherosclerotic disease. In children, TIAs are poorly understood and the exact incidence has not been described. TIA should be suspected in children with transient neurological deficits, in the context of risk factors for AIS, for example in children with a known vasculopathy such as moyamoya disease/syndrome, SCD, arterial dissection and congenital heart disease [8].

Clinical Presentation

TIAs can present as any focal neurological deficit depending on the vascular territory that is affected, i.e. hemiparesis, hemisensory deficit, visual deficits, aphasia, cerebellar, etc. The main feature is that these deficits may resolve before 24 h and that they are associated with the absence of radiological evidence of acute ischemia (restricted diffusion on MRI in the affected vascular territory) [8].

In the clinical setting, it is important to be cautious, and recognize other neurological disorders that may mimic TIAs, like postictal neurological deficits (Todd's paralysis) in the setting of epileptic seizures and hemiplegic or complicated migraine, particularly in patients with a positive past medical or family history. The attacks related to demyelinating disorders such as multiple sclerosis may also be confused with TIAs, since these can presented as a transient focal neurological deficit; however, they present with a more gradual symptom onset; and usually resolve after 24 or 48 h.

Diagnosis

The diagnosis of TIA can be made on the clinical basis, after excluding other common causes of acute neurological deficit in children (see above); and also when the acute focal neurological deficit happens in the context of a stroke or an existing stroke risk factor (cardiac, prothrombotic or vascular conditions).

Management

There is a lack of data regarding TIAs among the pediatric population, and none of the current available guidelines in pediatric stroke cover this issue in a separate fashion (American Heart Association Guidelines 2012, and American College of Chest Physicians, 2012) [8, 10]. It is nonetheless reasonable to follow adult guidelines in evaluating children with a high clinical suspicion of TIA, where other causes of transient neurological deficits have been ruled out. This would typically start with MRI/MRA of the brain, MRA of the neck, echocardiogram and a complete prothrombotic work up. For patients with TIAs, in the setting of any given risk factor for AIS, in the absence of previous strokes, treatment with ASA may be considered. In patients who are already on ASA, and present with further TIAs, the underlying etiology informs the decision whether to switch to clopidrogel or to start LMWH or VKA. For example, in patients with dissection and prior AIS who continue having TIAs while treated with ASA, switching to anticoagulation with LMWH or VKAs is reasonable. In patients with moyamoya and stroke who continue having TIAs while treated with ASA, switching to clopidrogel is preferred, due to the increased risk for ICH in this specific population.

Further long-term studies of pediatric patients with TIAs are warranted since there is currently insufficient data to support guidelines for this specific problem.

Conclusion

Pediatric cerebrovascular diseases are well recognized entities, and result mainly from cardiac, hematological and vascular disorders. The accurate and prompt diagnosis and treatment of these conditions can help to prevent death and neurological sequelae that interfere with the child's development and quality of life.

Acknowledgment

The authors would like to express their appreciation for the thoughtful comments provided by Drs. Paul Monagle (Melbourne, Vic., Australia) and Leslie Raffini (Philadelphia, Pa., USA) who reviewed this chapter.

References

1 Agrawal N, Johnston SC, Wu YW, Sidney S, Fullerton HJ: Imaging data reveal a higher pediatric stroke incidence than prior US estimates. Stroke 2009;40:3415–3421.
2 Golomb MR, Fullerton HJ, Nowak-Gottl U, Deveber G: Male predominance in childhood ischemic stroke: findings from the international pediatric stroke study. Stroke 2009;40:52–57.
3 deVeber G, Roach ES, Riela AR, Wiznitzer M: Stroke in children: recognition, treatment, and future directions. Semin Pediatr Neurol 2000;7:309–317.
4 Amlie-Lefond C, Bernard TJ, Sebire G, Friedman NR, Heyer GL, Lerner NB, et al: Predictors of cerebral arteriopathy in children with arterial ischemic stroke: results of the International Pediatric Stroke Study. Circulation 2009;119:1417–1423.
5 Bigi S, Fischer U, Wehrli E, Mattle HP, Boltshauser E, Burki S, et al: Acute ischemic stroke in children versus young adults. Ann Neurol 2011;70:245–254.
6 Mackay MT, Wiznitzer M, Benedict SL, Lee KJ, Deveber GA, Ganesan V. Arterial ischemic stroke risk factors: the International Pediatric Stroke Study. Ann Neurol 2011;69:130–140.
7 Kirton A, deVeber G: Advances in perinatal ischemic stroke. Pediatr Neurol 2009;40:205–214.
8 Roach ES, Golomb MR, Adams R, Biller J, Daniels S, Deveber G, et al: Management of stroke in infants and children: a scientific statement from a Special Writing Group of the American Heart Association Stroke Council and the Council on Cardiovascular Disease in the Young. Stroke 2008;39:2644–2691.
9 Bowers KJ, Deveber GA, Ferriero DM, Roach ES, Vexler ZS, Maria BL: Cerebrovascular disease in children: recent advances in diagnosis and management. J Child Neurol 2011;26:1074–1100.
10 Monagle P, Chan A, Goldenberg NA, Ichord R, Journeycake J, Nowak-Gottl U, et al: Antithrombotic therapy in neonates and children: American College of Chest Physicians Evidence-Based Clinical Practice Guidelines, ed 9. Chest 2012;141(suppl 2):e737S–e801S.
11 Schechter T, Kirton A, Laughlin S, Pontigon AM, Finkelstein Y, MacGregor D, et al: Safety of anticoagulants in children with arterial ischemic stroke. Blood 2012;119:949–956.
12 deVeber G: In pursuit of evidence-based treatments for paediatric stroke: the UK and Chest guidelines. Lancet Neurol 2005;4:432–436.
13 Rodan L, McCrindle BW, Manlhiot C, Macgregor DL, Askalan R, Moharir M, et al: Stroke recurrence in children with congenital heart disease. Ann Neurol 2012;72:103–111.
14 Domi T, Edgell DS, McCrindle BW, Williams WG, Chan AK, MacGregor DL, et al: Frequency, predictors, and neurologic outcomes of vaso-occlusive strokes associated with cardiac surgery in children. Pediatrics 2008;122:1292–1298.
15 Dlamini N, Freeman JL, Mackay MT, Hawkins C, Shroff M, Fullerton HJ, et al: Intracranial dissection mimicking transient cerebral arteriopathy in childhood arterial ischemic stroke. J Child Neurol 2011;26:1203–1206.
16 DeBaun MR, Armstrong FD, McKinstry RC, Ware RE, Vichinsky E, Kirkham FJ: Silent cerebral infarcts: a review on a prevalent and progressive cause of neurologic injury in sickle cell anemia. Blood 2012;119:4587–4596.
17 DeBaun MR. Secondary prevention of overt strokes in sickle cell disease: therapeutic strategies and efficacy. Hematology Am Soc Hematol Educ Program 2011;2011:427–433.
18 Hulbert ML, McKinstry RC, Lacey JL, Moran CJ, Panepinto JA, Thompson AA, et al: Silent cerebral infarcts occur despite regular blood transfusion therapy after first strokes in children with sickle cell disease. Blood 2011;117:772–779.
19 National institutes of Health Publication: The Mangement of Sickle Cell Disease, ed 4. No. 02–2117. Bethesda, National Institutes of Health Publication, 2002.

20 Ware RE, Helms RW: Stroke With Transfusions Changing to Hydroxyurea (SWiTCH). Blood 2012;119:3925–3932.
21 Adams RJ, Brambilla D: Discontinuing prophylactic transfusions used to prevent stroke in sickle cell disease. N Engl J Med 2005; 353:2769–2778.
22 Amlie-Lefond C, Gill JC: Pharmacology in childhood arterial ischemic stroke. Semin Pediatr Neurol 2010;17:237–244.
23 Dlamini N, Billinghurst L, Kirkham FJ: Cerebral venous sinus (sinovenous) thrombosis in children. Neurosurg Clin N Am 2010; 21:511–527.
24 Wasay M, Dai AI, Ansari M, Shaikh Z, Roach ES: Cerebral venous sinus thrombosis in children: a multicenter cohort from the United States. J Child Neurol 2008;23:26–31.
25 Kersbergen KJ, Groenendaal F, Benders MJ, de Vries LS: Neonatal cerebral sinovenous thrombosis: neuroimaging and long-term follow-up. J Child Neurol 2011;26:1111–1120.
26 Moharir MD, Shroff M, Stephens D, Pontigon AM, Chan A, MacGregor D, et al: Anticoagulants in pediatric cerebral sinovenous thrombosis: a safety and outcome study. Ann Neurol 2010;67:590–599.

Abbreviations

ACA	Anterior cerebral artery
AIS	Arterial ischemic stroke
APLA	Antiphospholipid antibody
aPTT	Activated partial thromboplastin time
ASA	Acetylsalicyclic acid
CBC	Complete blood count
CCAD	Cervicocephalic arterial dissection
CNS	Central nervous system
CSVT	Cerebral sinovenous thrombosis
CT	Computed tomography
CTA	Computed tomography angiography
CTV	Computed tomography venography
EEG	Electroencephalography
FCA	Focal cerebral arteriopathy
FVL	Factor V Leiden
ICH	Intracranial hemorrhage
INR	International normalized ratio
IVH	Intraventricular hemorrhage
LMWH	Low-molecular-weight heparin
MCA	Middle cerebral artery
MRA	Magnetic resonance angiography
MRI	Magnetic resonance imaging
MRV	Magnetic resonance venography
PFO	Patent foramen ovale
PT	Prothrombin time
RBC	Red blood cell
SCD	Sickle cell disease
TCD	Transcranial Doppler
TIA	Transient ischemic attack
t-PA	Tissue-plasminogen activator
UFH	Unfractionated heparin
VKA	Vitamin K antagonist
VWF	von Willebrand factor

Chapter 15: Bleeding and Clotting in Children with Cardiac Disease

Yaser Diab
Brian W. McCrindle
Leonardo R. Brandão

Introduction

Pediatric cardiac disease represents a major health burden affecting a large group of patients in tertiary pediatric centers. For example, congenital heart defects are 60 times more prevalent than pediatric cancer, constituting the leading cause of death in the first year of life. Besides mortality, disease- and treatment-related complications in children with cardiac conditions also impact morbidity, amongst which hemorrhagic and/or TEs are increasingly prevalent. The increased frequency of these complications is attributed to advances in medical and surgical care of this patient population with increased utilization of invasive cardiovascular procedures, indwelling vascular devices (i.e. catheters, stents, transvenous pacemakers, septal occluders, valves), and intensive antithrombotic therapies, as well as to increased awareness and recognition.

CHD affects about 1% of live births and accounts for the majority of cardiac pathologies in children. In the United States, more than 35,000 neonates are born with CHD annually and by the age of 5 years; approximately 80% of these children will undergo one or more cardiac surgical interventions. CHD can be classified, depending on the underlying lesion, into acyanotic and cyanotic. Common congenital heart disorders and their estimated distribution include [1] Acyanotic CHD: VSD 20%, PDA 10%, coarctation of the aorta 10%, critical aortic stenosis 5%, atrial septal defect 5%, interrupted aortic arch 1%, and cyanotic CHD: tetralogy of Fallot 10%, transposition of the great vessels 5%, tricuspid atresia 1%, pulmonary stenosis 1%, Ebstein anomaly 1%, hypoplastic left heart syndrome 1%.

Acquired heart disease is less common than CHD in children, but encompasses a number of disorders with significant morbidity and mortality. Important pediatric acquired heart disorders include: KD, IE, and cardiomyopathies.

Strong evidence-based recommendations addressing hemostatic/thrombotic disorders in pediatric cardiac patients are lacking, and current published guidelines are largely derived from small pediatric studies, single-center experiences and extrapolations from adult trials. Hence, current clinical practices may vary significantly according to provider preference, local policies and clinical needs. However, with the significant decreased mortality in children with CHD, more emphasis is being placed towards prevention and optimal management of complications, including bleeding and TE in this population. Given that in the USA alone around 1.3 million adults were born with CHD, it became imperative for referral centers to develop their own anticoagulation/hemostasis protocols to optimize the care of children with these conditions. In this chapter, an up-to-date overview of important hemostatic and thrombotic issues in pediatric cardiac patients, including the practices reflective of our local institutional protocols is presented, with particular emphasis on a practical diagnostic approach and therapeutic management.

Mechanical Circulatory Support for Pediatric Cardiac Disease

Overview

Mechanical circulatory support is used in children during CHD surgery using CPB and in children with cardiac or cardiorespiratory failure using ECMO and/or VAD.

In CPB, blood is aspirated from the venous system, passed to a reservoir, pumped through an oxygenator, and reinfused distal to the heart and/or site of surgery. Shed blood is aspirated through suckers in the surgical site and, after a few processing steps such as filtering or washing, is collected in the venous reservoir. Cardioplegic solution is typically added to venous reservoir blood and the mix refrigerated to 4°C and applied to the heart through the cardioplegia line.

The ECMO circuit includes a pump with console, an oxygenator and a heat exchanger, tubings, age- and size-appropriate cannulae, a flow and bubble sensor and pressure monitors. There are two main ECMO modalities – venoarterial and venovenous.

Venoarterial ECMO is the modality often used for patients requiring cardiac or cardiorespiratory support. Deoxygenated blood is removed from the venous circulation, oxygen and carbon dioxide are exchanged, and then the blood is pumped back into the patient's arterial circulation. This method supports both the heart and the lungs providing higher oxygenation levels than venovenous ECMO. Venoarterial ECMO involves ligation of the carotid artery and has a higher risk of systemic embolism compared to venovenous ECMO. Cannulation of vessels within the cervical region is obligatory in infants, while 'neck or femoral' access is possible in older children.

Venovenous ECMO is the modality used for patients who require respiratory support. In this mode, deoxygenated blood is taken from a major vein and returned to another major vein after oxygenation. Although there is no risk of cerebral arterial TE, venovenous ECMO requires aggressive anticoagulation due to lower flow in the venous system.

VADs are durable mechanical circulatory devices that are used for prolonged cardiac support as a bridge to transplantation in children with end-stage heart failure. The most widely used pediatric VAD is the Excor Pediatric VAD (Berlin Heart), a paracorporeal, pneumatically driven, pulsatile-flow mechanical circulatory support device available in a wide range of size. It consists of an external pumping chamber attached in parallel with the native ventricle via cannulae through the upper abdominal wall and can provide univentricular or biventricular support. Berlin Heart has been recently found to improve survival rates in children with severe heart failure awaiting heart transplantation [2]. Newer generation VAD devices with constant-flow circulatory support are emerging, but the practices summarized herein relate to the most commonly used Excor Pediatric VAD (Berlin Heart).

Important Coagulation Considerations

Contact of blood and its cellular components with the non-biologic surface of the extracorporeal circuit used during circulatory support results

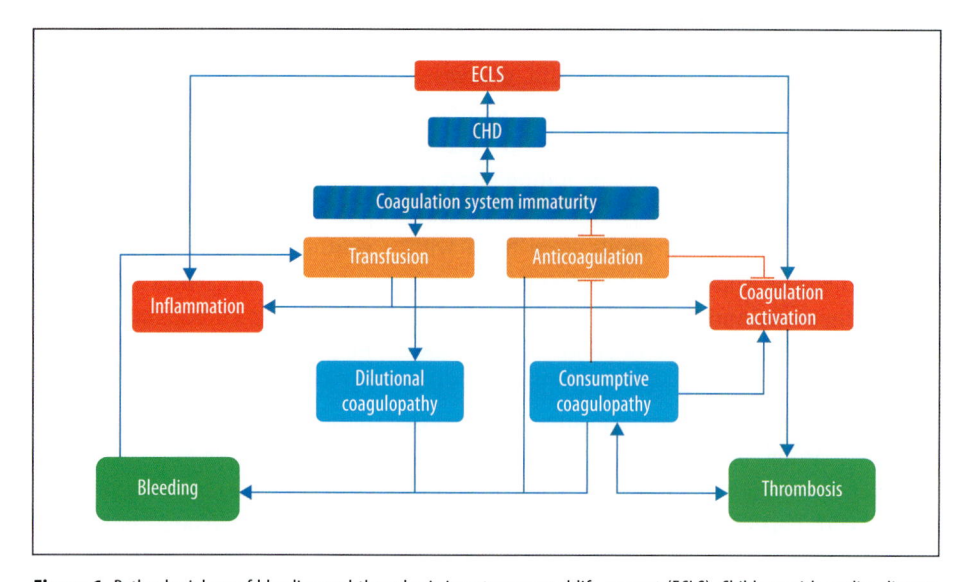

Figure 1. Pathophysiology of bleeding and thrombosis in extracorporeal life support (ECLS). Children with cardiac disease, especially CHD patients, often require ECLS. Exposure of blood to the extracorporeal circuits results in massive coagulation activation and inflammatory response. The inflammatory and coagulation systems interact at multiple levels which can lead to multiple hemostatic and/or prothrombotic derangements. As discussed elsewhere, CHD itself is associated with coagulation abnormalities which are more evident in cyanotic CHD especially in patients with single-ventricle physiology. In addition, some patients may be intrinsically prothrombotic due to an underlying inherited or acquire thrombophilia. Neonates and young infants are at higher risk for bleeding/thrombosis due to the immaturity of their hemostatic system which lacks adequate reserve under stress conditions such as ECLS. Further, because of these developmental hemostatic differences, achievement of optimal anticoagulation can be particularly challenging in pediatric patients. In addition, blood transfusion is required during ECLS for priming of the circuits, and dilution of coagulation factors may occur in infants due to their smaller blood volume increasing the risk of bleeding. Optimal anticoagulation that attenuates platelet and thrombin activation but provides sufficient clotting to prevent excessive bleeding is difficult to achieve and maintain during ECLS, and the efficacy of anticoagulation in suppressing coagulation activation seems to worsen with the duration of ECLS leading to microscopic and macroscopic clotting in the circuits, consumption of coagulation proteins and increased anticoagulation and blood product transfusion support. The resultant consumptive coagulopathy significantly increases the risk for TEs as well as bleeding complications.

in a significant inflammatory and thrombogenic response. Current heparin-coated extracorporeal circuit may reduce the inflammatory response and decrease the extracorporeal circuit thrombogenicity during extracorporeal circulation. Intensive antithrombotic therapy is mandatory to prevent device- and patient-related thrombosis during circulatory support but may increase the risk of bleeding. On the other hand, suboptimal anticoagulation during prolonged circulatory support will lead to excessive activation of coagulation on the surface of the extracorporeal circuit and within the patient's vasculature leading to circuit/systemic microscopic and/or macroscopic thrombosis, consumption of procoagulants and natural anticoagulants resulting in increasing blood transfusion support, as well as potential escalation of UFH dosage due to relative heparin resistance likely secondary to antithrombin consumption and to competitive heparin binding to inflammation-related circulating proteins. This issue may be further compounded in infants whose antithrombin levels are physiologically reduced at birth to <50% of adult levels and do not increase to adult levels until approximately 6 months of age. Circuit and systemic TE and increased usage of blood product transfusion will lead to further activation of coagulation, creating a vicious circle that may culminate into overt DIC (figure 1). Hence, achieving optimal anticoagulation during prolonged mechanical circulatory support may ultimately prevent both TEs and severe bleeding complications.

Because of the risk of TE and bleeding related to the narrow therapeutic window of standard UFH, particularly in critically ill infants, close coagulation monitoring is vital for management of children on circulatory support. This is primarily achieved by tests that can provide point of care monitoring of coagulation status and anticoagulation levels during mechanical circulatory support.

Activated Whole Blood Clotting Time

ACT is a point of care test that measures the integrity of the intrinsic and common coagulation pathways. To perform an ACT test, whole blood is placed in a test tube with 1 of 2 activators of the contact pathway, i.e. celite or kaolin. Typical target ACTs (ACT plus®, Medtronic Inc., Minneapolis, Minn., USA) are >480 s for CPB and 180–220 s for ECMO; however, there is considerable variation between devices, so results are not interchangeable from one device to another. Although the ACT remains the predominant test to manage UFH anticoagulation during ECMO and CPB in many centers, it has several limitations:

1. The ACT can be affected by factors unrelated to UFH anticoagulant activity, including hemodilution, hypothermia, immature coagulation system, severe hypocalcemia, and platelet dysfunction.
2. The reproducibility of ACT measurements can vary with the choice of activator, the operator, and the device.
3. During mechanical support, the correlation between ACT measurements and plasma heparin levels deteriorates over time.

Automated Protamine Titration Test

Automated protamine titration test is a point of care test that measures whole blood heparin concentration. This test is utilized in some centers in conjunction with ACT to monitor anticoagulation and determine the doses of UFH and protamine sulfate during CPB. At SickKids®, an individualized UFH and protamine management protocol based on heparin concentration measurement using a point of care analyzer (The HMS Plus Hemostasis Management System, Medtronic) was found to result in more reliable anticoagulation during CPB and improved postoperative outcomes [3].

Thromboelastography

TEG is a point of care test that measures the viscoelastic properties of the blood and provides overall assessment of hemostasis. TEG is used in some centers for monitoring coagulation during ECMO and for guiding transfusion after CPB. It is also part of the anticoagulation and platelet inhibition monitoring protocol for the Berlin Heart VAD.

Because of the complex coagulation changes that occur during pediatric mechanical support and the inherent limitations of any single test to monitor these coagulation changes, a detailed coagulation and anticoagulation monitoring strategy that utilizes a combination of assays is used at SickKids to better guide anticoagulation and blood product support during mechanical support (tables 1 and 2).

Cardiac Conduits, Shunts and Stents

Conduits used in pediatric cardiovascular surgery can be biologic (homografts or heterografts) or more often synthetic, which are more durable. Polytetrafluoroethylene (PTFE, or Gore-Tex®) grafts are currently the most widely used synthetic conduits. The Contegra® bioprosthetic valved conduit is a glutaraldehyde-preserved valve-containing bovine jugular vein graft (Contegra®, Medtronic) that has been used for reconstruction of a dysfunctional right ventricular outflow tract such as in patients with pulmonary atresia

Table 1. Antithrombotic regimen, laboratory monitoring and transfusion parameters for pediatric circulatory support

	CPB	ECMO	VAD (Berlin Heart Excor)
Anticoagulation monitoring	ACT, whole blood heparin concentration during CPB[1,2]	ACT, anti-Xa activity	Anti-Xa activity, TEG
Antithrombotic regimen	UFH during CPB (protamine reversal upon termination of CPB)[2]	UFH[3] AT supplementation to keep AT ≥60–70%[4] (while on UFH)	UFH 8–48 h following implantation of VAD[5] AT supplementation to keep AT ≥80% (while on UFH) Antiplatelet therapy (ASA and dipyridamole) within 72 h of VAD placement Once clinically stable, switch from UFH to therapeutic doses of LMWH (≤1 year) or VKA (>1 year) with target INR of 2.5–3.5 until transplanted or weaned from VAD
Coagulation monitoring	Whole blood heparin concentration[1], PT, aPTT, fibrinogen, platelet count upon termination of CPB	Platelet count, PT, aPTT, fibrinogen, AT, D-dimers	Platelet count, PT, TEG, aPTT, fibrinogen, AT, D-dimers
Transfusion parameters	After CPB[6], RBC (target HCT >28% if non-cyanotic; 35–40% if cyanotic or low cardiac output) Platelets (platelet count ≤100 × 10^9/l or bleeding >20 ml/kg/h) Cryoprecipitate (fibrinogen <1.0 g/l)	RBC (HCT <30%), platelets (platelet count <50–100 × 10^9/l, depending on age and/or active bleeding) Other blood products as clinically indicated	RBC (HCT <30%), platelets (platelet count <100 × 10^9/l) Other blood products as clinically indicated

Data from current practice in the Hospital for Sick Children, Toronto, Ont., Canada.
[1] Measured by point of care automated protamine titration test (The HMS Plus Hemostasis Management System).
[2] Refer to table 2 for details.
[3] Bolus of 75 U/kg at cannulation followed by infusion at an initial rate of 10 U/kg/h titrated to maintain ACT of 180–220 s (primary target) and anti-Xa of 0.35–0.7 IU/ml (secondary target).
[4] Dose of AT is calculated using the following formula: AT (U) = (desired AT level % – pretherapy AT level %) × bodyweight (in a patient receiving ECMO, an additional weight may be included to account for the amount of AT required for the ECMO circuits).
[5] Therapeutic infusion at standard age-appropriate doses titrated to maintain anti-Xa of 0.35–0.5 IU/ml.
[6] At initiation of CPB, RBC, frozen plasma and platelet units are added to prime.

Table 2. UFH and protamine management protocol during CPB

	<1 month	1 month to 1 year	>1 year
Prime UFH	4 U/ml prime solution	3 U/ml prime solution	3 U/ml prime solution
Bolus UFH	adjusted to target heparin concentration to 4.0 U/ml	adjusted to target heparin concentration to 3.5 U/ml	300 U/kg
CPB UFH	maintain heparin concentration at 3.0 U/ml (maximum total dose: 1,500 U/kg, <1 month; 900 U/kg, 1 month to 1 year)		150 U/kg if ACT <400 s 100 U/kg if ACT <400–480 s
Protamine reversal	total (patient + pump) protamine dose as calculated by the hemostasis management system × 1.5		3 mg/kg; administer an additional 1 mg/kg if ACT remained prolonged after the initial protamine dose

Data from Gruenwald et al. [3] and current practice in the Hospital for Sick Children, Toronto, Ont., Canada.

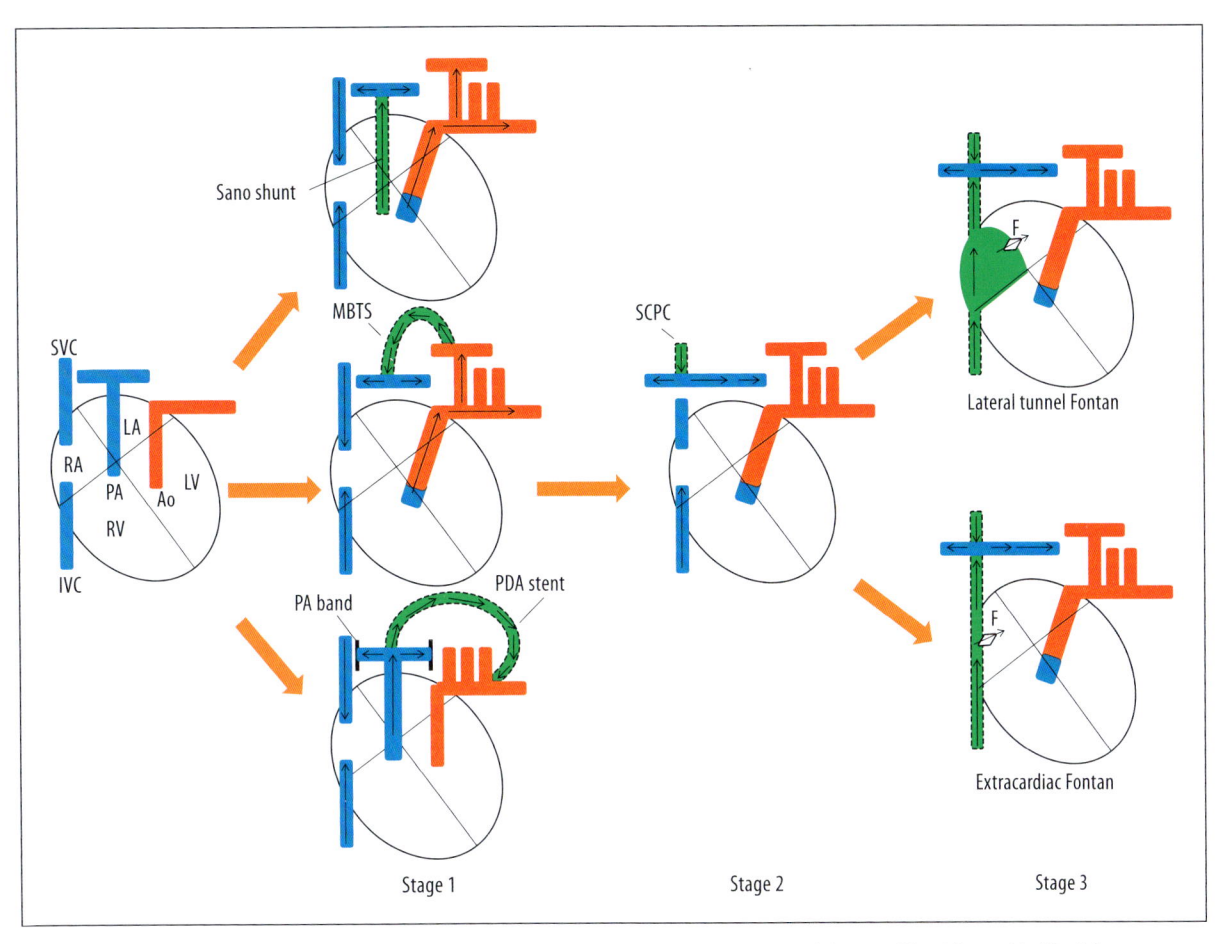

Figure 2. Staged repair for single-ventricle CHD. PA = Pulmonary artery; Ao = aorta; RA = right atrium; LA = left atrium; RV = right ventricle; LV = left ventricle, MBTS = modified BT shunt; F = fenestration. Surgery for CHD with single-ventricle physiology such as hypoplastic left heart syndrome consists of three stages. *Stage 1* is performed in the neonatal period (Norwood procedure) with the purpose of providing balanced systemic and pulmonary blood flow. In this first stage, the origin of the PA is connected to the aorta allowing the RV to pump blood to the systemic circulation, and a Gore-Tex graft connecting right innominate/subclavian artery and the right PA is created – 'modified BT shunt' (in 'Sano modification', the Gore-Tex graft connects the RV to the PA). Atrial septectomy is also performed during Norwood procedure to ensure an unobstructed connection between the pulmonary venous return and the systemic RV. Alternatively, in some high-risk patients, a hybrid procedure is sometimes performed in the first stage in which percutaneous PDA stenting and surgical bilateral PA banding are performed off bypass. *Stage 2* is performed at 4–6 months of age (Glenn procedure) in which a bidirectional cavopulmonary shunt is fashioned via an end-to-side anastomosis between the cranial end of the SVC and right PA. *Stage 3* is performed at 2–3 years of age (Fontan procedure) in which the IVC is connected to the right PA either by placement of a Gore-Tex baffle along the lateral aspect of the right atrium, which conveys IVC blood to the SVC orifice (lateral tunnel Fontan), or via a Gore-Tex conduit (extracardiac Fontan). A small fenestration is often also placed in the baffle or conduit to prevent the systemic venous pressure from reaching intolerably high levels during the intraoperative and early postoperative period. The end result is creation of a system with a single ventricle pumping blood into separate, in-series systemic and pulmonary circulations with the entire systemic venous return flowing passively into the pulmonary arteries.

and has also been used to construct the extracardiac Fontan connection between the IVC and the PA. Surgically created conduits and shunts are an integral part of the 3-stage palliative surgical approach to a heterogeneous group of complex CHD characterized by single-ventricle physiology (i.e. CHD with only one functional ventricle; figure 2).

Stents are increasingly used in pediatric cardiac disease to manage congenital obstructive lesions in the pulmonary or systemic circulations (e.g. tetralogy of Fallot or native/recurrent coarctation of the aorta), as well as acquired obstructive lesions after cardiac surgery or cardiac disease [4]. Balloon expandable stents, which can be redilated later, are preferred over self-expandable stents [4].

Thrombotic complications of cardiac conduits, shunts and stents and recommendations for thromboprophylaxis are discussed below.

Prosthetic Valves

Infants and children with valvular heart disease whose innate valves cannot be surgically repaired require valve replacement surgery. The three main types of prosthetic valves utilized in children are BVs, pulmonary autograft (Ross procedure), and MVs. While the risk of TE is low in BVs, their durability is poor. Hence, in most centers BVs are reserved for right-sided valve replacement or when there is contraindication to anticoagulation. MVs, on the other hand, are preferred for most children because of their durability. MVs, however, are thrombogenic necessitating lifelong anticoagulation. The three most commonly used MV designs are the caged ball (Starr-Edwards), the tilting disc (Bjork-Shiley, Medtronic-Hall) and the bi-leaflet (St. Jude) [5]. Thrombotic complications of MVs and recommendations for thromboprophylaxis are discussed below.

Bleeding in Children with Cardiac Disease

Pediatric cardiac patients are at increased risk for bleeding complications due to several intrinsic and extrinsic risk factors that are often present in this patient population. CHD in itself has been associated with several acquired hemostatic abnormalities including thrombocytopenia, platelet dysfunction, decreased coagulation proteins (e.g. AVWS), low-grade DIC, and primary hyperfibrinolysis. In addition, patients with evolving heart failure/dysfunction may also develop different degrees of acquired coagulopathy due to liver stasis and hypoperfusion. Moreover, certain syndromic forms of CHD can be associated with specific hemostatic defects, such as chromosome 22q11.2 microdeletion syndrome (DiGeorge/velocardiofacial syndrome) and Jacobsen syndrome (chapter 5). Similarly, Noonan syndrome can also be associated with thrombocytopenia, platelet dysfunction and multiple coagulation factor deficiencies, most commonly FXI deficiency [6].

Risk factors for perioperative bleeding include cyanotic CHD, young age (neonates and infants are at increased risk for hemodilution), CPB, deep hypothermic circulatory arrest, and complex surgical procedures. Longer storage duration of transfused RBC was recently identified as a risk factor for bleeding in children undergoing high-risk cardiac surgeries [7]. Lastly, higher intensity, combination regimens, and extended or even indefinite length of antithrombotic therapies are more often being utilized in pediatric cardiac patients, further increasing the bleeding risk.

Clinical Presentation

Bleeding can be classified with respect to severity into major bleeding (fatal, symptomatic involving a critical area such as intracranial or retroperitoneal, causing a fall in hemoglobin ≥2 g/dl over 24 h or leading to transfusion, or requiring surgical intervention) or minor bleeding (other than the above). Bleeding complications in the pediatric cardiac patient can be encountered in three main settings.

Intraoperative and Postoperative Bleeding in Cardiac Surgery
This type of bleeding presents in the form of persistent intraoperative oozing from the surgical field and/or excessive postoperative bleeding.

The most common causes of bleeding immediately after CPB are surgical causes, platelet abnormalities, hypofibrinogenemia, inadequate reversal of heparin with protamine, and combinations of these factors [8]. AVWS type 2A has also been increasingly recognized in children with CHD associated with high-velocity turbulent flow such as in patients with restrictive septal defects, stenotic or regurgitant valves, narrowed shunts or conduit, and VAD patients (chapter 9).

Bleeding during ECMO or VAD

Hemorrhage affects up to 45% of neonates, infants, and children on ECMO [9]. ICH occurs in at least 3–12% of patients, with the greatest risk in neonates, and this complication may, in fact, be present in up to 33% of patients (combined clinical and autopsy data). Bleeding rates are similarly high during VAD support. In the recent prospective study of Berlin heart VAD, major bleeding occurred in 50% of patients [2].

Bleeding while on Antithrombotic Therapy

The risk of antithrombotic therapy-related bleeding in pediatric cardiac patients is not known but is likely increased compared to non-cardiac pediatric patients given additional risk factors as outlined previously. A recent cohort study of 100 infants <6 months anticoagulated with UFH in the intensive care unit (~90% cardiac patients), targeting an anti-Xa range between 0.35 and 0.7 IU/ml, reported a major bleeding rate of 11% (as per ISTH criteria). Of 12/100 ECMO patients, 3 (25%) had major bleeding [10].

Diagnosis

The risk of perioperative bleeding in children with cardiac disease is difficult to ascertain given its complex multifactorial nature, and therefore requires a case-by-case assessment based on personal and family history of bleeding, specific risk factors for bleeding and laboratory findings. Children with cardiac disease who require surgery or invasive procedures should have a minimum preoperative hemostatic screening that ideally includes CBC count, PT, aPTT, TT and fibrinogen. Further laboratory investigations may be indicated if there is a history of bleeding or abnormal results on screening tests (chapter 3). Testing children at risk for AVWS should be considered in those with unexplained bleeding (chapter 9).

When sending coagulation testing on children with CHD, it is important to remember that cyanotic CHD is often associated with secondary polycythemia which if present will reduce the amount of plasma in a given volume of whole blood. Results in patients with high hematocrit (>55%) may be falsely prolonged. Therefore, when the hematocrit exceeds 55%, the reduced plasma volume requires a decrease in the volume of citrate anticoagulant used to maintain the recommended ratio of 9:1 using the following formula: $C = 1.85 \times 10^{-3} \times (100 - HCT) \times V$, where C = ml of 3.2% sodium citrate anticoagulant; HCT = hematocrit of the patient in %, and V = ml of whole blood in tube.

Children requiring circulatory support require close clinical and laboratory monitoring of their coagulation status as discussed earlier. In addition, surveillance for ICH with cranial ultrasound is routinely performed in infants receiving ECMO support given their heightened risk of ICH.

Management

Treatment of bleeding in cardiac patients is best guided by clinical assessment of the child's hemodynamic status, assessment of severity of bleeding and results of the hemostasis laboratory testing. An important challenge in this patient population is that anticoagulation is an indispensable part to prevent thrombus formation during CBP as well as after pediatric cardiac procedures with high thrombotic risk (for example after MV replacement). Hence, an individualized case-by-case assessment should be performed based on the risk of and gravity of TE complication (based on local and overall prevalence) versus severity of bleeding event. At SickKids, cardiac conditions considered high risk for TE include MVs, most cardiac stents, post-BT shunt, post-Fontan procedure, KD with significant CA involvement, ECMO and VAD, and history of previous TEs.

In general, minor bleeding events require only symptomatic management with no or minimal adjustment of antithrombotic therapy, while major bleeding will often require interruption or reversal of antithrombotic therapy and/or hemostatic interventions (as detailed below). Reversal of anticoagulation should follow the protocols detailed in chapter 16.

Empirical management based solely on clinical assessment of the patient is often employed for early postoperative bleeding since delaying treatment while awaiting diagnostic information may not be appropriate in many patients. Alternatively, targeted hemostatic interventions guided by clinical algorithms based on clinical and TEG parameters may be associated with decreased transfusions with equivalent or less bleeding in cardiac surgery [11]; however, this approach requires further validation in the pediatric population.

Management of bleeding in children receiving ECMO or VAD support can be quite challenging due to continued need for anticoagulation and the serious consequences of premature separation. The mainstay treatment is prevention by close laboratory monitoring and usage of blood product transfusion to optimize the hemostatic system (platelets, FP and cryoprecipitate). Surveillance for ICH with cranial ultrasound is routinely performed in infants receiving ECMO support given their risk of ICH. Bleeding during ECMO/VAD can be managed by local control of surgical bleeding using higher platelet transfusion threshold (>150 × 10^9/l) and decreasing intensity of anticoagulation (for example decreasing target ACT to 160–180 s in patients on ECMO).

Transfusion of blood products is used for children with thrombocytopenia, platelet dysfunction, coagulopathies, low plasma fibrinogen levels and AVWS. Suggested doses of platelet, FP and cryoprecipitate are detailed in the appendix. Treatment of AVWS is discussed in chapter 9. RBC transfusion is recommended to keep HCT of 28–30% for non-cyanotic CHD and 35–40% for cyanotic CHD or for patients with low cardiac output.

The use of desmopressin (DDAVP) may be considered for platelet dysfunction (chapter 5).

Antifibrinolytics, i.e. tranexamic acid or epsilon aminocaproic acid, are routinely used to decrease bleeding and transfusions in pediatric patients undergoing cardiac surgery involving CPB. Aprotinin, a polypeptide serine protease inhibitor which inhibits plasmin and other serine proteases, was the most commonly used antifibrinolytic medication in children undergoing heart surgery until it was taken off the market in 2007 after adult studies suggested increased mortality and renal failure.

The use of rFVIIa may be considered for severe bleeding refractory to other therapies. Suggested initial dosing is 20–45 µg/kg which can be escalated to 90 µg/kg every 4 h until bleeding is controlled; if no response, discontinue after maximum 3 doses. Importantly, the use of rFVIIa is associated with an increased risk of thrombosis [12].

Thromboembolism in Children with Cardiac Disease

Pediatric cardiac disease represents an important risk factor for TE in children. Importantly, TE complications in this patient population are associated with increased mortality, significant morbidity, increased hospital stay, and overall suboptimal clinical outcomes compared to children without cardiac disease.

VTE in the setting of pediatric cardiac surgery is observed in 19–40% of patients, depending on the nature of health care complexity of the local institution, with a 7% thrombosis-associated mortality, 15% recurrent VTE and 8–30% PTS frequency [13]. Up to a third of AIS in children result from cardiac disease with up to 26% mortality, 27% recurrence rate, and persistent neurologic deficits in 72% of patients [14]. CHD is directly responsible for non-CNS arterial TE in 22% of patients [15]. Strikingly, up to 28% of TEs in the setting of pediatric cardiac disease are extremely serious events (i.e. cardioembolic AIS, CSVT, PE, SVC syndrome) either requiring thrombectomy/thrombolytics, or leading to cardiopulmonary arrest or death [13].

Thromboembolism in Children with Congenital Heart Disease

TEs are a major cause of morbidity and mortality in children with CHD who require invasive surgical or catheter-based procedures. Historically, the frequency of TE in this patient population ranged from as low as 3% to as high as 30–40% depending on study design, imaging modality and patient population [13]. In a recent retrospective study of children requiring cardiac surgery at SickKids, among 1,195 procedures, the overall incidence of clinically evident TEs was 11%, which was likely an underestimate [13]. Neonatal age, baseline oxygen saturation <85%, previous thrombosis, heart transplantation, use of deep hypothermic circulatory arrest, longer cumulative time with central lines, and postoperative use of ECMO support were factors associated with increased risk of thrombosis [13].

Clinical Presentation

The presentation of TE in cardiac patients is highly variable depending on the location and extent of the thrombus, i.e. occlusive versus nonocclusive and long segment versus short segment (table 3). While most TEs present acutely in the early postoperative phase, children with prosthetic valves or shunts, or post-Fontan procedure can present with both early and/or late TE complications. Unexplained consumptive thrombocytopenia may be the primary manifestation of VTE in infants. Some patients with less extensive thrombi may have a late presentation with delayed sequelae such as PTS, portal hypertension and long-term complications associated with arterial thrombosis (chapters 11, 12, 13). In some patients, asymptomatic thrombi may be discovered incidentally on radiological studies performed for other reasons.

Diagnosis

It is important to maintain a high index of suspicion for TEs in children undergoing cardiac surgery given their increased propensity for thrombosis, variable and nonspecific presentation, and significant short-term and long-term complications. Confirmation of clinical suspicion requires radiological evidence and the choice of the radiologic modality (Doppler ultrasound, venography/angiography, echocardiography, neuroimaging, etc.) depends on the location of the thrombus (see chapters 10–14 for recommended diagnosis for the specific TE). New imaging modalities such contrast-enhanced MRV and multidetector CTA are emerging as useful imaging techniques for evaluation of TE in pediatric CHD.

Management

The management of TEs in pediatric cardiac patients does not, for the most part, differ from TE in other children and should follow published guidelines as discussed elsewhere [16] (see chapters 11–14 for recommended management). Anticoagulation alone is sufficient in most TEs in cardiac patients and should be continued beyond the standard treatment duration if the primary trigger for TE has not been eliminated (for example, uncorrected CHD in a patient with cardioembolic AIS). Some cardiac TEs can be life threatening and may require more aggressive therapeutic approaches (i.e. thrombolysis, catheter or surgical interventions). These treatment modalities

Table 3. TEs in children with CHD

TE location	Presentation
Extrathoracic venous thrombosis Cerebral venous sinuses	Seizures, neurological deficits
Neck, upper extremity veins (internal/external jugular, brachiocephalic, subclavian)	Upper extremity, facial swelling, catheter dysfunction
Intra-abdominal veins (portal/renal)	Abdominal swelling, specific organ dysfunction
Lower extremity veins (iliac, femoral, others)	Lower extremity swelling, catheter dysfunction
Extrathoracic arterial thrombosis Cerebral arterial circle of Willis (cardioembolic stroke)	Seizures, neurological deficits
Neck (internal/external carotid artery)	Seizures, neurological deficits
Lower extremity (iliac, femoral)	Color change (pallor to purple to black), decreased pulse, decreased temperature
Intrathoracic thrombosis IVC, SVC	Bilateral lower extremity swelling (IVC), facial swelling, SVC syndrome
Cardiac chambers/valves	Cardiac dysfunction, arrhythmia
Pulmonary veins/pulmonary arteries	Cardiac/respiratory dysfunction
Aorta	Same as peripheral arterial thrombosis above except potentially bilateral, discrepant upper and lower extremity blood pressures, hypertension (if renal artery is involved)
Fetal and surgically created shunts	Cardiac dysfunction
Mechanical valves	Acute pulmonary edema, cardiogenic shock, systemic embolism
VAD circuit/ECMO circuit	Visible circuit clots, circuit dysfunction, embolic phenomena

Data from Manlhiot et al. [13]. See also chapters 10–14 for further clinical presentations of TEs.

should be considered individually, balancing the risks and benefits.

Special Considerations

In addition to secondary erythrocytosis, infants with cyanotic CHD are at increased risk for iron deficiency anemia, which can increase the risk for cerebral thrombosis because of the poor deformability of the iron-deficient RBC, which further increases blood viscosity. To prevent this complication and to allow for maximal tissue oxygenation, all infants should have adequate dietary iron intake and should receive iron replacement therapy as needed to normalize RBC indices [17].

Following Fontan surgery, patients are sensitive to VKA and will require lower doses than what is recommended for other patients. This sensitivity to VKA is thought to be due to subclinical hepatic dysfunction that likely results from chronically elevated systemic venous pressure due to the absence of a right-sided pumping chamber in patients with Fontan physiology [18].

Thromboembolism in Children with Acquired Heart Disease

Kawasaki Disease

KD is the leading cause of pediatric acquired cardiac disease in North America. Up to 25% of untreated children (5% of treated children) develop CA aneurysms, which significantly increases the risk of CA thrombosis and consequently MI [19]. Recommendations for management of children with KD depend on the timing of presentation (acute phase vs. chronic phase), appearance and size of aneurysm and signs of coronary thrombosis [16]. In the acute phase, ASA in high dose (80–100 mg/kg) is recommended for up to 14 days and IVIG within 10 days of the onset of symptoms. At SickKids, children with large or giant CA aneurysms are given therapeutic doses of LMWH for 12–18 months before switching to VKA if clinically stable and free from TE based on data suggesting association between use of LMWH and favorable vascular remodeling in KD [20]. The antithrombotic management after the acute phase is outlined in figure 3.

Infective Endocarditis

IE is characterized by vegetations that typically involve native or prosthetic valves but can also affect other cardiac structures such as shunts, conduits, VSD, and PDA. Vegetations consist of a mass of platelets, fibrin, microcolonies of microorganisms and inflammatory cells which can cause significant damage to involved structure. Embolic complications, including AIS, cerebral mycotic aneurysms, pulmonary embolism, renal and splenic infarcts, retinal Roth spots, and osteomyelitis, can affect up to 40% of patients with IE [21]. Risk factors for TEs include larger size vegetations (>10 mm), mitral valve location of vegetations and staphylococcal and fungal infections. Most embolic episodes occur within the first 2–4 weeks after therapy.

IE was previously considered a formal contraindication for antithrombotic therapy. Currently, the role of antithrombotic therapy in IE remains controversial given the risk of ICH resulting from hemorrhagic transformation of ischemic infarcts, septic erosion of inflamed arteries or rupture of mycotic aneurysms and must, therefore, be considered individually based on assumed embolic risk, potential need for surgery, and bleeding risk [22]. A suggested strategy for management of anticoagulation in patients with valve-related IE is presented in table 4.

Cardiomyopathy

Cardiomyopathy encompasses a heterogeneous group of diseases of the myocardium associated with cardiac dysfunction that can be primary, acquired (e.g. viral myocarditis) or part of a multisystem disorder. Cardiomyopathies are classified according to cardiac physiology into dilated, hypertrophic, restrictive, arrhythmogenic right ventricular, and left ventricular noncompaction. Dilated cardiomyopathy is the most common type.

TEs, i.e. intraventricular thrombosis and cardioembolic strokes, are reported in up to 16% of children with dilated cardiomyopathy. These events can occur at any time in the patients' clinical course and are not related to clinical features or transplantation-free survival [23]. For children with dilated cardiomyopathy, VKA (target INR 2.0–3.0) is suggested no later than their activation on a cardiac transplant waiting list [16]. The risk of TE is also increased in restrictive cardiomyopathy and in left ventricular noncompaction cardiomyopathy [24]. At SickKids, both primary and secondary thromboprophylaxis is prescribed to selected children with cardiomyopathy (table 5).

Specific Thromboembolic Events in Pediatric Cardiac Disease

Mechanical Valve Thrombosis

MVT occurs at a rate of 0.1% per patient-year with the highest incidence during the first

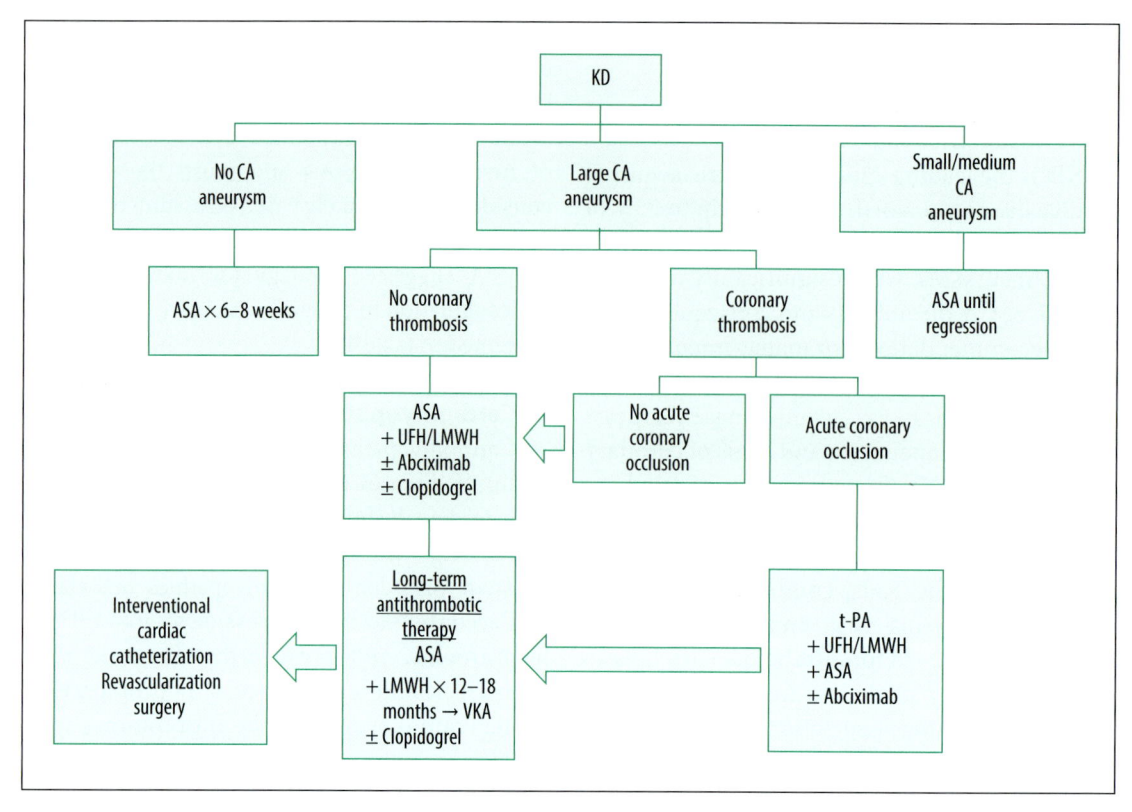

Figure 3. Antithrombotic therapy in KD. Abciximab is an intravenous glycoprotein IIb/IIIa receptor antagonist given as a bolus (250 µg/kg) followed by infusion (0.125 µg/kg per min for 12 h). Catheter interventions including balloon angioplasty, rotational ablation, and stent placement may be considered in patients presenting with ischemic symptoms, patients without ischemic symptoms but with reversible ischemia on stress test, and patients without ischemia but with ≥75% stenosis in the left anterior descending CA. Surgical revascularization may be considered in severe occlusion of the main trunk of the left main CA, severe occlusion of ≥1 major CA, severe occlusion in the proximal segment of the left anterior descending CA, if collateral coronary arteries in jeopardy, severe left ventricular dysfunction or recurrent MIs.

Table 4. Suggested strategy to antithrombotic therapy in IE

	Mechanical valve IE	**Native/bioprosthetic valve IE**
No clinical evidence of stroke	Continue anticoagulation and convert from VKA to i.v. UFH. Restart VKA when it is clear that invasive procedures will not be required and the patient has stabilized without signs of central nervous system involvement[1]	Antithrombotic therapy is not indicated
Clinical evidence of Stroke No radiological evidence for ICH	Hold VKA, resume anticoagulation with i.v. UFH within 1 week with serial brain imaging to exclude hemorrhagic transformation or ICH.	
Radiological evidence of ICH	Withhold anticoagulation, exclude mycotic aneurysms	

[1] Discontinuing anticoagulation until blood cultures are negative and the clinical signs of sepsis have resolved can be considered in patients with *Staphylococcus aureus* IE.

year after implantation and in patients with a mechanical tricuspid/mitral valve replacement. MVT can be obstructive, causing acute pulmonary edema, cardiogenic shock or systemic embolism, or non-obstructive, which are more likely to present with TEs, although almost 50% are asymptomatic. The diagnosis of MVT can be confirmed in most patients by the combination of transthoracic or transesophageal echocardiography and fluoroscopy. Current recommendations for acute treatment of MVT favor the use of systemic thrombolytic therapy as first-line treatment. Surgery is reserved for patients who have contraindication for or who fail thrombolysis [25]. Subsequently increasing the anticoagulation intensity (i.e. to a target INR 3.0–4.0) or adding ASA to VKA may be required in patients who develop MVT while on adequate anticoagulation to prevent further events.

Blalock-Taussig Shunt Thrombosis

Thrombotic occlusion of the BT shunt occurs in up to 17% of children and can compromise pulmonary blood flow requiring immediate intervention. Diagnosis is usually clinical, supported by echocardiographic and/or angiographic findings. Therapeutic options for children who develop acute BT shunt occlusion include catheter-directed thrombolytic therapy and/or angioplasty with stenting, and reoperation. Moreover, children with BT shunts may have reduced peripheral pulses in the ipsilateral arm, and may have measurably reduced growth of the arm. This can be of significance when assessing for PTS, which may also occur in the upper limbs secondary to VTE [26].

Thromboembolism after Superior Cavopulmonary Connection (Glenn Procedure)

Although TEs are thought to be relatively uncommon in infants after SCPC (Glenn procedure), thrombotic events were recently reported to occur in 28% after SCPC, suggesting that TEs are likely underappreciated in this patient population [27]. There are, additionally, several considerations related to the vascular anatomy after SCPC (Glenn procedure; figure 2) that could justify a more aggressive antithrombotic therapy in case of thrombosis (i.e. thrombolysis or surgery). First, following SCPC (Glenn procedure) blood flows directly from the SVC into the pulmonary arteries and the lungs; hence, any reduction in SVC flow to the lungs, due to thrombus occlusion, will dramatically reduce pulmonary blood flow. Second, increased pulmonary vascular resistance, due to pulmonary emboli, is of concern as the patient may become unsuitable for future Fontan surgery. Third, thrombus in the lower venous system or from collaterals (i.e. SVC → IVC → pulmonary veins) can give rise to paradoxical emboli as blood flow from the IVC bypasses the lungs. Finally, collaterals around thrombosis of central thoracic veins may interfere with the ability to complete the Fontan surgery [26].

Thromboembolism after Fontan Procedure

TEs remain a major complication after Fontan surgery. In a recent prospective study, the cumulative thrombosis rate was 23% in the first 2 years after surgery despite thromboprophylaxis with warfarin or ASA [28]. Further, TEs may occur any time following the Fontan procedure, but often present months to years later [29]. Similar to SCPC (Glenn) and Norwood procedures, thrombotic events after a Fontan procedure can have several important implications and may warrant an aggressive antithrombotic strategy in case of thrombosis, i.e. thrombolysis and surgery. First, the risk for paradoxical emboli continues to be a concern due to the presence of right to left communication. Second, because the pulmonary pressure cannot be increased in Fontan circuits, pulmonary emboli have an accentuated impact on pulmonary blood flow. Third, the Fontan circuit makes it difficult to obtain full lung perfusion during imaging,

Table 5. Thromboprophylaxis for pediatric cardiac disease/procedures

Procedure/condition	Thromboprophylaxis
Cardiac catheterization via an artery	UFH bolus dose (100 U/kg) and further doses (50 U/kg) in prolonged procedures (≥2 h)
Intravascular/intracardiac stents PDA stent	ASA and clopidogrel for 3 months
MBTS stent	Add ASA to LMWH until 2nd stage (SCPC)
Systemic venous system (includes pulmonary arteries in single ventricle patients)	LMWH for 3 months and ASA indefinitely
Pulmonary vein stent	LMWH for 3 months and ASA indefinitely
Pulmonary artery stent <5 mm	ASA indefinitely
ASD stent	LMWH and ASA until stent removal
RVOT and coarctation of the aorta stent	None
Coronary artery stents	Periprocedural UFH, ASA ± clopidogrel ± GP IIb/IIIa antagonist (eptifibatide is preferred) followed by ASA and clopidogrel for ≥1 month for bare metal stents and for ≥6 months for drug-eluting stents followed by indefinite ASA. Indefinite ASA and clopidogrel may be continued in high-risk patients
Staged surgery for single ventricle physiology MBTS (Norwood procedure)	Intraoperative UFH followed by therapeutic LMWH until Glenn procedure (note: no anticoagulation is given after Sano modification or hybrid procedure)
SCPC (Glenn procedure)	None for single shunt, therapeutic LMWH or VKA (target INR 2–3) for patients with bilateral shunts until the time of Fontan completion
Fontan procedure	VKA (target INR 2.0–3.0) for at least 6 months or until fenestration closure and ASA after VKA stopped
Prosthetic heart valves Mechanical prosthetic heart valves	VKA (target 2.5–3.5) for all mechanical valves
Bioprosthetic heart valves	No antithrombotic therapy as all bioprosthetic valves are placed in pulmonary position
Acquired cardiac disease Cardiomyopathy	Therapeutic LMWH or VKA (target INR 2.0–3.0) for all patients with dilated cardiomyopathy and LV shortening fraction <20% or qualitatively severely reduced function, left ventricular non-compaction, restrictive cardiomyopathy and history of TEs
Kawasaki disease	See figure 2
Primary pulmonary hypertension	VKA (target 1.5–2.0) when medical therapy is initiated

Data from Monagle et al. [16] and current practice at the Hospital for Sick Children, Toronto, Ont., Canada. ASD = Atrial septal defect; RVOT = right ventricular outflow tract; MBTS = modified BT shunt; LV = left ventricular; GP = glycoprotein.

rendering the radiological confirmation of pulmonary emboli particularly challenging.

Intracardiac Thrombosis

Intracardiac thrombosis can be encountered as a complication of CHD surgery, ECMO support or acquired cardiac disease. Right-sided and left-sided intracardiac thrombosis can lead to pulmonary embolism and AIS, respectively. Any cardiac chamber may be involved in children with CHD including hypoplastic chambers and blind stumps (right ventricle), aortic atresia, critical aortic stenosis, mitral atresia, pulmonary atresia with intact ventricular septum and Ebstein's anomaly. Right atrial thrombosis is most commonly due to indwelling central venous catheters. It may be rarely encountered in children with Eisenmenger syndrome (secondary pulmonary hypertension due to VSD). Left atrial thrombosis may rarely affect patients with significant mitral valve stenosis or cardiomyopathy. Thrombi in either atrium have been reported after a Fontan procedure. Anticoagulation is the main therapy for most cases of uncomplicated intracardiac thrombosis; however, thrombolytic therapy or surgical thrombectomy may be considered in selected cases of intracardiac thrombi causing flow obstruction, cardiac failure, or serious embolic phenomena [16].

Myocardial Infarction

Although rare in children, MI is a serious condition that results from critical decrease in CA perfusion. Causes for MI in children include [30]:
1. CA anomalies (anomalous origin of left CA from the PA, origin of a CA from the wrong aortic sinus with its course between the aorta and the PA)
2. CA complications associated with CHD or pediatric cardiac surgery (CA obstruction after arterial switch operation for D-transposition of the great arteries, CA complication after repair of tetralogy of Fallot, CA ostial stenosis associated with supravalvar aortic stenosis, CA obstruction associated with pulmonary atresia with intact ventricular septum)
3. CA sequelae of KD [thrombotic occlusion of large CA aneurysm, CA stenosis at ends of large aneurysm, obliterative coronary arteritis without large aneurysm (rare)]
4. Myocardial ischemia associated with hypertrophic cardiomyopathy
5. Myocardial ischemia associated with cocaine use
6. Atherosclerotic CA disease in children with homozygous familial hypercholesterolemia
7. Coronary allograft vasculopathy, an accelerated form of arteriopathy affecting the coronary vessels of heart transplant recipients

Children with MI rarely manifest with classic pressure-like chest pain. Presentation is more often nonspecific such as unusual irritability, nausea and vomiting, abdominal pain, shock, syncope, seizure, sudden unexpected cardiac arrest, or even silent. Diagnosis of clinically suspected cases can be confirmed by elevated cardiac enzymes (creatinine phosphokinase subfractions and troponin), ischemic changes on ECG and echocardiography, and in most cases an abnormal diagnostic coronary angiograph. Management requires early recognition and involvement of a pediatric cardiologist, and should be tailored depending on the underling etiology (see figure 3 for management of CA thrombosis in KD).

Thromboembolic Complications during Extracorporeal Membrane Oxygenation or Ventricular Assist Device Support

TE complications are frequent during support with ECMO and VAD and can manifest as circuit clots or systemic TE. Patients with CHD appear especially susceptible to thrombosis on ECMO [31]. With respect to coagulation changes during ECMO, three clinical phases may be observed in most but not all patients receiving prolonged ECMO support. In the first few days, there may be small minor clots that are seen in the circuits, UFH doses are relatively stable without significant fluctuation in ACTs or other anticoagulation measurements, and D-dimers are slightly elevated. After about 4–7 days of ECMO support, circuit clotting increases, UFH dose requirement increases, and it becomes more difficult to keep anticoagulation levels within target ranges. In addition, D-dimers become significantly elevated, platelet counts decrease, and there is increased need for blood product support. After approximately 7–10 days of ECMO support, particularly when anticoagulation has been suboptimal, circuit clotting becomes significant and may necessitate changing the circuits, UFH dosage requirements increase significantly and DIC-like state ensues leading to significant increase in blood product transfusions. Treatment options are limited in patients with ECMO/VAD-related TE, especially if the patient continues to require circulatory support, and include changing the circuits and increasing the intensity of anticoagulation.

Thromboprophylaxis in Pediatric Cardiac Disease

As described previously, the modern management of pediatric cardiac disease often requires complex surgical and/or transcatheter interventional procedures which can involve creation of extracardiac conduits and shunts and placement of intravascular or intracardiac stents, or MVs that can alter the blood flow shear stress, disrupt the endothelium and activate the coagulation system, increasing the risk for TEs and frequently necessitating primary thromboprophylaxis, i.e. use of antithrombotic therapy in patients who have not previously had TE. Moreover, as detailed earlier, TE is an important complication in pediatric cardiac patients and often necessitates continued thromboprophylaxis beyond the initial treatment of the thrombotic event if the underlying cardiac risk factor has not been corrected (secondary thromboprophylaxis). Primary and secondary thromboprophylaxis regimens in pediatric cardiac disease at SickKids are detailed in table 5. Important cardiac settings in which thromboprophylaxis is often required are discussed below.

Single-Ventricle Heart Palliation

There remains little conclusive evidence to support the optimal strategy to prevent thrombotic complications related to these procedures [29]. Published guidelines for thromboprophylaxis recommend intraoperative UFH followed by ASA or no further antithrombotic therapy after the Norwood procedure, postoperative UFH after SCPC (Glenn procedure), and ASA or therapeutic UFH followed by VKA (target INR 2.0–3.0) after the Fontan procedure [16]. However, due to previously stated limitations, these recommendations lack strong supportive evidence. Consequently, thromboprophylaxis practices vary considerably between centers. The thromboprophylactic regimen employed at SickKids was recently found to be associated with a reduction in early and long-term thrombotic complications in this patient population, suggesting that routine thromboprophylaxis across all 3 palliative stages may be warranted [27]. Primary thromboprophylaxis with ASA was reported to lower the risk of shunt thrombosis after Norwood procedure in a nonrandomized observational study [32]. There is no consensus regarding routine primary thromboprophylaxis for patients after Fontan procedure. In patients with fenestrated Fontan circuit, continued anticoagulation until fenestration closure either spontaneously or by transcatheter techniques is advocated by some because of the theoretical risk of paradoxical cardioembolic stroke [26]. While data from a recent randomized controlled study suggested that there was no significant difference between ASA and warfarin as primary thromboprophylaxis in the first 2 years after Fontan surgery, longer term data from SickKids indicates that warfarin may be associated with a superior outcome [27].

Cardiac Stents

Published guidelines for thromboprophylaxis for endovascular stents recommend UFH perioperatively but do not provide additional guidance due to the lack of data [16]. Thromboprophylaxis regimens used for cardiac catheterization via an artery, stents and cardiovascular shunts at SickKids are detailed in table 5.

Prosthetic Valves

Recommended thromboprophylaxis for pediatric prosthetic valves are based on adult guidelines and suggest VKA for MVs (target 2.0–3.0 for aortic MVs and 2.5–3.5 for mitral MVs), ASA (± clopidogrel) for 3 months for aortic BVs and VKA (target INR 2.0–3.0) for 3 months for mitral BVs, followed by long-term ASA for either aortic or mitral BVs [33]. Thromboprophylaxis regimens used for prosthetic valves at SickKids are detailed in table 5.

Primary Pulmonary Hypertension

Available evidence suggests that a prothrombotic state exists in patients with primary pulmonary hypertension which may led to in situ thrombosis in the pulmonary vasculature and disease progression and that anticoagulation therapy may improve outcome in these patients [34]. As such, anticoagulant prophylaxis is routinely given to children with primary pulmonary hypertension. Current guidelines recommend starting anticoagulation with VKAs (target INR 1.7–2.5 or 2.0–3.0) at the same time as other medical therapies [16]. The thromboprophylaxis regimen used at SickKids is detailed in table 5.

Conclusion

Both bleeding complications and TEs are significant morbidities in pediatric cardiac patients. Limited pediatric data are available on the best approach for prevention and optimal management of these serious events, and published guidelines provide only general recommendations that are based on low-quality evidence. As a result, there is a considerable practice variation among institutions. The management approaches presented here are based on available published data and the institutional experience at SickKids of managing a large number of pediatric cardiac patients over a span of several decades.

Acknowledgment

The authors would like to express their appreciation for the thoughtful comments provided by Drs. Leslie Raffini (Philadelphia, Pa., USA) and Paul Monagle (Melbourne, Vic., Australia) who reviewed this chapter.

References

1. Dolbec K, Mick NW: Congenital heart disease. Emerg Med Clin North Am 2011;29:811–827, vii.
2. Fraser CD Jr, Jaquiss RD, Rosenthal DN, Humpl T, et al: Prospective trial of a pediatric ventricular assist device. N Engl J Med 2012; 367:532–541.
3. Gruenwald CE, Manlhiot C, Chan AK, Crawford-Lean L, Foreman C, Holtby HM, Van Arsdell GS, Richards R, Moriarty H, McCrindle BW: Randomized, controlled trial of individualized heparin and protamine management in infants undergoing cardiac surgery with cardiopulmonary bypass. J Am Coll Cardiol 2010;56:1794–1802.
4. Okubo M, Benson LN: Intravascular and intracardiac stents used in congenital heart disease. Curr Opin Cardiol 2001;16:84–91.
5. Tong E: An overview of artificial heart valve replacement in infants and children. J Cardiovasc Nurs 1992;6:30–43.
6. Briggs BJ, Dickerman JD: Bleeding disorders in Noonan syndrome. Pediatr Blood Cancer 2012;58:167–172.
7. Manlhiot C, McCrindle BW, Menjak IB, Yoon H, Holtby HM, Brandao LR, Chan AK, Schwartz SM, Ben Sivarajan V, Crawford-Lean L, Foreman C, Caldarone CA, Van Arsdell GS, Gruenwald CE: Longer blood storage is associated with suboptimal outcomes in high-risk pediatric cardiac surgery. Ann Thorac Surg 2012;93:1563–1569.
8. Arnold P: Treatment and monitoring of coagulation abnormalities in children undergoing heart surgery. Paediatr Anaesth 2011;21:494–503.
9. Skinner SC, Hirschl RB, Bartlett RH: Extracorporeal life support. Semin Pediatr Surg 2006;15:242–250.
10. Schechter T, Finkelstein Y, Ali M, Kahr WH, Williams S, Chan AK, Deveber G, Brandao LR: Unfractionated heparin dosing in young infants: clinical outcomes in a cohort monitored with anti-factor Xa levels. J Thromb Haemost 2012;10:368–374.

11 Romlin BS, Wahlander H, Berggren H, Synnergren M, Baghaei F, Nilsson K, Jeppsson A: Intraoperative thromboelastometry is associated with reduced transfusion prevalence in pediatric cardiac surgery. Anesth Analg 2011;112:30–36.
12 McQuilten ZK, Barnes C, Zatta A, Phillips LE: Off-label use of recombinant factor VIIa in pediatric patients. Pediatrics 2012;129: e1533–e1540.
13 Manlhiot C, Menjak IB, Brandao LR, Gruenwald CE, et al: Risk, clinical features, and outcomes of thrombosis associated with pediatric cardiac surgery. Circulation 2011;124:1511–1519.
14 Rodan L, McCrindle BW, Manlhiot C, Macgregor DL, Askalan R, Moharir M, Deveber G: Stroke recurrence in children with congenital heart disease. Ann Neurol 2012;72:103–111.
15 Monagle P, Newall F, Barnes C, Savoia H, Campbell J, Wallace T, Crock C: Arterial thromboembolic disease: a single-centre case series study. J Paediatr Child Health 2008;44:28–32.
16 Monagle P, Chan AK, Goldenberg NA, Ichord RN, Journeycake JM, Nowak-Gottl U, Vesely SK: Antithrombotic Therapy in Neonates and Children: Antithrombotic Therapy and Prevention of Thrombosis, ed 9: American College of Chest Physicians Evidence-Based Clinical Practice Guidelines. Chest 2012;141(suppl 2):e737S–e801S.
17 Tempe DK, Virmani S: Coagulation abnormalities in patients with cyanotic congenital heart disease. J Cardiothorac Vasc Anesth 2002;16:752–765.
18 Streif W, Andrew M, Marzinotto V, Massicotte P, Chan AK, Julian JA, Mitchell L: Analysis of warfarin therapy in pediatric patients: a prospective cohort study of 319 patients. Blood 1999;94:3007–3014.
19 Paredes N, Mondal T, Brandao LR, Chan AK: Management of myocardial infarction in children with Kawasaki disease. Blood Coagul Fibrinolysis 2010;21:620–631.
20 Manlhiot C, Brandao LR, Somji Z, Chesney AL, MacDonald C, Gurofsky RC, Sabharwal T, Chahal N, McCrindle BW: Long-term anticoagulation in Kawasaki disease: initial use of low molecular weight heparin is a viable option for patients with severe coronary artery abnormalities. Pediatr Cardiol 2010;31:834–842.
21 Thom KE, Sivaprakasam P, Russel JL, Williams S, Allen U, Brandao LR: Abstracts of the XXIII Congress of the International Society on Thrombosis and Haemostasis with the 57th Annual SSC (Scientific and Standardization Committee) Meeting, July 23–28 2011, Kyoto, Japan, Abstract O-TU-046: Pediatric infective endocarditis over the last 30 years: thromboembolic complications and associations of vegetation and heart failure with mortality. J Thromb Haemost 2011;9(suppl 2):274.
22 Baddour LM, Wilson WR, Bayer AS, Fowler VG Jr, et al: Infective endocarditis: diagnosis, antimicrobial therapy, and management of complications: a statement for healthcare professionals from the Committee on Rheumatic Fever, Endocarditis, and Kawasaki Disease, Council on Cardiovascular Disease in the Young, and the Councils on Clinical Cardiology, Stroke, and Cardiovascular Surgery and Anesthesia, American Heart Association: endorsed by the Infectious Diseases Society of America. Circulation 2005;111:e394–e434.
23 McCrindle BW, Karamlou T, Wong H, Gangam N, Trivedi KR, Lee KJ, Benson LN: Presentation, management and outcomes of thrombosis for children with cardiomyopathy. Can J Cardiol 2006;22:685–690.
24 Williams GD, Hammer GB: Cardiomyopathy in childhood. Curr Opin Anaesthesiol 2011;24:289–300.
25 Sun JC, Davidson MJ, Lamy A, Eikelboom JW: Antithrombotic management of patients with prosthetic heart valves: current evidence and future trends. Lancet 2009;374:565–576.
26 Monagle P: Thrombosis in children with BT shunts, Glenns and Fontans. Prog Pediatr Cardiol 2005;21:17–21.
27 Manlhiot C, Brandao LR, Kwok J, Kegel S, Menjak IB, Carew CL, Chan AK, Schwartz SM, Sivarajan VB, Caldarone CA, Van Arsdell GS, McCrindle BW: Thrombotic complications and thromboprophylaxis across all three stages of single ventricle heart palliation. J Pediatr 2012;161:513–519.e3.
28 Monagle P, Cochrane A, Roberts R, Manlhiot C, Weintraub R, Szechtman B, Hughes M, Andrew M, McCrindle BW: A multicenter, randomized trial comparing heparin/warfarin and acetylsalicylic acid as primary thromboprophylaxis for 2 years after the Fontan procedure in children. J Am Coll Cardiol 2011;58:645–651.
29 Thom KE, Hanslik A, Male C: Anticoagulation in children undergoing cardiac surgery. Semin Thromb Hemost 2011;37:826–833.
30 Takahashi M: Cardiac ischemia in pediatric patients. Pediatr Clin North Am 2010;57:1261–1280.
31 Reed RC, Rutledge JC: Laboratory and clinical predictors of thrombosis and hemorrhage in 29 pediatric extracorporeal membrane oxygenation nonsurvivors. Pediatr Dev Pathol 2010;13:385–392.
32 Li JS, Yow E, Berezny KY, Rhodes JF, et al: Clinical outcomes of palliative surgery including a systemic-to-pulmonary artery shunt in infants with cyanotic congenital heart disease: does aspirin make a difference? Circulation 2007;116:293–297.
33 Whitlock RP, Sun JC, Fremes SE, Rubens FD, Teoh KH: Antithrombotic and Thrombolytic Therapy for Valvular Disease: Antithrombotic Therapy and Prevention of Thrombosis, 9th ed: American College of Chest Physicians Evidence-Based Clinical Practice Guidelines. Chest 2012;141(suppl 2):e576S–e600S.
34 Johnson SR, Granton JT, Mehta S: Thrombotic arteriopathy and anticoagulation in pulmonary hypertension. Chest 2006;130:545–552.

Abbreviations

ACT	Activated clotting time
AIS	Arterial ischemic stroke
Anti-Xa	Anti-factor Xa
aPTT	Activated partial prothrombin time
ASA	Acetylsalicyclic acid
AT	Antithrombin
AVWS	Acquired von Willebrand syndrome
BT Shunt	Blalock-Taussig Shunt
BV	Bioprosthetic valve
CA	Coronary artery
CBC	Complete blood count
CHD	Congenital heart disease
CNS	Central nervous system
CPB	Cardiopulmonary bypass
CSVT	Cerebral sinovenous thrombosis
CTA	Computed tomography angiography
DDAVP	1-Deamino-8-D-arginine vasopressin (desmopressin)

DIC	Disseminated intravascular coagulation	PDA	Patent ductus arteriosus
ECMO	Extracorporeal membrane oxygenation	PE	Pulmonary embolism
FP (FFP)	Frozen plasma (Fresh frozen plasma)	PT	Prothrombin time
FXI	Factor XI	PTS	Postthrombotic syndrome
HCT	Hematocrit	RBC	Red blood cell
ICH	Intracranial hemorrhage	rFVIIa	Recombinant activated factor VII
IE	Ineffective endocarditis	SCPC	Superior cavopulmonary connection
INR	International normalized ratio	SVC	Superior vena cava
ISTH	International Society on Thrombosis and Haemostasis	TE	Thromboembolism/thromboembolic event
IVC	Inferior vena cava	TEG	Thromboelastography
IVIG	Intravenous immunoglobulin	t-PA	Tissue-plasminogen activator
KD	Kawasaki disease	TT	Thrombin time
LMWH	Low-molecular-weight heparin	UFH	Unfractionated heparin
MI	Myocardial infarction	VAD	Ventricular assist device
MRV	Magnetic resonance venography	VKA	Vitamin K antagonist
MV	Mechanical valve	VSD	Ventricular septal defect
MVT	Mechanical valve thrombosis	VTE	Venous thromboembolism/thromboembolic event
PA	Pulmonary artery		

Chapter 16 Antithrombotic Therapy in Children

Tina Biss
Paul Monagle

Introduction

The requirement for antithrombotic therapy for the treatment and prevention of TEs in children is increasing. This increase is likely multifactorial but certainly involves the improvement in survival from complex diseases being complicated by a rising incidence of thromboembolic complications.

Antithrombotic therapy has many specific challenges in infants and children, related to the changes that occur in the hemostatic system during normal development (chapter 4), the difficulty in administering anticoagulant therapy that arises from the lack of suitable preparations and the often small doses required, and the difficulties in monitoring due to physiologically abnormal baseline tests and problematic venipuncture.

There is also a relative lack of evidence to guide dosing and monitoring of antithrombotic therapy in children. There are far fewer randomized controlled studies of antithrombotic therapy in children than there are in adults, and much of the guidance for dosing and monitoring is extrapolated from data obtained from adult studies. Treatment is often led by the experience of the treating physician and individualized according to the child being treated. The most comprehensive and globally accepted guidelines currently available are those published by the American College of Chest Physicians [1].

Unfractionated Heparin

Mechanism of Action and Pharmacokinetics

Heparin acts as an anticoagulant by binding to and potentiating the effect of AT (chapter 2). UFH is usually administered intravenously by continuous infusion but can also be given subcutaneously. UFH is metabolized by the liver and is renally excreted. If a bolus dose of heparin is administered, followed by a continuous infusion, the anticoagulant effect plateaus after 4 h. Without a bolus dose, it plateaus after 6 h. The half-life of UFH is short (although the actual half-life seems age dependent) [2], meaning that reversal of the anticoagulant effect is rapid if the infusion is stopped.

Indications

UFH, administered by continuous infusion, is the anticoagulant of choice for situations where rapid onset of anticoagulant effect and/or rapid reversal are required, e.g. for postoperative anticoagulation or anticoagulation in patients with a high risk of bleeding due to other causes. It is also useful as a short-term anticoagulant agent, such as during renal dialysis or CPB surgery.

Dosing

The use of a loading dose and the choice of initial maintenance dose mainly depend on clinical situation and age. A loading dose should be avoided or reduced in neonates, children with stroke or if the risk of bleeding is high.

Loading dose: 75 U/kg as an i.v. infusion over 10 min.

Initial maintenance dose: <1 year of age, 28 U/kg/h; ≥1 year of age, 20 U/kg/h.

Monitoring

UFH treatment requires monitoring to ensure that the anticoagulant effect is within the desired range. Monitoring classically should occur 6 h after commencing a heparin infusion and 4 h after any change in infusion rate, although in children this is often not feasible. A blood sample for monitoring should be taken at least every 24 h once therapeutic levels are achieved. UFH can be monitored using several different laboratory assays.

Activated Clotting Time

This is a bedside test that measures the time taken for whole blood to clot after the addition of kaolin, often used for heparin monitoring during CPB surgery or ECMO. The target range is analyzer dependent. The ACT may be prolonged by other factors such as thrombocytopenia, hypothermia and hemodilution.

Table 1. Adjustment of heparin infusion according to monitoring of aPTT, aPTR and anti-Xa levels

aPTT	aPTR	Anti-Xa level IU/ml[1]	Bolus U/kg	Hold min	Rate change %
<50 s	<1.2	<0.1	50	–	↑20
50–59 s	1.2–1.4	0.1–0.34	–	–	↑10
60–85 s	1.5–2.5	0.35–0.70	–	–	no change
86–95 s	2.6–3.0	0.71–0.89	–	–	↓10
96–120 s	3.1–3.5	0.9–1.2	–	30	↓10
>120 s	>3.5	>1.2	–	60	↓15

[1] This assumes that the aPTT range of 60–85 s correlates to an anti-factor Xa level of 0.35–0.70 IU/ml. This will depend on the reagent and analyzer used in the laboratory.

Activated Partial Thromboplastin Time or Activated Partial Thromboplastin Ratio

The aPTT measures clotting via the intrinsic pathway (chapter 2) and is prolonged by UFH. The target range is analyzer and reagent dependent. The aPTR is a ratio of patient aPTT/normal aPTT for age and an aPTR of 1.5–2.5 is usually the desired range, although there have been specific recommendations against using aPTR in children (see table 1 for details of UFH infusion adjustment according to aPTT/aPTR). Levels of aPTT/aPTR may be difficult to monitor in the presence of a prolonged baseline aPTT such as might be due to physiological factor deficiency in infants <6 months, the presence of a coagulation inhibitor (e.g. lupus anticoagulant) or a consumptive coagulopathy.

Anti-Factor Xa Activity Assay

Anti-Xa activity assay measures the degree of inhibition of activated factor X by UFH. The target range is usually 0.35–0.7 IU/ml anti-Xa level (see table 1 for details of UFH infusion adjustment according to anti-Xa levels). If UFH therapy is being monitored using aPTT/aPTR, some would advise requesting an anti-Xa level within the first 24 h of therapy to see if this correlates with the aPTT/aPTR. If the correlation is poor, it may be necessary to monitor using anti-Xa levels in place of aPTT/aPTR. For children <12 months of age, monitoring of UFH therapy using anti-Xa levels is often advocated, although there are no clinical outcome data to support one means of monitoring over another in a pediatric population.

When UFH therapy is being monitored, care must be taken to avoid heparin contamination of blood samples. This can be done by withdrawing a minimum of 8 ml of 'dead space' blood before taking a sample from a peripheral catheter for monitoring. To avoid significant blood loss, a common practice is to withdraw the 'dead space' blood in a sterile fashion and return it back. There are no published recommendations for the minimum amount of blood to discard prior to taking a sample from a central venous catheter, but it is likely that a greater volume would be required due to the greater volume of dead space. Wherever possible, drawing a blood sample from a peripheral vein in the contralateral arm to the heparin infusion is preferred.

Problems

Antithrombin Deficiency

Response to UFH can be reduced by the presence of AT deficiency. Infants <6 months have relative 'heparin resistance' due to a physiological deficiency of AT. Thus, in infants who cannot reach the required level of anticoagulation with UFH therapy, some suggest administration of AT concentrate [3]. However, this concentrate is expensive, not commonly available and no safety data exist for its use in infants. In addition, some studies raise the possibility of AT concentrates in neonates causing harm [4]. Acquired causes for AT deficiency, e.g. nephrotic syndrome, protein-losing enteropathy, L-asparaginase chemotherapy, may also result in heparin resistance which can respond to replacement of AT using AT concentrate. Again, it should be used with caution.

Heparin-Associated Thrombocytopenia

Heparin-associated thrombocytopenia is a benign fall in platelet count, rarely below $100 \times 10^9/l$. It is not associated with increased bleeding risk or thrombotic risk.

Heparin-Induced Thrombocytopenia

HIT is detailed below (p. 222).

Osteopenia

Osteopenia was reported secondary to prolonged administration of subcutaneous UFH in pregnant women. Only three cases of osteopenia have been reported in children treated with UFH.

Reversal

UFH can be rapidly reversed by stopping the infusion. Within 2–4 h, reversal will be adequate for the patient to undergo surgery. If more rapid reversal is required, e.g. major hemorrhage, protamine sulphate can be administered. This is given at a dose of 1 mg per 100 U of heparin received within the previous 2 h to a maximum of 50 mg, as a slow i.v. infusion. Care must be taken when giving protamine as high doses can be anticoagulant rather than procoagulant. Allergic reactions to the drug are not uncommon, particularly in children with fish allergy.

Low-Molecular-Weight Heparin

Mechanism of Action and Pharmacokinetics

LMWH have a similar mode of action to UFH, although they have a higher ratio of anti-factor Xa/IIa activity. They are given by s.c. injection, either once or twice daily, and peak levels occur at around 2–4 h after administration. The half-life is 2–4 h, i.e. longer than UFH. LMWH is excreted renally.

Indications

LMWH is the preferred agent for relatively short-term anticoagulant therapy (up to 3 months' duration) in stable children with a low bleeding risk. LMWH may be preferred to oral VKAs in children who have dietary problems, multiple interacting medications, need frequent reversal of anticoagulation for invasive procedures such as lumbar punctures and in infants who often have poor stability of VKA. LMWH is the preferred long-term therapy for adult cancer patients [5], but no specific advice exists for children with malignancy. It should be remembered that there are few safety data to support the use of LMWH for periods longer than 3 months in children in contrast to VKAs which are established as long-term anticoagulant agents.

Dosing

The dose of LMWH differs according to the age of the child and the clinical indication, i.e. therapeutic or prophylactic (table 2). There remains some debate over the optimal doses of LMWH in neonates [6].

When children are switched from UFH infusion to LMWH injections, the UFH infusion should be stopped at the same time that the first dose of LMWH is given.

Monitoring

LMWH therapy is monitored using the anti-Xa activity assay. The recommended therapeutic target range is 0.5–1.0 IU/ml in a sample taken 4–6 h after s.c. injection or 0.5–0.8 IU/ml in a sample taken 2–6 h after s.c. injection [1]. The anti-Xa assay is taken after the first dose for once daily regimes and after the second dose for twice daily regimes. Monitoring frequency will vary according to the age of the child but will usually occur after every change in dose and at least once weekly while the child is in hospital and once monthly when he/she is an outpatient, although there are no specific recommendations available in terms of the frequency of monitoring. LMWH doses are increased or reduced by varying increments depending on the degree of deviation from the therapeutic target range (table 3). Trough levels are monitored if there is a concern about accumulation of the drug, such as due to renal impairment, or to monitor efficacy in once daily dosing (trough level of ≥0.1 IU/ml) [7].

Table 2. Therapeutic and prophylactic dosing of enoxaparin, tinzaparin and dalteparin according to age

	Therapeutic dose	Prophylactic dose
Enoxaparin		
≤2 months of age	1.5 mg/kg s.c. bid	1.5 mg/kg s.c. od
>2 months of age	1 mg/kg s.c. bid	1 mg/kg s.c. od
Tinzaparin		
≤2 months of age	275 U/kg s.c. od	75 U/kg s.c. od
2–12 months of age	250 U/kg s.c. od	75 U/kg s.c. od
1–5 years	240 U/kg s.c. od	75 U/kg s.c. od
5–10 years	200 U/kg s.c. od	75 U/kg s.c. od
10–16 years	175 U/kg s.c. od	50 U/kg s.c. od
Dalteparin		
≤2 months of age	150 U/kg s.c. bid	150 U/kg s.c. od
>2 months of age	100 U/kg s.c. bid	100 U/kg s.c. od

Problems

Renal Impairment

LMWH can accumulate in the presence of significant renal impairment, i.e. glomerular filtration rate <30 ml/min. A 50% reduction in LMWH dose and more frequent monitoring is recommended for adults with significant renal impairment (as defined above), but no guidance for children exists.

Administration

Daily s.c. injections are poorly tolerated by some children. Bruising, hematoma formation and skin infection may occur at the injection sites. Some centers recommend the use of an s.c. port, such as the Insuflon™ device, into which the LMWH is injected. This port can be replaced every 5–7 days, avoiding daily needles. The occurrence of hematoma at the Insuflon injection site in low birthweight neonates has led some to avoid their use in neonates <3 kg in weight [8].

Heparin-Induced Thrombocytopenia

HIT is detailed below (p. 222).

Table 3. Adjustment of LMWH according to monitoring of anti-Xa levels

Anti-Xa level	Withhold next dose?	Dose change	Timing of next anti-Xa level
<0.35 IU/ml	no	increase by 25%	after next dose
0.36–0.49 IU/ml	no	increase by 15%	after next dose
0.5–1.0 IU/ml	no	no	after one week if hospitalized, one month if outpatient
1.01–1.25 IU/ml	no	decrease by 15%	after next dose
1.26–1.5 IU/ml	no	decrease by 25%	after next dose
1.51–2.0 IU/ml	yes	decrease by 30%	when next dose is due; if >1.5, continue to withhold dose and repeat after 12 h
>2.0 IU/ml	yes	decrease by 40%	when next dose is due; if >1.5, continue to withhold dose and repeat after 12 h

Reversal

Stopping LMWH therapy results in return to a non-anticoagulated state within 18–24 h of the last dose of tinzaparin (once daily dosing) and 8–12 h of the last dose of enoxaparin (twice daily dosing). If more rapid reversal is required, protamine sulphate may be given. LMWH is not as readily reversed by protamine sulphate as UFH (≈40–50%). The dose of protamine sulphate is estimated according to the degree of reversal required and the time elapsed since the last LMWH dose was given. If protamine sulphate is given within 8 h of the LMWH, then the maximum neutralizing dose is 1 mg protamine sulphate per 100 U (or 1 mg) of LMWH given in the last dose. If more than 8 h have elapsed, the dose is 0.5 mg protamine sulphate per 100 U (or 1 mg) of LMWH given. Repeated measurements of anti-Xa level may be necessary to monitor the efficacy of reversal using protamine sulphate, with further aliquots being given until the desired reduction in anti-Xa level is achieved. The maximum dose of protamine sulphate is 50 mg.

Vitamin K Antagonists

Mechanism of Action and Pharmacokinetics

Coumarin derivatives produce an anticoagulant effect by interfering with the cyclic conversion of vitamin K to its reduced form (vitamin K hydroquinone). VKA inhibits the regeneration of vitamin K hydroquinone from vitamin K epoxide by inhibiting the VKOR enzyme in the vitamin K cycle. Vitamin K hydroquinone is an essential cofactor for the post-ribosomal activation (γ-carboxylation) of coagulation factors II, VII, IX and X without which they are unable to bind calcium and become active in the coagulation cascade.

Coumarin derivatives are given orally and are rapidly absorbed from the gastrointestinal tract. However, the anticoagulant effect takes several days to develop due to the time taken for the circulating γ-carboxylated coagulation factors to undergo degradation. Warfarin is given as a once daily dose, preferably in the evening to allow dose adjustments to be made in response to monitoring. Warfarin is metabolized by the liver. The half-life of warfarin is approximately 40 h causing its anticoagulant effect to last for 3–5 days.

Indications

VKAs are used for children who require long-term anticoagulation therapy such as children with cardiac disease requiring chronic anticoagulation and children with a history of venous TE and persisting risk factors for recurrence. Warfarin is also occasionally used for shorter-term anticoagulant therapy in those who prefer to

Table 4. Adjustment of warfain dose according to INR during initiation and maintenance phases of therapy

	INR	Action
Initiation		
Day 1		If the baseline INR is 1.0–1.3, give 0.2 mg/kg orally (maximum 10 mg)
Days 2–4	1.1–1.3	repeat initial loading dose
	1.4–1.9	50% of initial loading dose
	2.0–3.0	50% of initial loading dose
	3.1–3.5	25% of initial loading dose
	>3.5	hold until INR <3.5 then restart at 50% of initial loading dose
Maintenance	1.1–1.4	increase dose by 20%
	1.5–1.9	increase dose by 10%
	2.0–3.0	no change
	3.1–3.5	decrease dose by 10%
	>3.5	hold until INR <3.5 then restart at 20% less than previous dose

receive treatment via an oral route as it is the oral anticoagulant for which there is the most safety data and experience in children.

Dosing

Warfarin is the most commonly used VKA in children. Acenocoumarol and phenprocoumon are used in some European and South American countries. Guidelines for the administration of warfarin are presented in table 4. Age-related loading doses of acenocoumarol are: 2 months to 1 year, 0.2 mg/kg; 1–5 years, 0.09 mg/kg; 6–10 years, 0.07 mg/kg; 11–18 years, 0.06 mg/kg [9]. The INR was developed for monitoring patients treated with a VKA (see below). The INR is the ratio of a patient's PT to a normal control sample, raised to the power of the International Sensitivity Index value for the analytical system used: (observed PT/control PT)^{ISI}, where ISI = international sensitivity index (sensitivity of thromboplastin). There is a marked variability between children in response to loading doses, and factors other than weight, such as liver disease, nutritional status and concurrent medications, are often taken into consideration when deciding a starting dose as these may all influence response to a VKA. The VKORC1 and CYP2C9 genotypes have also been shown to have a significant impact on warfarin dose requirements, and pharmacogenetics-based dosing of VKAs may become a reality in the future [10].

In the case of a newly diagnosed TE or thromboprophylaxis for high risk of thrombosis, VKA loading should begin when the child is on therapeutic doses of UFH or LMWH. UFH or LMWH therapy should be continued until the child has had 2 consecutive INRs that are within the desired therapeutic range.

Monitoring

The anticoagulant effect of VKA is monitored using the PT which becomes prolonged when the levels of active coagulation factors II, VII, IX and X fall. The degree of prolongation is proportional to the degree of anticoagulant effect. When used for monitoring VKA therapy, the PT is expressed as the INR, which is a means of standardizing results from different laboratories that may use different thromboplastin reagents and equipment. The INR is maintained within a desired therapeutic range that is dependent upon the clinical indication for anticoagulation (see relevant chapters). VKAs have a narrow therapeutic window and a deviation from the desired INR target range can result in a reduction in efficacy (if the INR is too low) or a hemorrhagic event (if the INR is too high).

Children receiving a VKA have regular INR checks. These can be done at a hospital anticoagulant clinic or a private laboratory. However, many children use point-of-care INR monitors, such as the Coaguchek® monitor. This allows a parent/carer to test the INR on a capillary blood sample and receive an immediate result. The result is then telephoned to the team managing the anticoagulant therapy who will advise on the warfarin dose required and when the INR should next be checked. Most studies in children have described home monitoring supported by anticoagulant clinics which have dosed the child, as distinct from self-management, and all had strong education components. The benefits of using a home monitoring device include less time taken off school/work and rapid response to situations that may result in deviation from target INR range, such as fever, diarrhea and interactions with other medications. The use of a point-of-care device, alongside appropriate education of the child and family, has been shown to improve anticoagulation control in children [11].

Interactions and Problems
Poor INR Control

Control of VKA in children is complicated by numerous factors such as complexity of the underlying health problem(s), multiple intercurrent viral illnesses and variation in the vitamin K content of the child's diet. In infants, additional problems include the challenge of accurate dosing (VKA is often only available in tablet form), increased sensitivity due to physiologically low levels of the vitamin-K dependent clotting factors and differences in vitamin K content of formula (more vitamin K) vs. breast milk (less vitamin K). Adolescents can also experience variability in INR due to alcohol intake. VKAs interact with many medications and herbal remedies that may potentiate or reduce the anticoagulant effect [12].

These problems mean that maintenance of INR within target range in children is often poor, with as few as 50% of measurements within range in some studies. This can be improved by close monitoring and awareness of the described problems.

Adolescent females taking a VKA should be aware of the risk of teratogenicity in the fetus should they become pregnant. This issue should be raised in a sensitive manner, but they should be aware that the VKA needs to be stopped immediately on discovery of pregnancy and that an alternative anticoagulant may be required.

Osteopenia

Long-term use of VKAs in children was associated with osteopenia in some studies. These studies lacked adequate control groups, and so the true cause of the osteopenia (VKAs vs. underlying disease vs. multifactorial) remains unclear. Still, some advise monitoring of bone mineral density with DEXA scanning on an annual or bi-annual basis in children receiving long-term VKA.

Reversal

The management needed for the reversal of a VKA depends on the INR, the presence or absence of bleeding symptoms and the indication for anticoagulant therapy.

The options for VKA reversal differ in the time of response:
- Stopping VKA: 3–5 days.
- Vitamin K: oral vitamin K, 24 h; i.v. vitamin K, 4–6 h. Doses of 30 µg/kg have been used i.v. in children [13]. Although there are no published data on the efficacy of VKA reversal using oral vitamin K in children, 1–2 mg as a single dose is often recommended, with a further dose 24 h later if the degree of reversal is inadequate. For children with active bleeding, particularly those who are unlikely to restart a VKA soon, 5 mg oral/i.v. vitamin K may be given.
- FP: 15 ml/kg – immediate effect.
- PCC: e.g. Octaplex, Beriplex, 25–50 U/kg – immediate effect.

For VKA associated with major hemorrhage (e.g. ICH; major gastrointestinal hemorrhage; other significant hemorrhage with >2 g/dl fall in hemoglobin or hemodynamic instability) or the need for urgent surgery, rapid reversal of VKA with PCC and i.v. vitamin K is indicated. If PCC is not available, FP should be used with i.v. vitamin K.

For VKA associated with minor hemorrhage – slower reversal with i.v. or oral vitamin K.

Table 5. Recommended dosing and monitoring for new anticoagulant agents in children

Anticoagulant agent	Mode of administration	Dose	Monitoring test	Target range
Bivalirudin	i.v.	0.125 mg/kg bolus, followed by 0.125 mg/kg/h infusion	aPTT	60–85 s
Argatroban	i.v.	0.75 µg/kg/min	aPTT	60–85 s
Fondaparinux	s.c.	0.1 mg/kg once daily	anti-Xa levels[1], although routine monitoring not required	0.5–1.0 IU/ml

[1] This assay must be calibrated with fondaparinux.

Raised INR without hemorrhage is usually managed conservatively by omission of one or more VKA doses and monitoring of INR unless there are significant risk factors for bleeding.

New Anticoagulant Agents

Introduction

In recent years, there has been much interest in the development of novel anticoagulants. These include oral and parenteral preparations; they are broadly divided into two groups according to their target for inhibition: direct thrombin inhibitors and FXa inhibitors. There is the potential for advantages of these agents over standard anticoagulant therapy in children with UFH, LMWH and VKAs, all of which can be problematic in this patient population for various reasons (refer to chapters above). Ideally, an oral agent would have advantages over a VKA, the major advantage being a predictable anticoagulation response when given as a fixed dose or dosed according to bodyweight that would obviate the need for monitoring. Other advantages would include a lack of interaction with other drugs and a lack of influence of diet and alcohol. Parenteral agents would have advantages over heparin with its risk of development of HIT (see p. 222) and potential heparin resistance resulting from AT deficiency in infants (see p. 213).

Many alternative oral anticoagulants have now been developed, and studies in adults are promising. There have been few studies of these agents in children, but this is an area in which we are likely to see significant advances in the relatively near future [14].

Direct Thrombin Inhibitors

The three DTIs that have been used in children are lepirudin, bivalirudin and argatroban.

Mechanism of Action

DTIs directly bind to and inhibit thrombin. They inhibit both thrombin that is within clot and circulating thrombin, in comparison to UFH and LMWH which only inhibit circulating thrombin.

Parenteral Preparations

Bivalirudin has been evaluated as an anticoagulant for the treatment of venous and arterial TEs in children <6 months of age, and dosing recommendations are shown in table 5. It has also been evaluated in the prevention of TEs during percutaneous coronary intervention, and safety was confirmed in children 0–16 years of age. Argatroban has been studied in children requiring alternative anticoagulation to heparin for HIT and was found to prevent TEs: dosing guidance is shown in table 5. The dose should be reduced in the presence of hepatic failure as argatroban is metabolized exclusively by the liver. Anticoagulation with lepirudin is associated with high bleeding rates in children, so it is not discussed here further.

Oral Preparations

The oral DTI that has shown the most promise in the anticoagulation of adults is dabigatran. It has a predictable dose-response and therefore does not require monitoring. Dabigatran is currently in early clinical trials in children, and its use cannot be recommended until studies of dosing, efficacy and safety are reported.

Monitoring

Bivalirudin and argatroban are monitored using the aPTT or aPTR in a similar way to UFH. Monitoring should occur 4 h after an initial bolus followed by an infusion or 6 h after starting an infusion without a bolus, should be repeated 4 h after each change in dose, and should be requested a minimum of 24 hourly.

Factor Xa Inhibitors

Mechanism of Action

These agents are highly selective inhibitors of FXa. They work independently of AT and do not inhibit thrombin.

Parenteral Preparations

Fondaparinux is a synthetic pentasaccharide FXa inhibitor which is administered s.c. as a once daily dose. There have been only a few reports of fondaparinux cross-reacting with HIT antibodies, so it can be safely used in patients with HIT or who are at risk of HIT. A prospective dose-finding and safety study of fondaparinux in children aged 1–18 years led to the dosing recommendations shown in table 5.

Oral Preparations

Rivaroxaban is an oral FXa inhibitor that is licensed for several indications in adults. International multi-center trials are currently underway and, until they are completed, rivaroxaban cannot be recommended for use in children.

In summary, Argatroban is currently the agent of choice for the anticoagulation of children with HIT. There is evidence base to support the use of bivalirudin during percutaneous coronary intervention. The DTIs may be useful, in preference to UFH, for the anticoagulation of children with low AT levels. Fondaparinux shows promise as a once-daily s.c. agent for the treatment of TEs in children.

Reversal

One of the major disadvantages of the new anticoagulant agents is the lack of available antidotes to reverse their anticoagulant effect. Suggested approaches to the reversal of new anticoagulant agents in the event of hemorrhage or the need for urgent surgery are as follows [15]:

Stop the Drug

Once stopped, the time taken for reversal of the anticoagulant effect depends on the half-life of the agent. For the parenteral DTIs, the half-life is short, particularly for bivalirudin which has a half-life of approximately 25 min. The half-life of fondaparinux is 17–21 h.

Treat Mechanical Causes of Bleeding

This may require endoscopy, invasive radiological procedures (such as vessel embolization) or surgery.

Antifibrinolytic Agents/DDAVP

Antifibrinolytic agents/DDAVP may reduce bleeding.

Consider FP/rFVIIa/PCCs/aPCCs

Although these agents have no specific effect against the new anticoagulant agents, they may be useful. PCCs and aPCCs (e.g. FEIBA) are helpful in the reversal of DTIs but rFVIIa is not as its hemostatic effect relies on the generation of a 'thrombin burst'. Due to their high content of FX (refer to the appendix for details), PCCs and aPCCs may be useful in the reversal of direct FXa inhibitors.

Dialysis

Although this has not been well studied, hemodialysis probably adequately removes dabigatran from the circulation because it is the least protein bound of the novel oral DTIs.

Antiplatelet Therapy

Mechanism of Action and Pharmacokinetics

Antiplatelet agents inhibit platelet aggregation and therefore prevent them from performing their role in primary hemostasis. The mechanism of action varies according to the specific agent. Typical antiplatelet agents and their mechanisms of action are listed below.

Acetylsalicylic Acid

Inhibition of the cyclooxygenase enzyme prevents the formation of thromboxane via the cyclooxygenase pathway (chapter 2). The enzyme is irreversibly inhibited, so the effect of ASA can last for 5–7 days after the last dose as this is the duration of time that it takes for new platelets to be generated.

Dipyridamole

Inhibition of adenosine deaminase and phosphodiesterase results in an accumulation of adenosine and cAMP, which causes a reduction in platelet aggregation in response to ADP (chapter 2). The effect of dipyridamole lasts for only 12–24 h after the last dose is given.

Clopidogrel

Inhibition of the P_2Y_{12} subtype of the ADP receptor inhibits platelet aggregation by blocking activation of the GP IIb/IIIa pathway (chapter 2).

It is a pro-drug, so its effects can be seen for as long as 14 days after the last dose is given due to ongoing conversion of pro-drug to active drug.

Indications

Antiplatelet agents are usually used to treat and prevent arterial thrombosis. In children, they are most frequently used for the prevention of recurrent ischemic stroke, thrombosis of endovascular stents and for the treatment of Kawasaki disease.

Dosing

The doses for the common antiplatelet agents for children are: ASA, 1–5 mg/kg/day; dipyridamole, 2–5 mg/kg/day; clopidogrel, 0.2 mg/kg/day [rounded to one quarter or one half tablets (75-mg tablets)]. All are given as a single daily dose.

Monitoring

The efficacy of antiplatelet agents is usually monitored clinically, i.e. by the assessment of their ability to prevent TEs. The clinical utility of laboratory monitoring of antiplatelet therapy is debated. Platelet aggregation studies may be performed to demonstrate a reduction in platelet response to agonists, including arachidonic acid (inhibited in the presence of ASA) and ADP (inhibited in the presence of dipyridamole or clopidogrel). A newer technique, known as platelet-mapping thromboelastography, uses a global hemostatic test (thromboelastography) to demonstrate inhibition of platelet response to arachidonic acid and ADP.

Problems

Bleeding

Antiplatelet agents can result in hemorrhagic complications. These usually take the form of mucocutaneous bleeding, i.e. bruising, epistaxis, oral cavity bleeding, but can result in gastrointestinal bleeding and posttraumatic bleeding. Gastrointestinal bleeding is a particular problem with ASA due to its tendency to cause gastric inflammation and ulceration.

Reye's Syndrome

Reye's syndrome is a rare complication of ASA therapy in children usually associated with doses >40 mg/kg. This dose is much higher than that required for antiplatelet therapy, and is more consistent with ASA doses when used as an antipyretic or analgesic. ASA should not be used for these indications in children. Reye's syndrome may be temporally associated with viral illness and results in hepatitis and encephalopathy with the potential for long-term morbidity and mortality in relation to brain damage.

Reversal

Stopping the antiplatelet agent will reverse the antiplatelet effect within 24 h for dipyridamole, 5–7 days for ASA, and 7–14 days for clopidogrel. In the case of ongoing or major hemorrhage associated with antiplatelet therapy or the need for urgent surgery, transfusion of platelet concentrate 15 ml/kg should be considered. Transfused platelets will not be sensitive to the effects of ASA or dipyridamole once the agent is stopped, but repeated platelet transfusions may be required for clopidogrel-related bleeding due to the ongoing production of active drug from pro-drug. In life-threatening bleeding, administration of off label rFVIIa could be considered.

Thrombolysis

Mechanism of Action and Pharmacokinetics

The most frequently used thrombolytic agent in pediatric practice is rt-PA (Alteplase®) [16]. rt-PA catalyzes the conversion of plasminogen to plasmin which in turn converts fibrin to FDPs (chapter 2). rt-PA is rapidly metabolized by the liver with a half-life of only 5 min.

Indications and Contraindications

Thrombolysis is reserved for cases of severe arterial or venous thrombosis in which rapid restoration of blood flow is likely to improve outcome either in the short-term or long-term, particularly where there is risk of loss of life, limb or organ (see relevant chapters).

Thrombolysis is contraindicated in the presence of active bleeding, head injury, recent trauma/surgery, recent childbirth, recent cardiopulmonary resuscitation, congenital bleeding disorder and uncontrolled systolic hypertension.

If there are concerns that there may be ICH, e.g. in a premature neonate, imaging must be performed to rule this out before commencing thrombolysis.

The decision to administer thrombolytic therapy is often a multidisciplinary one and should involve discussion with the child and/or their parents due to the risk of bleeding complications. Many of the contraindications are 'relative', and the potential benefits of thrombolysis may still outweigh the risks even if contraindications are present.

Dosing

Due to its short half-life, rt-PA is administered by continuous i.v. infusion.

Systemic Thrombolysis

While a number of dosing regimens have been reported, most commonly, rt-PA is administered at a dose of 0.5 mg/kg/h as a continuous infusion for 6 h. A low-dose UFH infusion is administered concurrently at 10 U/kg/h to prevent further thrombus formation. If the child was previously receiving full-dose UFH, the infusion rate must be reduced 30 min prior to starting thrombolytic therapy. The rate is increased to full dose 30 min after completion of a 6-hour infusion of rt-PA.

Response to thrombolysis is assessed after 6 h using appropriate imaging, and the course may be repeated if indicated.

Due to physiological deficiency of plasminogen, children <1 year of age receiving thrombolytic therapy are pre-treated with 15 ml/kg FP in order to provide a source of plasminogen. Administration of FP can be considered for older children who fail to respond to thrombolysis.

Catheter-Directed Thrombolysis

This may be an option if the site of the thrombus can be accessed, e.g. placement of a catheter adjacent to the site of a vascular thrombus. The dose of rt-PA for local thrombolysis varies between centers and can range from 0.01 mg/kg/h to 0.05 mg/kg/h. The dose may be increased if lysis is not achieved.

Preparation and Monitoring

Children receiving thrombolysis are frequently nursed on a pediatric intensive care unit. All staff should be made aware that thrombolytic therapy is being administered. Baseline bloods include CBC, PT, aPTT, fibrinogen, D-dimer. A crossmatch sample should be sent in case blood transfusion is required.

During thrombolysis, the risk of hemorrhage can be reduced by the avoidance of arterial puncture, catheterization, intramuscular injections, physiotherapy, excessive handling/personal care, ASA/nonsteroidal anti-inflammatory agents.

Most protocols suggest that the CBC, PT, aPTT, fibrinogen and D-dimer should be repeated after 4 h and every 8 h thereafter. The fibrinogen level is expected to fall, and the D-dimer levels are expected to rise. If this does not occur, it may mean that the lysis is not optimal. Aim to maintain a platelet count of >50 × 10^9/l using infusion of 15 ml/kg platelet concentrate (refer to the appendix for details of platelet dosing).

Management of Thrombolysis-Related Bleeding

Major bleeding during thrombolytic therapy occurs in 10–30% of children. Management depends on the severity of the bleeding. The following should be considered: stopping infusion of rt-PA and UFH; use of local measures to achieve hemostasis, such as pressure at wound site or nasal packing; administration of cryoprecipitate to reverse the thrombolytic effect of rt-PA and administration of protamine sulphate to reverse the UFH effect. In major life-threatening bleeding, administration of off label rFVIIa should be considered.

Heparin-Induced Thrombocytopenia

Introduction

HIT is a complication of UFH and LMWH that results in thrombocytopenia and a predisposition to the occurrence of TEs [17].

Incidence

HIT is a very infrequent occurrence in childhood, with rates ranging from almost zero in unselected heparinized children to 2.3% of children in the pediatric intensive care unit setting. Reports suggest the incidence in children is much less than expected if the rate of developing HIT relative to heparin exposure was the same as that observed in adults, raising the possibility that children are protected from developing HIT through as yet undefined mechanisms.

Clinical Presentation

HIT presents with a fall in platelet count of >50% from the highest platelet count that immediately precedes the HIT-associated platelet count fall, usually to around a median of 50 × 10^9/l. Thrombosis can be venous or arterial. There can be an anaphylactoid reaction to i.v. bolus UFH administration or following s.c. LMWH injections; some patients develop necrotizing skin reactions at the sites of s.c. injection. Thrombosis occurs in 50–70% of adults within one month of diagnosis of HIT and can be fatal. The data available in a pediatric population are limited [18].

Table 6. Calculation of pre-test probability score (the 4 Ts score) for suspected HIT

Criterion	Points
Degree of **T**hrombocytopenia	
>50% fall and platelet nadir >20 × 10⁹/l	2
30–50% fall or platelet nadir 10–19 × 10⁹/l	1
Fall <30% or platelet nadir <10 × 10⁹/l	0
Timing of thrombocytopenia	
Onset between days 5–10 of heparin or <1 day if recent heparin exposure	2
Consistent with days 5–10 fall, but not clear or onset after day 10	1
Platelet count fall <4 days and no recent heparin exposure	0
Presence of **T**hrombosis	
New thrombosis (confirmed)/skin necrosis/systemic reaction	2
Progressive/recurrent/suspected thrombosis	1
None	0
Presence of o**T**her causes for thrombocytopenia	
None	2
Possible	1
Definite	0

Low score, 0–3; intermediate score, 4–5; high score, 6–8.

Diagnosis

The diagnosis of HIT is dependent upon the presence of suggestive clinical features in association with abnormal laboratory tests. The criteria used in adults to assess the pre-test probability of HIT are the 4Ts (table 6), although it should be noted that this score has not been validated in a pediatric population.

Most laboratories will provide an ELISA test for the detection of anti-PF4/heparin antibodies. These tests have a high sensitivity for HIT but a low specificity as anti-PF4/heparin antibodies are often present in the absence of HIT, i.e. there is a high rate of false-positive results. A serotonin-release assay provides a more specific result, but samples may need to be sent to a reference laboratory.

Management

The management of children with HIT is currently extrapolated from adult data and should always involve the advice of a hematologist. Given the apparent very low rate of HIT in children, specific testing for HIT should be limited as the rate of false positives is high, and it is often difficult not to act on a positive test. However, substitution of all heparin for an alternative anticoagulant (argatroban, danaparoid, fondaparinux, lepirudin, bivalirudin) that does not cross-react with HIT antibodies has considerable risks. Hence, in all cases the diagnosis should be confirmed and risk-benefit ratio considered.

Management of Anticoagulant Therapy during Surgery

Introduction

Anticoagulation during the perioperative period can increase the risk of surgical bleeding. For all anticoagulated children undergoing a surgical procedure, it is essential that there is close communication between the hematology/thrombosis and surgical teams. Anticoagulated children and their parents/carers should be advised to inform the hematology/thrombosis team if a surgical or dental procedure is scheduled.

The perioperative management of anticoagulation prior to surgery will depend on the risk of TE whilst off anticoagulant therapy, the type of anticoagulant drug and the nature of the surgery in terms of the bleeding risk (table 7).

These lists are not comprehensive, and clinical scenarios will often need to be assessed on an individual basis prior to deciding on a plan for the management of anticoagulation therapy during surgery.

Major Risk of Bleeding

Management of Anticoagulation during Surgery with a Major Risk of Bleeding and Low Risk of Thrombosis

Anticoagulant therapy can safely be stopped prior to surgery and restarted postoperatively when the bleeding risk is acceptable. The exact

Table 7. Assessment of risk of thrombosis and bleeding during interruption of anticoagulant therapy for surgery

Risk of thrombotic event whilst off anticoagulation	
High risk	Recent VTE (within the previous 6 weeks), recurrent VTE, metal prosthetic heart valve (especially mitral), major thrombophilic abnormality[1], antiphospholipid syndrome, stroke
Low risk	Fontan procedure, distant history of VTE, central venous catheter-associated DVT
Risk of bleeding from surgical procedure	
Major bleeding risk	Neuro-/spinal surgery, intra-abdominal surgery, major orthopedic surgery
Minor bleeding risk	Dental extractions, excision of small skin lesion, grommet insertion

[1] Antithrombin deficiency; protein S deficiency; protein C deficiency; combined thrombophilic defect, e.g. double heterozygosity for FVL mutation and Prothrombin gene mutation.

schedule will depend upon the type of anticoagulant therapy due to the variation in half-life between different agents.

Vitamin K Antagonist

In order to allow the INR to fall to <1.5, warfarin is stopped 4–5 days prior to the surgical procedure. The INR is checked on the morning of surgery to ensure that it is safe to proceed. VKA can be restarted within 24 h of surgery if the bleeding risk is felt to be low. In this situation, VKA is usually restarted at the child's usual maintenance dose.

Low-Molecular-Weight Heparin

The last therapeutic dose of tinzaparin or enoxaparin should be given at least 24 h prior to surgery. In patients who are not at excessive risk of thrombosis, it is usual practice to start a prophylactic daily dose of LMWH the evening following surgery (provided that there is no bleeding) and to continue this until the bleeding risk is felt to be low and therapeutic anticoagulation can be restarted.

Unfractionated Heparin

This is stopped 4 h prior to a major surgical procedure and is restarted once the bleeding risk is low, usually at least 24 h after surgery.

Management of Anticoagulation during Surgery with a Major Risk of Bleeding and High Risk of Thrombosis

'Bridging anticoagulant therapy' is needed to ensure that the period of time that the child is not anticoagulated is as short as is safe in terms of the bleeding risk associated with surgery.

Vitamin K Antagonist

The INR should be measured 2–3 days after stopping the VKA and an alternative anticoagulant agent administered if the INR is below the desired therapeutic INR range. This can be a therapeutic dose of LMWH up until 12–18 h prior to surgery or UFH as an infusion that is stopped 4 h prior to surgery. Postoperatively, a UFH infusion may be started 4–6 h after surgery if there is no active bleeding, and this is continued until it is safe to restart LMWH and/or VKA.

Low-Molecular-Weight Heparin

The last dose of LMWH should be given at least 12 h prior to surgery for a twice daily dosing regime or 18 h prior to surgery for a once daily dosing regime. A previous study of a small number of children on a twice daily dosing regime with LMWH has showed residual anti-factor Xa activity was present 12 h after a dose in the majority of those children, so omission of LMWH for at least 24 h may be safer for procedures which carry a high risk of hemorrhage-associated morbidity/mortality, e.g. neuro-/spinal surgery, lumbar puncture [19]. Postoperatively, an UFH infusion may be started 4–6 h after surgery if there is no active bleeding, and this is continued until it is safe to restart the LMWH.

Unfractionated Heparin
The UFH infusion should be stopped 4 h prior to surgery and may be restarted 4–6 h after surgery if there is no active bleeding.

In children with an extremely high risk of pulmonary embolism, e.g. in the case of a recent proximal DVT, who are undergoing a surgical procedure with a major risk of bleeding, e.g. brain tumor resection, it may not be safe to allow the child to remain without anticoagulant therapy for the duration of time that is required to prevent surgical bleeding. In this situation, it is appropriate to insert an IVC filter in order to prevent further thromboembolism. Anticoagulation can be deferred for up to 14 days after IVC filter insertion. It is recommended that a temporary IVC filter is inserted and that it is removed as soon as practical as long-term complications of IVC filters can include filter migration (to the heart or pulmonary vessels) and erosion of the IVC wall. Thrombus may form proximal and/or distal to the filter, resulting in PE or significant lower limb swelling.

Minor Risk of Bleeding

Management of Anticoagulation during Surgery with a Minor Risk of Bleeding
Vitamin K Antagonist
It may not be necessary to stop VKA for some procedures, e.g. dental extraction. An INR measurement on the day of the procedure is advised to ensure that it is not above the desired therapeutic INR range. For other procedures, halving the warfarin dose for 2–3 days prior to the procedure will allow the INR to drift down to the lower part of the therapeutic range allowing the surgery to proceed safely. The usual maintenance dose is reinstated or a loading dose is given on the evening following surgery.

Low-Molecular-Weight Heparin
It may not be necessary to stop LMWH therapy, but the timing of the dose should be altered so that surgery occurs at the trough level and the LMWH dose is given immediately after the procedure provided that there is no bleeding.

Management of Antithrombotic Therapy in Children with Thrombocytopenia

Introduction
Children requiring anticoagulant, antiplatelet or thrombolytic therapy may become thrombocytopenic for other reasons, most commonly chemotherapy or sepsis. The risk of continuing antithrombotic therapy in thrombocytopenic children is increased risk of bleeding. However, thrombocytopenia in itself is not protective in terms of thrombosis. Generally speaking, children with thrombocytopenia who require antithrombotic therapy fall into two categories: (a) Those in whom antithrombotic therapy may be reduced in relation to the degree of thrombocytopenia as the risk of thrombosis is relatively low; (b) Those in whom antithrombotic therapy must be continued due to a high risk of thrombosis and in whom a 'safe' platelet count may need to be maintained using transfusion of platelet concentrates. Management decisions will often need to be individualized according to the particular needs of the child. There is no published evidence on this topic, and the recommendations below are based on consensus opinion.

Anticoagulant Therapy
UFH or LMWH therapy may be given at a reduced intensity in children with thrombocytopenia. Doses are often halved when the platelet

Table 8. Risk factors for thrombosis and bleeding in hospitalized children

Risk factors for thrombosis
Patient-related factors: Adolescent/post-pubertal, obesity, central venous catheter, malignancy, congenital heart disease, nephrotic syndrome, inflammatory bowel disease, sickle cell disease, known thrombophilic abnormality, estrogen-containing contraceptive pill, pregnancy or post-partum, previous VTE, family history of VTE
Admission-related factors: Immobility, major abdominal/pelvic surgery, major orthopedic surgery (especially lower limb), sepsis, severe trauma, severe burns

Risk factors for bleeding
Thrombocytopenia, recent head injury, recent neurosurgery/eye surgery, recent spinal surgery, congenital or acquired bleeding disorder, acute stroke, uncontrolled systolic hypertension, recent lumbar puncture or spinal/epidural anesthesia

count is $<50 \times 10^9/l$ and UFH/LMWH is stopped when the platelet count is $<30 \times 10^9/l$. Daily monitoring of the platelet count allows for UFH/LMWH to be restarted at half or full dose once the platelet count recovers to the desired threshold. For children who are at a particularly high risk of a TE, e.g. recent TE (within the last 6 weeks), it may be necessary to continue therapeutic doses of UFH/LMWH. In this situation, platelet concentrates may be transfused in order to maintain a platelet count of $>50 \times 10^9/l$. Oral anticoagulant therapy is often avoided in children who are thrombocytopenic or who are likely to become thrombocytopenic, e.g. children receiving chemotherapy. LMWHs are preferred due to their shorter half-life.

Thrombolytic Therapy

Thrombolytic therapy is usually reserved for a significant TE that threatens life, limb or organ. A platelet count threshold of $>50 \times 10^9/l$ is sometimes recommended prior to thrombolysis. It may be necessary to transfuse platelet concentrates in order to achieve this prior to or concurrent to commencing thrombolytic therapy, depending on the clinical urgency of thrombolysis. In other cases a surgical approach, e.g. embolectomy, may be preferred in a child with thrombocytopenia and a high risk of bleeding.

Antiplatelet Therapy

A platelet count threshold of $>50 \times 10^9/l$ is considered by some to be adequate for antiplatelet therapy. Children with a lower platelet count may continue antiplatelet therapy if the risk of thrombosis is considered to be higher than the risk of bleeding. These children should be monitored closely for the occurrence of hemorrhagic symptoms.

Thromboprophylaxis

Indications

Thromboprophylaxis refers to measures taken to reduce the risk of TE. Successful thromboprophylaxis relies on the identification of children who are at significant risk for TEs (table 8) and who therefore have the potential to benefit from preventative measures. These risk factors must be balanced against the risk of bleeding (table 8).

General Measures

Adequate hydration, early mobilization after surgery and prompt removal of central venous and arterial catheters, when possible, are important to reduce the risk of TE in hospitalized children.

Mechanical Thromboprophylaxis

Graduated compression stockings may be used to prevent lower limb DVT in hospitalized children. Pneumatic calf compression devices may be used during surgery in children who are at risk of DVT.

Chemical Thromboprophylaxis

The usual agents for short-term thromboprophylaxis are the LMWHs and the doses are shown in table 2. Monitoring is not usually required but a trough anti-Xa activity level after 2–3 doses can be useful to rule out accumulation in children with significant renal impairment.

Long-term thromboprophylaxis may involve the use of a VKA. This is particularly the case for the prevention of catheter-related thrombosis in children with indwelling central catheters for total parenteral nutrition. Some studies have supported the administration of warfarin, with an INR target range of 1.5–1.9.

Travel-Related Thromboembolism

In children who have had a previous VTE and/or have significant risk factors, it is appropriate to offer advice regarding prevention of VTE for flights of >6 hours' duration and for long journeys using other modes of transport that involve immobility. This general advice includes adequate hydration and frequent mobilization in addition to early reporting of symptoms of VTE. The use of chemical thromboprophylaxis to prevent travel-related VTE is not currently recommended in adults [20], and there is no evidence for this practice in children.

Acknowledgment

The authors would like to express their appreciation for the thoughtful comments provided by Drs. Laura Avila (Toronto, Ont., Canada), Mattia Rizzi (Toronto, Ont., Canada) and Leonardo R. Brandão (Toronto, Ont., Canada), Ted Warkentin (Hamilton, Ont., Canada) and Yaser Diab (Washington, D.C., USA) who reviewed this chapter.

References

1 Monagle P, Chan AKC, Goldenberg NA, Ichord RN, Journeycake JM, Nowak-Göttl U, Vesely S: Antithrombotic therapy in neonates and children: Antithrombotic therapy and prevention of thrombosis, ed 9: American College of Chest Physicians Evidence-Based Clinical Practice Guidelines. Chest 2012;141:e737S–e801S.
2 Newall F, Barnes C, Ignjatovic V, Monagle P: Heparin-induced thrombocytopenia in children. J Paediatr Child Health 2003;39:289–292.
3 Manco-Johnson MJ: How I treat venous thrombosis in children. Blood 2006;107:21–29.
4 Schmidt B, Gillie P, Mitchell L, Andrew M, Caco C, Roberts R: A placebo-controlled randomized trial of antithrombin therapy in neonatal respiratory distress syndrome. Am J Respir Crit Care Med 1998;158:470–476.
5 Aki EA, Vasireddi SR, Gunukula S, Barba M, Sperati F, Terrenato I, Muti P, Schünemann H: Anticoagulation for the initial treatment of venous thromboembolism in patients with cancer. Cochrane Database Syst Rev 2011;CD006649.
6 Malowany JI, Monagle P, Knoppert DC, Lee DS, Wu J, McCusker P, Massicotte MP, Williams S, Chan AK, Canadian Paediatric Thrombosis and Hemostasis Network: Enoxaparin for neonatal thrombosis: a call for a higher dose for neonates. Thromb Res 2008;122:826–830.
7 Trame MN, Mitchell L, Krümpel A, Male C, Hempel G, Nowak-Göttl U: Population pharmacokinetics of enoxaparin in infants, children and adolescents during secondary thromboembolic prophylaxis: a cohort study. J Thromb Haemost 2010;8:1950–1958.
8 Dix D, Andrew M, Marzinotto V, Charpentier K, Bridge S, Monagle P, deVeber G, Leaker M, Chan AKC, Massicotte MP: The use of low molecular weight heparin in pediatric patients: a prospective cohort study. J Pediatr 2000;136:439–445.
9 Bonduel M, Sciuccati G, Hepner M, Feliu Torres A, Pieroni G, Frontroth JP, Serviddio RM: Acenocoumarol therapy in pediatric patients. J Thromb Haemost 2003;1:1740–1743.
10 Biss TT, Avery PJ, Brando LR, Chalmers EA, Williams MD, Grainger JD, Leathart JBS, Hanley JP, Daly AK, Kamali F: VKORC1 and CYP2C9 genotype and patient characterics explain a large proportion of the variability in warfarin dose requirement among children. Blood 2012;119:868–873.
11 Bauman ME, Black K, Kuhle S, Wand L, Legge L, Callen-Wicks D, Mitchell L, Bajzar L, Massicotte MP: KIDCLOT©: The importance of validated educational intervention for optimal long term warfarin management in children. Thromb Res 2009;123:707–709.
12 Bonduel MM: Oral anticoagulation therapy in children. Thromb Res 2012;118:85–94.
13 Bolton-Maggs P, Brook L: The use of vitamin K for reversal of over-warfarinization in children. Br J Haematol 2002;118:924.
14 Young G: New anticoagulants in children: a review of recent studies and a look to the future. Thromb Res 2011;127:70–74.

15 Crowther MA, Warkentin TE: Bleeding risk and the management of bleeding complications in patients undergoing anticoagulant therapy: focus on new anticoagulant agents. Blood 2008;111:4871–4879.
16 Williams MD: Thrombolysis in children. Br J Haematol 2010;148: 26–36.
17 Klenner A, Greinacher A: Heparin-induced thrombocytopenia in children; in Warkentin T, Greinacher A (eds): Heparin-Induced Thrombocytopenia, ed 4. New York, Informa Healthcare USA, 2007, pp 503–517.
18 Newall F, Ignjatovic V, Johnston L, Summerhayes R, Lane G, Cranswick N, Monagle P: Age is a determinant factor for measures of concentration and effect in children requiring unfractionated heparin. Thromb Haemost 2010;103:1085–1090.
19 Dix D, Charpentier K, Sparling C, Massicotte MP: Determination of trough anti-factor Xa levels in pediatric patients on low molecular weight heparin (LMWH). J Pediatr Hematol Oncol 1998;20: 667.
20 Kahn SR, Lim W, Dunn AS, Cushman M, Dentali F, Akl EA, Cook DJ, Balekian AA, Klein RC, Le H, Schulman S, Murad MH: Prevention of VTE in nonsurgical patients: antithrombotic therapy and prevention of thrombosis, ed 9: American College of Chest Physicians Evidence-Based Clinical Practice Guidelines. Chest 2012;141: e195S–e226S.

Abbreviations

ACT	Activated clotting time
ADP	Adenosine 5′-diphosphate
Anti-Xa	Anti-factor Xa
aPCC	Activated prothrombin complex concentrate
aPTT	Activated partial prothrombin time
aPTR	Activated partial thromboplastin ratio
ASA	Acetylsalicyclic acid
AT	Antithrombin
CBC	Complete blood count
CPB	Cardiopulmonary bypass
CYP2C9	Cytochrome P450 2C9
DDAVP	1-deamino-8-D-arginine vasopressin (desmopressin)
DTI	Direct thrombin inhibitor
DVT	Deep vein thrombosis
ECMO	Extracorporeal membrane oxygenation
ELISA	Enzyme-linked immunosorbent assay
FDP	Fibrin degradation product
FEIBA	FVIII inhibitor bypass activity
FP (FFP)	Frozen plasma (Fresh frozen plasma)
FII	Factor II (prothrombin)
FVII	Factor VII
FVIII	Factor VIII
FIX	Factor IX
FX	Factor X
FVL	Factor V Leiden
GP	Glycoprotein
HIT	Heparin-induced thrombocytopenia
ICH	Intracranial hemorrhage
INR	International normalized ratio
IVC	Inferior vena cava
LMWH	Low-molecular-weight heparin
PCC	Prothrombin complex concentrate
PF4	Platelet factor 4
PT	Prothrombin time
rFVIIa	Recombinant activated factor VII
rt-PA	Recombinant tissue-plasminogen activator
TE	Thromboembolism/thromboembolic event
UFH	Unfractionated heparin
VKA	Vitamin K antagonist
VKOR	Vitamin K epoxide reductase
VKORC1	Vitamin K epoxide reductase complex subunit 1
VTE	Venous thromboembolism/thromboembolic event

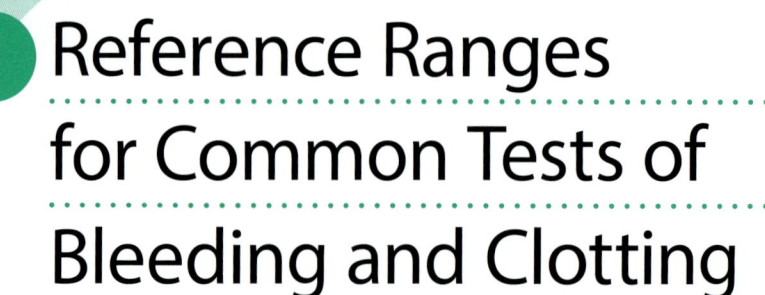

Appendix I: Reference Ranges for Common Tests of Bleeding and Clotting

Vicky R. Breakey

Reference Ranges for Common Tests of Bleeding and Clotting

In order to assist the clinician, the following table of reference ranges is included (table 1). These are the current reference ranges reported by the laboratory at The Hospital for Sick Children (Toronto, Ont., Canada). They are provided as an example of normal ranges for common tests in pediatric thrombosis and hemostasis. It is important for the reader to note that the generation of local normal ranges is suggested by a recent formal ISTH SSC report [1]. The main recommendation of the consensus report was that all diagnostic laboratories processing pediatric samples for hemostasis assays should use age, analyzer and reagent specific reference ranges. Suggested age ranges were specified. Aware of the difficulty of each laboratory to perform its own reference levels, hemostasis test results can be compared across laboratories provided the population, reagent and analyzer are identical.

Variations of Reference Values Based on Age

As discussed in detail in chapter 4, there is some variation in normal ranges for coagulation factors based on the age of the patient. Landmark work done by Dr. Maureen Andrew and colleagues studied this variation and tables 2 and 3 show their findings with values shown representing 95% of the population (mean ± 2 SD) [2–4]. Additional investigations provided similar ranges for preterm infants [5]. More recent work by Dr. Paul Monagle and colleagues [6] demonstrates that the absolute values of reference ranges for coagulation tests vary with analyzer and reagent systems. This emphasizes the importance of laboratories developing age-related reference ranges specific to local equipment [1].

Table 1. Common blood product dosing [1, 2]

Blood component	Dosage	Description
Red cell concentrates	10–15 ml/kg BW (increases hemoglobin 20–30 g/l)	- approximately 250–300 ml/U - hematocrit approximately 0.6 - in patients >20 kg the transfusion volume is rounded to the nearest number of packed RBC concentrate
Frozen plasma	10–20 ml/kg BW (max. 3–4 U)	- approximately 200 ml/U - contains all coagulation factors and complement
Cryoprecipitate	1 U/7–10 kg BW raises fibrinogen 0.5 g, to a maximum of 10 U	- approximate volume 10 ml/unit - contains fibrinogen (average 200 mg/U) - contains FVIII, VWF, FXIII
Cryosupernatant	10–50 ml/kg BW	- approximately 250 ml/unit - plasma deficient in high-molecular-weight multimers of VWF
Platelet concentrates	10–15 ml/kg BW or 1 U whole blood-derived platelets/5–10 kg BW, up to the equivalent of 1 U of apheresis platelet or 5–6 U of whole blood derived platelets	- whole blood-derived platelets 50–60 ml/U - buffy coat pool (300 ml) - apheresis platelets (single donor platelets) (300 ml)

Adapted from 'The Hospital for Sick Children Transfusion Medicine Blood and Blood Product Information' pocketcard, Department of Pediatric Laboratory Medicine, July, 2008.

used for fractionation then it is tested by nucleic acid testing for parvovirus B19 by the fractionation facility.

In most developed countries, the safety of plasma-derived products is further achieved by pathogen inactivation of plasma-derived coagulation factors using solvent-detergent treatment, pasteurization, methylene blue, psoralen and/or nano-filtration. There are rarer and emerging pathogens, including prions, zoonotic viruses, protozoa that are not routinely screened for whose risk of blood-borne transmissibility and overall prevalence must still be clarified.

The processing of whole blood donation involves separation into components. These components include RBCs, platelets, frozen plasma, cryoprecipitate and cryosupernatant. Fractionated blood products from plasma include albumin, intravenous immunoglobulin, subcutaneous immunoglobulin, various factor concentrates and PCC.

Blood Components (table 1)

Red Blood Cell Concentrates

Transfusion of RBCs may be needed to support excessive blood loss to ensure adequate tissue oxygen delivery. Standard pediatric dosing is 10–15 ml/kg (increases hemoglobin 20–30 g/l) [1, 2]. It is generally recommended to round the volume needed to the nearest unit to limit exposure and minimize wastage.

Frozen Plasma

Fresh frozen plasma (FFP, frozen within 8 h of whole blood collection) and frozen plasma (FP, frozen within 24 h of whole blood collection) contain all clotting factors. Levels of FV and FVIII may be reduced in FP as compared to FFP. FP is the product currently used in clinical practice.

The current recommendations for the use of FP [2] include:
1 The treatment of active bleeding, or prior to surgery or an invasive procedure, in patients

Appendix II

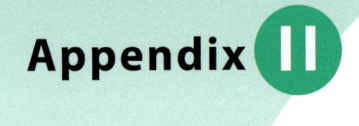

Common Products Used to Manage Bleeding and Clotting

Ewurabena Simpson
Mira Liebman

Disclaimer: Dosing guidelines are suggestions based on the current practices at the Hospital for Sick Children, Toronto, Ont., Canada. Doses do not necessarily conform to the manufacturer's recommendations and not all products are licensed for use in children. It is essential that the reader be aware of product monographs and verifies the indications, contraindications and recommended doses.

Blood and Blood Product Information

Blood components that are commonly used for the treatment of pediatric bleeding disorders include RBC concentrates, platelet concentrates, frozen plasma, cryoprecipitate, cryosupernatant and plasma-derived components, including factor concentrates.

Transfusion Basics

Blood Product Collection and Testing

Blood products are prepared from blood obtained through voluntary donations. Blood donation centers are run by agencies who oversee processing, distribution and administration of blood products. Blood is collected as whole blood or as plasma, RBCs or platelets in the case of apheresis donation. Once blood is collected, it is tested, processed and made into various blood products.

Before an individual can donate blood they undergo screening using a questionnaire, vital sign assessment and a hemoglobin measurement. The units collected are tested for blood groups, RBC antibodies and assessment for blood borne infections. There is variation in this testing internationally. For example, in Canada, testing is done for HIV 1 (including group O), HIV2 and HCV through antibody and nucleic acid testing, hepatitis B using surface antigen, core antibody and nucleic acid testing, HTLV I and II with antibody testing and West Nile Virus using nucleic acid testing. Bacteria tested for are syphilis via serology and bacterial culture is done on platelet products only. Chagas disease is tested for in at risk donors by antibody testing. If plasma is

Table 2. Reference values for coagulation tests by age compared to adults (bold values are significantly different to adults)

	Day 1	Day 5	Day 30	Day 90	Day 180	1–5 years	6–10 years	11–16 years	Adult (>16 years)
PT, s	10.1–15.9	10.0–15.3	10.0–14.3	10.0–14.2	10.7–13.9	10.6–11.4	10.1–12.1	10.2–12	11.0–14.0
aPTT, s	**31.3–54.5**	**25.4–59.8**	**32.0–55.2**	29.0–50.1	28.1–42.9	24–36	26–36	26–37	27–40
FII, U/ml	**0.26–0.70**	**0.33–0.93**	**0.34–1.02**	**0.45–1.05**	**0.60–1.16**	**0.71–1.16**	**0.67–1.07**	**0.61–1.04**	0.70–1.46
FV, U/ml	**0.34–1.08**	**0.45–1.45**	**0.62–1.34**	**0.48–1.32**	**0.55–1.27**	0.79–1.27	**0.63–1.16**	**0.55–0.99**	0.62–1.50
FVII, U/ml	**0.28–1.04**	**0.35–1.43**	**0.42–1.38**	**0.39–1.43**	**0.47–1.27**	**0.55–1.16**	**0.52–1.20**	**0.58–1.15**	0.67–1.43
FVIII, U/ml	0.61–1.39	0.55–1.21	0.58–1.24	0.56–1.02	0.55–0.91	0.59–1.42	0.58–1.32	0.53–1.31	0.50–1.49
VWF-Ag, U/ml	**0.50–2.87**	**0.50–2.54**	**0.50–2.46**	**0.50–2.06**	**0.50–1.97**	0.60–1.20	0.44–1.44	0.46–1.53	0.50–1.58
FIX, U/ml	**0.15–0.91**	**0.15–0.91**	**0.21–0.81**	**0.21–1.13**	**0.36–1.36**	**0.47–1.04**	**0.63–0.89**	**0.59–1.22**	0.55–1.63
FX, U/ml	**0.12–0.68**	**0.19–0.79**	**0.31–0.87**	**0.35–1.07**	**0.38–1.18**	**0.58–1.16**	**0.55–1.01**	**0.50–1.17**	0.70–1.52
FXI, U/ml	**0.10–0.66**	**0.23–0.87**	**0.27–0.79**	**0.41–0.97**	**0.49–1.34**	0.56–1.50	**0.52–1.20**	**0.50–0.97**	0.67–1.27
FXII, U/ml	**0.13–0.93**	**0.11–0.83**	**0.17–0.81**	**0.25–1.09**	**0.39–1.15**	0.64–1.29	0.60–1.40	**0.34–1.37**	0.52–1.64
PK, U/ml	**0.18–0.69**	**0.20–0.76**	**0.23–0.91**	**0.41–1.05**	**0.56–1.16**	0.65–1.30	0.66–1.31	0.53–1.45	0.62–1.62
HMWK, U/ml	**0.06–1.02**	**0.16–1.32**	**0.33–1.21**	0.30–1.46	0.36–1.28	0.64–1.32	0.60–1.30	0.63–1.19	0.50–1.36
FXIII-a, U/ml	**0.27–1.31**	0.44–1.44	0.39–1.47	0.36–1.72	0.46–1.62	**0.72–1.43**	**0.65–1.51**	0.57–1.40	0.55–1.55
FXIII-b, U/ml	**0.30–1.22**	0.32–1.80	0.39–1.73	0.48–1.84	0.50–1.70	**0.69–1.56**	**0.77–1.54**	0.60–1.43	0.57–1.37

Table 3. Reference values for the inhibitors of coagulation in healthy babies and children compared to adults (bold values are significantly different to adults)

	Day 1	Day 5	Day 30	Day 90	Day 180	1–5 years	6–10 years	11–16 years	Adult (>16 years)
AT, U/ml	**0.39–0.87**	**0.41–0.93**	**0.48–1.08**	0.73–1.21	0.84–1.24	0.82–1.39	0.90–1.31	0.77–1.32	0.77–1.30
Protein C, U/ml	**0.17–0.53**	**0.20–0.64**	**0.21–0.65**	**0.28–0.80**	**0.37–0.81**	**0.40–0.92**	**0.45–0.93**	**0.55–1.11**	0.70–1.80
Protein S, U/ml	**0.12–0.60**	**0.22–0.78**	**0.33–0.93**	0.54–1.18	0.55–1.19	0.21–0.69	0.22–0.62	0.26–0.55	0.24–0.62

References

1. Ignjatovic V, Kenet G, Monagle P: Perinatal and Paediatric Haemostasis Subcommittee of the Scientific and Standardization Committee of the International Society on Thrombosis and Haemostasis. J Thromb Haemost 2012;10:298–300.
2. Andrew M, Vegh P, Johnston M, Bowker J, Ofosu F, Mitchell L: Maturation of the hemostatic system during childhood. Blood 1992;80:1998–2005.
3. Andrew M, Paes B, Milner R, Johnston M, Mitchell L, Tollefsen DM, Powers P: Development of the human coagulation system in the full-term infant. Blood 1987;70:165–172.
4. Andrew M, Paes B, Johnston M: Development of the hemostatic system in the neonate and young infant. Am J Pediatr Hematol Oncol 1990;12:95–104.
5. Andrew M, Paes B, Milner R, Johnston M, Mitchell L, Tollefsen DM, et al: Development of the human coagulation system in the healthy premature infant. Blood 1988;72:1651–1657.
6. Monagle P, Barnes C, Ignjatovic V, et al: Developmental haemostasis. Impact for clinical haemostasis laboratories. Thromb Haemost 2006;95:362–372.

Abbreviations

aPTT	Activated partial thromboplastin time
aPC	Activated protein C
AT	Antithrombin
FII	Factor II (prothrombin)
FV	Factor V
FVIII	Factor VIII
FIX	Factor IX
FX	Factor X
FXI	Factor XI
FXII	Factor XII
FXIII	Factor XIII
HMWK	High-molecular-weight kininogen
INR	International normalized ratio
ISTH	International Society on Thrombosis and Haemostasis
PK	Prekallikrein
PT	Prothrombin time
PTT	Partial thromboplastin time
VWF	von Willebrand factor
VWF:Ag	VWF antigen
VWF:RCo	VWF activity (ristocetin cofactor assay)

Table 1. Normal ranges for common tests in the work-up of children with bleeding or clotting disorders as reported in the laboratory at the Hospital for Sick Children (as of December 2012)

Test	Reference intervals
INR	
<3 months	0.90–1.60
>3 months to 21 years	0.8–1.20
aPTT, s	
<3 months	25–45
>3 months to 21 years	24–36
Fibrinogen, g/l	
<3 months	1.6–4.0
>3 months to 21 years	1.9–4.4
D-dimer, µg/ml FEU	
<3 days	<2.50
4 days to 21 years	<0.50
FII, IU/ml	
<3 days	0.41–0.73
4 days to 21 years	0.83–1.47
FV, IU/ml	
<3 days	0.64–1.54
4 days to 21 years	0.71–1.68
FVIII activity, IU/ml	
<3 days	0.83–3.29
4 days to 21 years	0.56–1.72
FIX activity, IU/ml	
<3 days	0.35–0.97
4 days to 21 years	0.74–1.66
FX, IU/ml	
<3 days	0.46–0.75
4 days to 21 years	0.69–1.54
FXI activity, IU/ml	
<3 days	0.07–0.79
4 days to 21 years	0.63–1.52
FXII,	
<3 days	0.13–0.97
4 days to 21 years	0.40–1.49
FXIII	for details of FXIII testing, see chapter 9
VWF:Ag, IU/ml	
Patients with blood group O	0.47–1.39
Patients with blood group non-O	0.84–1.92
VWF:RCo, IU/ml	
>3 months, blood group O	0.38–1.22
>3 months, blood group non-O	0.73–1.81

Test	Reference intervals
Protein C activity, IU/ml	
1–3 days	0.24–0.51
4 days to 1 year	0.28–1.24
>1–21 years	0.64–1.77
Protein S antigen, IU/ml	
1–3 days	0.28–0.67
4 days to 1 year	0.29–1.62
>1–21 years	0.67–1.94
AT, U/ml	0.80–1.30
Reptilase time, s	<20
Thrombin time, s	<21
aPC resistance	>2.4
Antiphospholipid antibody screen	tests done include: lupus sensitive aPTT, DRVVT (diluted Russell's viper venon test) screen and confirm, and hexagonal phase test
Anticardiolipin antibody (IgG), U/ml	anticardiolipin antibody by ELISA technique
Negative	<10
Equivocal	10–15
Positive	>15
Lipoprotein (a), mg/dl	
Male	<36
Female	<35
Homocysteine, µmol/l	
<5 years	0.5–11.0
6–12 years	5.0–12.0
13–59 years	5.0–15.0
>60 years	5.0–20.0

Acknowledgment: Dr. William Brien, Department of Pediatric Laboratory Medicine, The Hospital for Sick Children.

with acquired deficiencies of one or more coagulation factors when no alternative therapies are available or appropriate.
2. Active bleeding, or prior to surgery, or an invasive procedure in patients with a congenital factor deficiency when no alternative therapies are available or appropriate.
3. Reversal of VKAs (e.g. warfarin) effect or immediate correction of vitamin K deficiency in patients with active bleeding, or prior to surgery, or an invasive procedure (if PCC is not available).
4. Consumptive coagulopathy or DIC with active bleeding.
5. TTP (if plasmapheresis is not available immediately).

See chapter 8 for more information on the management of rare coagulation factor deficiencies and chapter 9 for management of TTP and DIC.

Cryoprecipitate

Cryoprecipitate describes several insoluble proteins that are separated from liquid plasma after partial thawing of one unit of frozen plasma at a temperature between 1 and 6°C for 24 h. These proteins include fibrinogen, fibronectin, FVIII, FXIII as well as VWF [1, 2].

The relative content of coagulation factors within any given unit of cryoprecipitate depends on the original level of these factors prior to blood/plasma donation. Approximately 40–70% of the FVIII and VWF that was originally present in the donor plasma will remain in a single unit of cryoprecipitate, which is approximately 70–100 IU of FVIII/VWF. Each unit of cryoprecipitate will also contain a minimum of 150 mg of fibrinogen and 40–60 IU of FXIII [2].

Cryosupernatant

After the separation of cryoprecipitate, the residual liquid plasma is known as cryoprecipitate-poor plasma or cryosupernatant. This residual plasma can be frozen for ultimate transfusion or further processed to separate its albumin and gamma globulin (intravenous immunoglobulin) components. Cryosupernatant may be indicated for the treatment of TTP and HUS as it does not contain high weight multimers of VWF (see chapter 9) [2].

Platelet Concentrates

Transfusion of platelets is necessary in cases of bleeding due to thrombocytopenia or platelet function abnormality (see chapter 5). Transfusion of platelets may also be given prophylactically for platelets counts of less than $10 \times 10^9/l$ and for prophylaxis prior to invasive procedures at the discretion of the surgeon.

Whenever possible, platelets should be ABO compatible. Dosing of platelets at 5–10 ml/kg should increase platelet count by $30–60 \times 10^9/l$ [1, 2]. HLA-matched whole blood-derived platelets can be considered for patients who are refractory to random platelets [1].

Factor Concentrates

Factor concentrates are either derived from human plasma or produced using recombinant cell lines. Purified plasma-derived factor concentrates are obtained from large pools of donated plasma or cryoprecipitate, which are separated and reduced. The concentrated product is subsequently treated using the methods described above to inactivate pathogens.

Specific information about FVIII and FIX deficiencies can be found in chapter 6, about VWF deficiency in chapter 7 and about rare congenital factor deficiencies in chapter 8. In addition, a 'Registry of Clotting Factor Concentrates' has been developed by the World Federation of Hemophilia can be found at http://www1.wfh.org/publication/files/pdf-1227.pdf. The registry provides an overview of the products available internationally and clarifies the differences between them.

Fibrinogen Concentrates

Fibrinogen concentrates (e.g. RiaSTAP® and Haemocomplettan P®; CSL Behring), are currently indicated for routine or surgical prophylaxis and for the management of hemorrhage in patients with congenital or acquired fibrinogen deficiencies (chapter 8). These fibrinogen concentrates are usually available in 1 and 2 g freeze-dried formulations, which contain approximately 900–1,300 and 1,800–2,600 mg of human fibrinogen, respectively [2, 3].

Factor VII Concentrates

Purified plasma-derived FVII concentrates, e.g. Factor VII (Baxter), Factor VII (BPL, UK), Provertin-Um TIM3 (Baxter), are indicated for the treatment of congenital FVII deficiency (chapter 8). It is important to note that FVII concentrates are associated with an increased risk of thrombosis when administered at high doses.

rFVIIa (e.g. Novoseven, Novo Nordisk) is indicated for the treatment of bleeding in patients with congenital FVII deficiency (chapter 8) and for the prophylaxis and management of acute bleeding in patients with hemophilia A or B, who have developed inhibitors to FVIII and FIX (chapter 6). It may also be used in patients with platelet dysfunction, like GT who are refractory to platelet transfusion (chapter 5) [1–3]. rFVIIa has a short half-life and is generally administered every 2–6 h to achieve hemostasis [2].

Factor VIII Concentrates

FVIII concentrates are indicated for the treatment and prevention of bleeding episodes, perioperative prophylaxis as well as routine bleeding prophylaxis in adults and children with hemophilia A (chapter 6). Recombinant FVIII products are either full-length (e.g. Advate®, Kogente-FS®) or B-domain deleted molecules (e.g. Xyntha®) that are produced in mammalian cell culture and subsequently purified using immunoaffinity methods. Details on the dosing for FVIII in patients with hemophilia are available in chapter 6 [4].

Factor IX Concentrates

FIX concentrates are indicated for the treatment and prevention of bleeding episodes as well as perioperative prophylaxis in adult and pediatric patients with hemophilia B (chapter 6).

von Willebrand Factor Concentrates

There are plasma-derived FVIII products which contain significant quantities of VWF. A new recombinant VWF is under development. When available, these preparations are used instead of cryoprecipitate for the treatment of significant bleeding in patients with VWD (chapter 7).

Prothrombin Complex Concentrates

PCCs are human plasma-derived FIX complexes, which contain coagulation factors II, VII, IX and X as well as human-derived protein S and protein C. Some forms of PCCs also contain antithrombin. PCCs can be divided into two categories based on their composition. All PCCs contain factors II, IX and X (3-factor PCC) and some contain higher levels of FVII (4-factor PCC). 4-factor PCC is a newer product and may not be easily available.

PCC is indicated for the treatment of bleeding episodes and peri-operative prophylaxis of bleeding in acquired deficiencies of the prothrombin complex coagulation factors, such as deficiency caused by treatment or overdose with VKA (chapter 16). Some studies suggest that the 4-factor PCC is more effective in the reversal of VKA effects (normalization of INR) due to the higher content of FVII. The second licensed indication for the use of PCC is for the treatment of bleeding and perioperative prophylaxis in patients with congenital deficiencies of the coagulation factors II, VII and X when purified specific factor concentrates are not available (chapter 8). Due to the large number of PCCs availably internationally, it is recommended to consult the drug monograph for specifics of administration and dosing.

Table 2. Protein C concentrate

	Initial dose	Subsequent 3 doses	Maintenance dose
Acute episode/short-term prophylaxis	100–120 IU/kg BW	60–80 IU/kg BW q6 h	45–60 IU/kg BW q6 or 12 h
Long-term prophylaxis	NA	NA	45–60 IU/kg BW q12 h

Activated Prothrombin Complex Concentrates

Activated prothrombin complex (FEIBA®, Baxter) is a human plasma-derived FIX complex that contains FIX and various amounts of factors II and X, mainly activated FVII and trace levels of FVIII. FEIBA bypasses FVIII activity in patients who cannot respond normally to FVIII due to the presence of FVIII inhibitors. FEIBA is indicated for the treatment and prophylaxis of bleeding episodes in patients with hemophilia A and inhibitor to FVIII, in hemophilia B patients with inhibitor to FIX and in nonhemophiliac patients with acquired inhibitors to factors VIII, IX and XI. For specific recommendations on the management of hemophilia patients with inhibitors, see chapter 6.

Factor XI Concentrates

Human plasma-derived FXI concentrate (Hemoleven® LFB, France) is indicated only for the treatment of patients with significant FXI deficiency (chapter 8). The plasma-derived product is heat treated.

Factor XIII Concentrates

A human plasma-derived FXIII product (Fibrogammin® P, CSL Behring; Corifact®, CSL Behring) has been developed and licensed for the prophylactic treatment of congenital FXIII deficiency (chapter 8). A recombinant FXIII (Catridecacog®, Novo Nordisk) is currently available in Europe for patients >6 years of age.

Protein C Concentrate

Protein C concentrate (Ceprotin®, Baxter) is a highly purified plasma-derived product which may be indicated for the treatment of patients with congenital protein C deficiency for the prevention and treatment of VTE and for the treatment of purpura fulminans in pediatric patients with meningococcemia [4] (table 2).

Antithrombin Concentrate

Antithrombin concentrate is available in plasma-derived (Thrombate®, Grifols) and recombinant (ATryn, GCT Biotherapeutics) formulations. It may be indicated for patients with acquired or congenital antithrombin deficiency in a high-risk situation for thrombosis [5] (see chapter 16 for discussion on the use of antithrombin concentrate in children with acquired antithrombin deficiency and heparin resistance).

To calculate the dose (IU) = desired % increase × BW (kg) (usual dose is approximately 100 IU/kg body weight).

Dosage should be individualized for each patient, but recommendation is that initial loading dose is calculated to achieve a target plasma antithrombin level of 120% (1.2 IU/ml). Treatment goal is to achieve and maintain antithrombin activity levels between 80 and 120% (0.8–1.2 IU/ml) of normal [2].

After antithrombin therapy has been initiated, close monitoring of antithrombin activity levels is required for effective treatment. Measure preinfusion and postinfusion (20 min peak) plasma antithrombin levels. Then measure levels 12 h after initial dose and then at the trough prior to subsequent dosing to ensure therapeutic target plasma antithrombin levels of 80–120% (0.8–1.2 IU/ml) of normal [2].

Other Agents for Achieving Hemostasis

Desmopressin

Patients with mild type 1 VWD or mild hemophilia A (with FVIII coagulant activity >5%) with minor bleeding can be managed with DDAVP. DDAVP test is usually recommended for type 1 VWD and mild hemophilia A prior to its use in the clinical setting (see chapters 6 and 7 for details). DDAVP may be used for mild-to-moderate bleeding in patients with platelet function defects (chapter 5). Intravenous dosing of DDAVP has led to hyponatremia and severe decreases in plasma osmolality especially in young children, which can lead to coma, seizures and death. Fluid restriction during administration and close monitoring of serum sodium levels and urine output are necessary (table 3).

Antifibrinolytics

Antifibrinolytics are drugs which exert their effect through inhibition of fibrinolysis. They interfere with the production of plasmin from plasminogen. They are used for excessive bleeding and are particularly useful for surgical bleeding and mucocutaneous bleeding.

Tranexamic acid and ε-aminocaproic acid are synthetic derivatives of the amino acid lysine. They competitively inhibit the activation of plasminogen to plasmin and bind to specific sites on both plasminogen and plasmin which prevents the degradation of fibrin [2]. These drugs should be used with caution in patients with renal insufficiency and/or genitourinary hemorrhage (table 4).

Topical Hemostatic Agents

Topical hemostatic agents are used in various surgical scenarios to aid in clot formation. There are various products available. These include physical agents such as bone wax, ostene, and dry matrix, biologically active agents like topical thrombin (human or bovine) and fibrin sealants and tissue adhesives such as cyanoacrylate and bovine albumin-glutaraldehyde tissue adhesive [2] (table 5).

Table 3. DDAVP/desmopressin

Dosing

Intravenous/subcutaneous
Children ≥3 years: 0.3 µg/kg BW (maximum dose 20 µg slow intravenous infusion) (over 20–30 min in 50 ml of isotonic saline) beginning 30–90 min before procedure; may repeat dose if needed. Fluid restriction should be observed.

Intranasal
Children >12 years: ≤50 kg: 150 µg (1 spray); >50 kg: 300 µg (1 spray each nostril). Repeat intranasal use is determined based on the patient's clinical status and laboratory investigations; if used pre-operatively, should be administered 2 h prior to surgery.

Table 4. Antifibrinolytics

Product	Dose
Tranexamic acid	
Intravenous	10 mg/kg/dose preprocedure and tid-qid after until able to take p.o.
Oral	25 mg/kg/dose tid-qid beginning evening prior to procedure and for up to 3–10 days after tranexamic acid 5% mouthwash: qid starting on the day of dental/oral surgery beginning 5–10 min before the extraction.
ε-Aminocaproic acid	
Oral, intravenous	loading dose: 100–200 mg/kg BW maintenance dose: 100 mg/kg/dose every 6 h maximum daily dose: 30 g

Table 5. Topical hemostatic agents

Product	Indications
Physical agents	
Bone wax, ostene	blood oozing from the cut surface of medullary bone (e.g. following median sternotomy, orthopedic and neurosurgery procedures)
Dry matrix	
Gelatin matrix	applied directly to sites of low flow bleeding; absorbs water and concentrates hemostatic factors at the site of bleeding, and tamponades bleeding vessels by exerting pressure
Oxidized regenerated cellulose	
Microporous polysaccharide spheres	
Microfibrillar collagen	
Biologically active agents	
Topical thrombin	may be used for the management of diffuse bleeding from pleural and/or peritoneal, or for localized areas of bleeding
Fibrin sealants	

Acknowledgment

The authors would like to express their appreciation for the thoughtful comments provided by Drs. Wendy Lau (Toronto, Ont., Canada), Nancy Robitaille (Montreal, Que., Canada) and Jeremy Robertson (Sydney, N.S.W., Australia) who reviewed this chapter.

References

1. Callum JL, Ontario Regional Blood Coordinating Network: Bloody Easy 3. Blood Transfusions, Blood Alternatives, and Transfusion Reactions: A Guide to Transfusion Medicine. Toronto, Ontario Regional Blood Coordinating Network, 2011.
2. Canadian Blood Services: Circular of Information for the Use of Human Blood and Blood Components. Ottawa, Canadian Blood Services, 2009.
3. World Federation of Hemophilia: Registry of Factor Concentrates, ed 9. Available online at: http://www1.wfh.org/publication/files/pdf-1227.pdf.
4. Veldman A, Fischer D, Wong FY, Kruez W, Sasse M, Eberspacher B, Mansmann U, Schosser R: Human protein C concentrate in the treatment of purpura fulminans: a retrospective analysis of safety and outcome in 94 pediatric patients. Crit Care 2010;14:R156.
5. Rodgers GM: Role of antithrombin concentrate in treatment of hereditary antithrombin deficiency. An update. Thromb Haemost 2009;101:806–812.

Abbreviations

BW	Body weight
DDAVP	1-Deamino-8-D-arginine vasopressin (desmopressin)
DIC	Disseminated intravascular coagulation
FP (FFP)	Frozen plasma (Fresh frozen plasma)
FVII	Factor VII
FVIII	Factor VIII
FIX	Factor IX
FXIII	Factor XIII
GT	Glanzmann thrombasthenia
HCV	Hepatitis C
HIV	Human immunodeficiency virus
HLA	Human leukocyte antigens
HUS	Hemolytic uremic syndrome
PCC	Prothrombin complex concentrate
RBC	Red blood cell
rFVIIa	Recombinant activated factor VII
TTP	Thrombotic thrombocytopenic purpura
VKA	Vitamin K antagonist
VTE	Venous thromboembolism/thromboembolic event
VWD	von Willebrand disease
VWF	von Willebrand factor

Abbreviations

	International Standards
p.o.	Per oral
s.c.	Subcutaneous
i.m.	Intramuscular
i.v.	Intravascular
U	Unit
EU	Equivalent unit
IU	International unit
l	Liter
dl	Deciliter
ml	Milliliter
fl	Femtoliter
kg	Kilogram
g	Gram
mg	Milligram
µg	Microgram
µmol	Micromole
qid	Four times a day
tid	Three times a day
bid	Twice a day
od	Once a day
h	Hour
min	Minute
s	Second

A

ABI	Ankle-brachial index
ACA	Anterior cerebral artery
ACLA	Anticardiolipin antibodies
ACT	Activated clotting time
ADAMTS13	A disintegrin and metalloproteinase with a thrombospondin type 1 motif, member 13
ADP	Adenosine 5′-diphosphate
aHUS	Atypical hemolytic uremic syndrome
AIS	Arterial ischemic stroke
$α_2$-AP	$α_2$-Antiplasmin
Anti-Xa	Anti-factor Xa
aPC	Activated protein C
aPCC	Activated prothrombin complex concentrate
APLA	Antiphospholipid antibodies
APLS	Antiphospholipid syndrome
aPTR	Activated partial thromboplastin ratio
aPTT	Activated partial thromboplastin time
ARC	Arthrogryposis-renal dysfunction-cholestasis
ASA	Acetylsalicylic acid
AT	Antithrombin
ATE	Arterial thromboembolism/thromboembolic event
ATP	Adenosine triphosphate
AVWS	Acquired von Willebrand syndrome

B

BCS	Budd-Chiari syndrome
$β_2$-GPI	Anti-$β_2$-glycoprotein antibody
BSS	Bernard-Soulier syndrome
BT shunt	Blalock-Taussig shunt
BU	Bethesda unit
BV	Bioprosthetic valve
BW	Body weight

C

CA	Coronary artery
CAMT	Congenital amegakaryocytic thrombocytopenia
CBC	Complete blood count
CCAD	Cervicocephalic arterial dissection
CFB	Complement factor B
CFH	Complement factor H
CFHR	Complement factor H-related proteins
CFI	Complement factor I
CHD	Congenital heart disease
CLD	Chronic liver disease
CNS	Central nervous system
COX	Cyclooxygenase
CPB	Cardiopulmonary bypass
CRF	Chronic renal failure
CSVT	Cerebral sinovenous thrombosis
CT	Computed tomography
CTA	Computed tomography angiography
CTPA	Computed tomography pulmonary angiography
CTPH	Chronic thromboembolic pulmonary hypertension
CTV	Computed tomography venography
CVC	Central venous catheter
CYP2C9	Cytochrome P450 2C9

D

DDAVP	1-deamino-8-D-arginine vasopressin (desmopressin)
DIC	Disseminated intravascular coagulation
DTI	Direct thrombin inhibitor
DUS	Doppler ultrasonography
DVT	Deep vein thrombosis

E

EACA	Epsilon-aminocaproic acid (Amicar)
ECMO	Extracorporeal membrane oxygenation
EEG	Electroencephalography
ELISA	Enzyme-linked immunosorbent assay
EN-RBD	European Network of Rare Bleeding Disorders

F

FCA	Focal cerebral ateriopathy
FDPs	Fibrin degradation products
FEIBA	FVIII inhibitor bypass activity
FNAIT	Fetal and neonatal alloimmune thrombocytopenia
FP (FFP)	Frozen plasma (Fresh frozen plasma)
FPD/AML	Familial platelet disorder and predisposition to acute myelogenous leukemia
FII	Factor II (prothrombin)
FV	Factor V
FVII	Factor VII
FVIII	Factor VIII
FIX	Factor IX
FX	Factor X
FXI	Factor XI
FXIII	Factor XIII
FVL	Factor V Leiden
FVIII:C	Factor VIII coagulant

G

GA	Gestational age
GGCX	γ-Glutamyl carboxylase
GI	Gastrointestinal
GP	Glycoprotein
GPS	Gray platelet syndrome
GT	Glanzmann thrombasthenia

H

HAT	Hepatic artery thrombosis
HCT	Hematocrit
HCV	Hepatitis C virus
HIT	Heparin-induced thrombocytopenia
HIV	Human immunodeficiency virus
HLA	Human leukocyte antigens
HLAS	Hypoprothrombinemia-lupus anticoagulant syndrome
HMWK	High-molecular-weight kininogen
HPA	Human platelet alloantigens
HSCT	Hematopoietic stem cell transplantation
HTC	Hemophilia treatment center
HUS	Hemolytic uremic syndrome

I

ICH	Intracranial hemorrhage
IE	Infective endocarditis
INR	International normalized ratio
ISTH	International Society on Thrombosis and Haemostasis
ITI	Immune tolerance induction
ITP	Immune thrombocytopenia
IVC	Inferior vena cava
IVH	Intraventricular hemorrhage
IVIG	Intravenous immunoglobulin

K

KD	Kawasaki disease
KMP	Kasabach-Merritt phenomenon

L

LAC	Lupus anticoagulant
LDH	Lactate dehydrogenase
LDL	Low-density lipoprotein
LMWH	Low-molecular-weight heparin
Lp(a)	Lipoprotein(a)
LTA	Light transmission aggregometry

M

MCA	Middle cerebral artery
MCP	Membrane cofactor protein
MDS	Myelodysplastic syndrome
MI	Myocardial infarction
MMR	Measles, mumps, rubella
MPV	Mean platelet volume
MRA	Magnetic resonance angiography
MRI	Magnetic resonance imaging
mRNA	Messenger RNA
MRPA	Magnetic resonance pulmonary angiography
MRV	Magnetic resonance venography
MTHFR	Methylenetetrahydrofolate reductase
MV	Mechanical valve
MVT	Mechanical valve thrombosis
MYH9	Myosin heavy chain 9

N

NA	Not available
NAT	Neonatal autoimmune thrombocytopenia
NEC	necrotizing enterocolitis
NS	Normal saline
NSAIDs	Nonsteroidal anti-inflammatory drugs

P

PA	Pulmonary artery
PAI-1	Plasminogen activator inhibitor type 1
PBQ	Pediatric Bleeding Questionnaire
PCC	Prothrombin complex concentrate
PCR	Polymerase chain reaction
PDA	Patent ductus arteriosus
PE	Pulmonary embolism
PFA-100®	Platelet function analyzer-100
PFD	Platelet function defect
PFO	Patent foramen ovale
PICC	Peripheral inserted central catheter
PIOPED	Prospective investigation of pulmonary embolism diagnosis
PISAPED	Prospective investigation study of acute pulmonary embolism diagnosis
PF4	Platelet factor 4

PRP	Platelet-rich plasma		**U**	
PT	Prothrombin time		UAC	Umbilical artery catheter
PTS	Postthrombotic syndrome		UFH	Unfractionated heparin
PVT	Portal vein thrombosis		ULVWF	Unusually large von Willebrand factor
			UVC	Umbilical vein catheter
	R		u-PA	Urokinase plasminogen activator
RAT	Renal artery thrombosis			
RBC	Red blood cell			**V**
rFVIIa	Recombinant activated factor VII		VAD	Ventricular assist device
rFXIII	Recombinant factor XIII		VK	Vitamin K
Rh	Rhesus		VKA	Vitamin K antagonist
RIPA	Ristocetin-induced platelet aggregation		VKDB	Vitamin K deficiency bleeding
rt-PA	Recombinant tissue-plasminogen activator		VKOR	Vitamin K epoxide reductase
RVT	Renal vein thrombosis		VKORC1	Vitamin K epoxide reductase complex subunit 1
			V/Q scan	Ventilation-perfusion scan
	S		VSD	Ventricular septal defect
SaO_2	Oxygen saturation		VT	Vascular thrombosis
SCD	Sickle cell disease		VTE	Venous thromboembolism/thromboembolic event
SCPC	Superior cavopulmonary connection			
SLE	Systemic lupus erythematosus		VWD	von Willebrand disease
SOS	Sinusoidal obstruction syndrome		VWF	von Willebrand factor
SpVT	Splenic vein thrombosis		VWF:Ag	VWF antigen
SVC	Superior vena cava		VWF:CBA	VWF collagen binding activity
			VWF:RCo	VWF activity (ristocetin cofactor assay)
	T			
TAFI	Thrombin-activatable fibrinolysis inhibitor			**W**
			WAS	Wiskott-Aldrich syndrome
TAR	Thrombocytopenia with absent radii		WBC	White blood cell
TCD	Transcranial Doppler			
TE	Thromboembolism/thromboembolic event			**X**
			XLT	X-linked thrombocytopenia
TEG	Thromboelastography			
TEM	Transmission electron microscopy			
TF	Tissue factor			
TFPI	Tissue factor pathway inhibitor			
TIA	Transient ischemic attack			
t-PA	Tissue-plasminogen activator			
TT	Thrombin time			
TTP	Thrombotic thrombocytopenic purpura			
TxA_2	Thromboxane A_2			

In the algorithms, **bold** type denotes diagnoses and *italics* denote treatments, unless otherwise stated.

Subject Index

Activated clotting time (ACT)
    heparin monitoring 215
    mechanical circulatory support coagulation considerations 197
Activated partial thromboplastin time (aPTT)
    bleeding child evaluation 20
    disseminated intravascular coagulation 106
    heparin monitoring 215
    thrombosis 131
    von Willebrand disease 82
ADAMTS13, thrombotic thrombocytopenic purpura pathophysiology 111, 112
Afibrinogenemia 96
Aggregometry, see Platelet aggregometry
ε-Aminocaproic acid (EACA)
    acquired von Willebrand disease management 120
    overview 240
    platelet function defect management 54, 55
    von Willebrand disease management 85
Ankle-brachial index (ABI), peripheral arterial insufficiency 161
Anti-cardiolipin antibodies (ACLA), thrombophilia testing 134, 135
Anti-D, immune thrombocytopenia management 49
Anti-factor Xa activity assay, heparin monitoring 215, 217, 219
$α_2$-Antiplasmin, functional overview 11, 12
Antithrombin
    coagulation regulation 9
    deficiency 134, 216
    transfusion 239, 240
Aortic thrombosis
    clinical presentation 159
    diagnosis 159
    management 159
    overview 158
Argatroban, see Direct thrombin inhibitors

Arterial ischemic stroke (AIS)
    clinical presentation 180
    diagnosis 180–182
    management
        antithrombotic therapy 182, 183
        cardiogenic stroke 183
        cervicocephalic arterial dissection as cause 183–185
        endovascular intervention 187
        moyamoya disease 185, 186
        neonates 183
        neuroprotection 182
        sickle cell disease 186, 187
        thrombolysis 187
    overview 179, 180
Arterial thromboembolism (ATE), see also specific diseases
    complications 160, 161
    epidemiology 154
    non-catheter causes 160
    renal artery stents 160
Arthropathy, hemophilia association 75
Asphyxia, thrombocytopenia in neonates 37
Aspirin
    cardiac procedure thromboprophylaxis 210
    complications 223, 224
    dosing 223
    indications 223
    mechanism of action 223
    monitoring 223
    reversal 224
    transient ischemic attack management 192

Bernard-Soulier syndrome (BSS), thrombocytopenia 30, 31, 51, 53
Bivalirudin, see Direct thrombin inhibitors
Blalock-Taussig shunt, thromboembolism 207
Budd-Chiari syndrome (BCS)
    clinical presentation 175

diagnosis 175
management 175
overview 175

Candidiasis, thrombocytopenia 32
Cardiomyopathy, thromboembolism 205
Cardiopulmonary bypass (CPB), coagulation considerations 195–197
Catheter-related thrombosis
  arterial
    clinical presentation 155
    diagnosis 155
    differential diagnosis 155, 156
    management 156
    overview 154, 155
    umbilical artery catheter-related thrombosis
      clinical presentation 158
      diagnosis 158
      management 158
      overview 156, 158
  venous
    clinical presentation 144
    diagnosis 144
    management 144, 145
    occlusion 145, 146
    overview 144
    prophylaxis 145
Central venous catheter (CVC), *see also* Catheter-related thrombosis
  hemophilia considerations 63
  occlusion 145, 146
Cerebral sinovenous thrombosis (CSVT)
  clinical presentation 188
  diagnosis 188–190
  management
    children 190, 191
    neonates 190
    principles 190
  overview 187, 188
Cervicocephalic arterial dissection, *see* Arterial ischemic stroke
Chest X-ray, thrombosis 131
Chronic fetal hypoxia
  clinical findings 26
  thrombocytopenia 25, 26
Chronic renal failure bleeding
  diagnosis 116, 117
  management 117, 118
  overview 116

Chronic thromboembolic pulmonary hypertension (CTPH) 147, 148
Clopidogrel
  complications 223, 224
  dosing 223
  indications 223
  mechanism of action 223
  monitoring 223
  reversal 224
Coagulation
  amplification 9
  initiation 8, 9
  propagation 9
  regulation
    antithrombin 9
    protein C 10, 11
    tissue factor pathway inhibitor 9
Coagulopathy of chronic liver disease, *see* Liver failure
Complete blood count (CBC)
  bleeding child evaluation 18
  chronic renal failure bleeding 116
  disseminated intravascular coagulation 106
  hemolytic uremic syndrome 110
  thrombosis 131
  thrombotic thrombocytopenic purpura 113
  von Willebrand disease 82
Compression stockings, deep vein thrombosis management 143
Computed tomography (CT)
  arterial ischemic stroke 180
  cerebral sinovenous thrombosis 188, 189
  deep vein thrombosis 142
  thrombosis 130, 131
Congenital amegakaryocytic thrombocytopenia (CAMT) 30, 32
Congenital heart disease (CHD)
  bleeding, perioperative
    clinical presentation 200, 201
    diagnosis 201
    management 201, 202
    overview 200
  conduits, shunts, and stents 197, 199, 200, 211
  mechanical circulatory support
    coagulation considerations 195–197
    thromboembolism 209, 210
  thromboembolism
    Blalock-Taussig shunt 207
    clinical presentation 203
    diagnosis 203

Fontan procedure 207, 209
Glenn procedure 207
intracardiac thrombosis 209
management 203, 204
overview 202, 203
prophylaxis 208, 210, 211
special considerations 204
types 194
valve prosthesis
overview 200
thromboembolism 205, 207
Cryoprecipitate
chronic renal failure bleeding management 117
disseminated intravascular coagulation
management 107
transfusion 237
von Willebrand disease management 86, 87
Cryosupernatant, transfusion 237

D-dimer test, thrombosis 131, 132
Deep vein thrombosis (DVT), *see also* Venous thromboembolism
clinical presentation 141, 142
diagnosis 142
epidemiology 1
management 142, 143
post-thrombotic syndrome 149–152
prophylaxis 143
Desmopressin (DDAVP)
acquired hemophilia management 119
acquired von Willebrand disease management 120
chronic renal failure bleeding management 117
hemophilia management 60, 61, 68
overview 240
platelet function defect management 55
von Willebrand disease management 85–87
Developmental hemostasis, overview 23, 24
Dialysis
chronic renal failure bleeding management 117
hemodialysis-related thrombosis
clinical presentation 167
diagnosis 167
management 167
overview 166, 167
prophylaxis 167, 168
Dipyridamole
complications 223, 224
dosing 223
indications 223

mechanism of action 223
monitoring 223
reversal 224
Direct thrombin inhibitors (DTIs)
mechanism of action 221
monitoring 222
oral preparations 222
parenteral preparations 221, 222
Disseminated intravascular coagulation (DIC)
clinical presentation 105, 106
diagnosis 106, 107
management 107–109
neonates 37
pathophysiology 105, 106
Doppler ultrasonography (DUS)
arterial catheter-related thrombosis 155
deep vein thrombosis 142
thrombosis 128–130
Drug-induced thrombocytopenia 32, 33
Dysfibrinogenemia 96, 97

Endocarditis, *see* Infective endocarditis
Estrogens, *see also* Oral contraceptives
chronic renal failure bleeding management 117, 118
Extracorporeal membrane oxidation (ECMO)
bleeding 201
coagulation considerations 195–197
thromboembolism 209, 210

Factor II, *see* Prothrombin
Factor V, deficiency
clinical presentation 99
diagnosis 99, 100
factor VIII deficiency combination 100
management 100
overview 98
Factor VII
deficiency
clinical presentation 93
diagnosis 93
management 93–95
overview 93
transfusion 95, 96, 238
Factor VIIa
acquired hemophilia management 118, 119
acquired von Willebrand disease management 120
coagulopathy of chronic liver disease
management 115, 116

Subject Index

247

disseminated intravascular coagulation
management 108
platelet function defect management 55, 56
Factor VIII
acquired hemophilia management 119
deficiency
clinical presentation 98
diagnosis 98
factor V deficiency combination 100
management 98, 99
overview 97, 98
elevation in thrombophilia 133
hemophilia management 60
history of use 2
inhibitors in therapy
bypassing agents 64, 65
definitions 64
factor dosing in patients with inhibitors 68, 69
factor dosing in patients without inhibitors 66–68
immune tolerance induction 65
prophylaxis 65
risk factors in development 64
transfusion 238
von Willebrand disease management 88
Factor IX
hemophilia management 60
history of use 2
inhibitors in therapy
bypassing agents 64, 65
definitions 64
factor dosing in patients with inhibitors 68, 69
factor dosing in patients without inhibitors 66–68
immune tolerance induction 65
prophylaxis 65
risk factors in development 64
transfusion 238
Factor X
deficiency
clinical presentation 101
diagnosis 101, 102
management 102
overview 101
transfusion 102
Factor Xa inhibitors
mechanism of action 222
oral preparations 222
parenteral preparations 222
reversal 222, 223
Factor XI
deficiency
clinical presentation 91
diagnosis 91
management 92, 93
overview 90, 91
transfusion 93, 239
Factor XIII, transfusion 239
Fetal and neonatal alloimmune thrombocytopenia (FNAIT)
diagnosis 26
genetic counseling 27
imaging 27
management 27
overview 26
Fibrinogen
degradation products 12
disorders
afibrinogenemia 96
diagnosis 97
dysfibrinogenemia 96, 97
hypofibrinogenemia 96
management 97
transfusion 238
Fibrinolysis
degradation products 12
regulation 11, 12
Flow cytometry, citrated blood analysis in platelet disorders 46
Fontan procedure, thromboembolism 207, 209
Frozen plasma (FP), fresh frozen plasma (FFP)
coagulopathy of chronic liver disease management 115
thrombotic thrombocytopenic purpura management 113
transfusion 236, 237

GATA-1, mutations and thrombocytopenia 31
Genetic testing
bleeding child 21
thrombotic thrombocytopenic purpura 113
vitamin K-dependent clotting factor deficiency 84
Glanzmann thrombasthenia (GT) 51
Glenn procedure, thromboembolism 207
Gray platelet syndrome 31

Hemodialysis, *see* Dialysis
Hemolytic uremic syndrome (HUS)
    atypical disease 110, 111
    clinical presentation 109, 110
    diagnosis 110
    management 110, 111
    overview 109
Hemophilia
    acquired disease
        diagnosis 118
        management
            acute bleeding 118, 119
            inhibitor eradication 119
        overview 118
    chronic complications
        arthropathy 75
        pseudotumor 75
        synovitis 73, 74
    classification 59, 60
    history of care 2, 3
    inhibitors
        bypassing agents 64, 65
        definitions 64
        immune tolerance induction 65
        prophylaxis 65
        risk factors in development 64
    management in children and adolescents
        adjuvant therapy 60, 61
        bleeding episodes
            factor dosing in patients with inhibitors 68, 69
            factor dosing in patients without inhibitors 66–68
            initial assessment 66
        factor replacement 60
        prophylaxis 61, 62
        site-specific bleeding and management
            gastrointestinal bleeding 72
            hematuria 73
            intracranial hemorrhage 72
            joints 69, 70
            mucosa 71
            muscle 70, 71
            vital structure compression 71, 72
        supportive care 62–64
    neonates and infants
        delivery considerations 35
        index cases 35, 36
        management 35, 76
    surgery and procedure precautions 73, 74
Hemostasis, *see* Developmental hemostasis; Primary hemostasis; Secondary hemostasis
Heparin
    aortic thrombosis management 159
    arterial catheter-related thrombosis management 156, 158
    arterial ischemic stroke management 182–184
    cerebral sinovenous thrombosis management 190
    deep vein thrombosis management 142
    disseminated intravascular coagulation management 108
    hemodialysis-related thrombosis management and prophylaxis 167, 168
    hepatic artery thrombosis management 173
    low-molecular-weight heparin
        complications 217
        dosing 217
        half-life 216
        indications 216, 217
        mechanism of action 216
        monitoring 217, 218
        reversal 218
    nephrotic syndrome-associated thrombosis management 168, 169
    renal vein thrombosis management 164, 165
    sinusoidal obstruction syndrome management 174
    surgical management 227, 228
    thrombocytopenia patients 228, 229
    transient ischemic attack management 192
    unfractionated heparin
        complications 216
        dosing 215
        half-life 214, 215
        indications 215
        mechanism of action 214
        monitoring 215, 216
        reversal 216
Heparin-induced thrombocytopenia (HIT)
    clinical presentation 225
    diagnosis 226
    incidence 225
    low-molecular-weight heparin 217
    management 226
    unfractionated heparin 216
Hepatic artery thrombosis (HAT)
    clinical presentation 170, 173

diagnosis 173
management 173
overview 170
History, *see* Medical history
Homocysteine, thrombophilia testing 135
Human immunodeficiency virus (HIV), thrombocytopenia in neonates 33
Hypofibrinogenemia 96
Hypothrombinemia lupus anticoagulant syndrome (HLAS) 121

Immune thrombocytopenia (ITP)
clinical presentation 47
diagnosis 47, 48
management
emergency management 50, 51
first-line treatment 49
persistent disease 49, 50
principles 48, 49
neonates
clinical findings 28
management 28
overview 28
overview 46, 47
Immunoadsorption, acquired hemophilia management 119
Infective endocarditis (IE), thromboembolism 205, 206
Inferior vena cava filter, pulmonary embolism prevention 149
International normalized ratio (INR)
bleeding child evaluation 18
testing, *see* Prothrombin time
Intracranial hemorrhage (ICH)
cerebral sinovenous thrombosis 191
hemophilia 72
Intravenous immunoglobulin (IVIG)
acquired hemophilia management 119
acquired von Willebrand disease management 120
immune thrombocytopenia management 49

Jacobsen syndrome, thrombocytopenia 31

Kasabach-Merritt phenomenon (KMP), thrombocytopenia in neonates 38
Kawasaki disease, thromboembolism 205

Lepirudin, *see* Direct thrombin inhibitors
Lipoprotein(a) [Lp(a)], thrombophilia testing 135
Liver failure

coagulopathy of chronic liver disease
clinical presentation 114, 115
diagnosis 115
management 115, 116
overview 114
thrombocytopenia in neonates 38
Low-molecular-weight heparin, *see* Heparin
Lupus anticoagulant (LAC), thrombophilia testing 134, 135
Lupus anticoagulant syndrome, *see* Hypothrombinemia lupus anticoagulant syndrome

α-Macroglobulin, functional overview 12
Magnetic resonance imaging (MRI)
arterial ischemic stroke 180, 181
cerebral sinovenous thrombosis 188, 189
deep vein thrombosis 142
thrombosis 131
Medical history
bleeding child
age 14, 15
bleeding history 15, 16
family history 16
sex 15
symptom scoring 16, 17
thrombosis
family history 126
medical history 126
risk factors 125, 126
von Willebrand disease 81, 82
Menorrhagia
platelet function defect management 56
von Willebrand disease management 87, 88
Mesenteric vascular thrombosis
clinical presentation 175
diagnosis 176
management 176
overview 175
Mitral valve prosthesis
cardiac procedure thromboprophylaxis 211
overview 200
thromboembolism 205, 207
Moyamoya disease, arterial ischemic stroke management 185, 186
Myocardial infarction (MI), children 209

Necrotizing enterocolitis, thrombocytopenia 32
Nephrotic syndrome-associated thrombosis
clinical presentation 168

diagnosis 168
management 168, 169
overview 168

Oral contraceptives, von Willebrand disease
management 85, 88
Osteopenia
heparin induction 216
vitamin K antagonist induction 220

Pain management, hemophilia considerations 63, 64
Peripheral arterial insufficiency, arterial thrombosis 161
Peripheral blood film
bleeding child evaluation 18
coagulopathy of chronic liver disease 115
disseminated intravascular coagulation 106
Physical examination
bleeding child 16, 18
thrombosis 126–128
Plasmapheresis, thrombotic thrombocytopenic purpura management 113
Plasmin, inhibitors 11, 12
Plasminogen
activators 11
inhibition of activation 11
Plasminogen activator inhibitor-1 (PAI-1)
deficiency
clinical presentation 103
diagnosis 103
management 103
overview 103
functional overview 11
Platelet
activation 6, 7
adhesion 6
aggregation 7
count and morphology 43, 45
disorder diagnosis in children 43–46
function defects
classification 52
glycoprotein disorders 51, 53
granule disorders 53, 54
treatment
bleeding episodes 56, 57
hemostatic agents 54–56
function testing 20, 21
transfusion
children 55, 237

disseminated intravascular coagulation 107
neonatal thrombocytopenia 34, 35
Platelet aggregometry
light transmission aggregometry 45, 46
lumiaggregometry 46
overview 45
whole blood aggregometry 46
Platelet function analyzer (PFA-100)
bleeding child evaluation 20, 21
von Willebrand disease evaluation 82, 83
Portal vein thrombosis (PVT)
clinical presentation 169
diagnosis 169
management 169–172
overview 169
Post-thrombotic syndrome (PTS)
clinical presentation 150
diagnosis 150
management 150, 151
organ thrombosis 177
overview 149, 150
prevention 151, 152
Primary hemostasis
laboratory testing 21
platelet activation 6, 7
platelet adhesion 6
platelet aggregation 7
vasoconstriction 6
Primary pulmonary hypertension, thromboprophylaxis 211
Protein C
activated protein C resistance 134
coagulation regulation 10, 11
deficiency 133, 134
disseminated intravascular coagulation management 109
transfusion 239
Protein S, deficiency 133, 134
Prothrombin
deficiency
clinical presentation 101
diagnosis 101
management 101
overview 100, 101
elevation in thrombophilia 132, 133
transfusion 239
Prothrombin complex concentrate (PCC)
acquired hemophilia management 118, 119

coagulopathy of chronic liver disease
  management 116
  transfusion 238, 239
  vitamin K antagonist reversal 220
Prothrombin time (PT)
  bleeding child evaluation 18
  coagulopathy of chronic liver disease 115
  disseminated intravascular coagulation 106
  hemolytic uremic syndrome 110
Pseudotumor, hemophilia association 75
Pulmonary embolism (PE), *see also* Venous thromboembolism
  chronic thromboembolic pulmonary hypertension 147, 148
  clinical presentation 146, 147
  diagnosis 147
  epidemiology 1
  inferior vena cava filter for prevention 149
  management 147
  overview 146
Pulmonary hypertension, *see* Primary pulmonary hypertension
Purpura fulminans 138

Red cell concentrate, transfusion 236
Reference values, bleeding and clotting tests 232–234
Renal artery stent, thrombosis 160
Renal artery thrombosis (RAT)
  clinical presentation 166
  diagnosis 166
  management 166
  overview 166
Renal failure, *see* Chronic renal failure bleeding
Renal vein thrombosis (RVT)
  clinical presentation 163, 164
  diagnosis 164
  management 164, 165
  outcomes 165, 166
  overview 163
Reperfusion injury, arterial thrombosis 161
Reye's syndrome 224
Rituximab
  acquired hemophilia management 119
  immune thrombocytopenia management 49, 50

Secondary hemostasis
  coagulation
    amplification 9
    initiation 8, 9

propagation 9
    contact system 9
    overview 7, 8
Sepsis, thrombocytopenia 37
Sickle cell disease (SCD), arterial ischemic stroke management 186, 187
Sinusoidal obstruction syndrome (SOS)
  clinical presentation 173
  diagnosis 173, 174
  management 174
  overview 173
Splenectomy
  immune thrombocytopenia management 50
  splenic vein thrombosis 176
  thrombotic thrombocytopenic purpura management 114
Splenic vein thrombosis (SpVT)
  clinical presentation 176
  diagnosis 176
  management 176
  overview 176
Stroke, *see* Arterial ischemic stroke; Cerebral sinovenous thrombosis; Intracranial hemorrhage; Transient ischemic attack
Synovitis, hemophilia association 73, 74

Thrombin
  bovine thrombin and acquired inhibitors 121, 122
  inhibitors, *see* Direct thrombin inhibitors
Thrombin time (TT), bleeding child evaluation 20
Thrombocytopenia, *see also specific diseases*
  antithrombotic therapy 228, 229
  genetic syndromes 28–32
  heparin induction, *see* Heparin-induced thrombocytopenia 216, 217
  neonates
    definition 24, 25
    diagnostic algorithm 38, 39
    etiology 25
    platelet transfusion 34, 35
Thrombocytopenia with absent radii (TAR) 29, 30, 32
Thromboelastography (TEG), mechanical circulatory support coagulation considerations 197
Thromboembolism (TE), *see* Arterial thromboembolism; Congenital heart disease; Venous thromboembolism
Thrombolysis
  arterial ischemic stroke management 187

deep vein thrombosis management 143
thrombocytopenia patients 229
tissue plasminogen activator
   bleeding complication management 225
   contraindications 224
   dosing 224, 225
   half-life 224
   indications 224
   mechanism of action 224
   monitoring 225
Thrombophilia
   anatomical thrombophilia 138, 139
   anticoagulation factor deficiency 133, 134
   endothelial damage mediators 134, 135
   factor VIII elevation 133
   impact in childhood thrombosis 135, 136
   laboratory testing guidelines 137, 138
   overview 132
   prothrombin elevation 132, 133
   purpura fulminans 138
Thromboprophylaxis
   cardiac procedures 210, 211
   indications 229, 230
Thrombosis, *see also specific diseases*
   etiology 125
   history
      family history 126
      medical history 126
      risk factors 125, 126
   imaging
      chest X-ray 131
      computed tomography 130, 131
      Doppler ultrasonography 128–130
      magnetic resonance imaging 131
      venography 130
      ventilation/perfusion lung scan 131
   laboratory testing 131, 132
   overview 124, 125
   physical examination 126–128
Thrombotic thrombocytopenic purpura (TTP)
   clinical presentation 112, 113
   diagnosis 113
   genetic testing 113
   management
      idiopathic disease 113, 114
      Upshaw-Schülman syndrome 113
   pathophysiology 111, 112
Tissue factor pathway inhibitor (TFPI), coagulation regulation 9

Tissue plasminogen activator (t-PA)
   functional overview 11
   thrombolysis, *see* Thrombolysis
Topical hemostasis, overview of agents 240, 241
TORCH, thrombocytopenia 33
Tranexamic acid
   acquired von Willebrand disease management 120
   coagulopathy of chronic liver disease management 116
   overview 240
   platelet function defect management 54
Transfusion, *see also specific blood products*
   blood product collection and testing 235, 236
   dosing 236
Transient ischemic attack (TIA)
   clinical presentation 191
   diagnosis 191
   management 191, 192
   overview 191

Umbilical artery catheter-related thrombosis
   clinical presentation 158
   diagnosis 158
   management 158
   overview 156, 158
Unfractionated heparin, *see* Heparin
Upshaw-Schülman syndrome, management 113
Urea clot lysis test, bleeding child evaluation 20

Vasoconstriction, overview 6
Venography, thrombosis 130
Venous thromboembolism (VTE), *see also* Deep vein thrombosis; Pulmonary embolism
   cancer patients 148, 149
   neonates 148
   overview 141
   travel-related thromboembolism 230
   venous stenting 149
Ventilation/perfusion scan
   pulmonary embolism 147
   thrombosis 131
Ventricular assist device (VAD)
   bleeding 201
   coagulation considerations 195–197
   thromboembolism 209, 210
Vitamin K, coagulopathy of chronic liver disease management 115
Vitamin K antagonists (VKA)
   arterial ischemic stroke management 182–184

cardiac procedure thromboprophylaxis 210, 211
complications 220
deep vein thrombosis management 142, 143
dosing 219
indications 218, 219
mechanism of action 218
monitoring 219, 220
reversal 220, 221
surgical considerations 227, 228
transient ischemic attack management 192
warfarin half-life 218
Vitamin K deficiency bleeding (VKDB)
diagnosis 36
management 36, 37
overview 36
Vitamin K-dependent clotting factor deficiency
clinical presentation 102
diagnosis 102
management 102, 103
overview 102
von Willebrand disease (VWD)
acquired disease
diagnosis 120
management 120, 121
overview 119, 120
classification 36, 79, 81
diagnosis
type 1 disease 83
type 1C disease 83
type 2 disease 83, 84
type 3 disease 84
genetic testing 84
laboratory testing 82, 83
management
cryoprecipitate 86, 87
desmopressin 85, 86
factor concentrates 86
menorrhagia 87, 88
nonspecific adjunctive therapy 85
perioperative management 87
principles 84, 85
medical history 81, 82
pathophysiology 79–81
platelet-type disease 31, 32
prophylaxis 88
von Willebrand factor (VWF), transfusion 86, 238

Warfarin, *see* Vitamin K antagonists
Wiskott-Aldrich syndrome (WAS), thrombocytopenia 28, 29